Study Guide

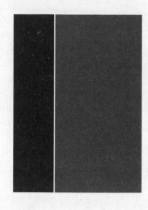

# Linton

# Introduction to Medical-Surgical Nursing

## Fourth Edition

**Nancy K. Maebius, PhD, RN**
Faculty
Galen Health Institute
San Antonio, Texas

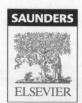

SAUNDERS

ELSEVIER

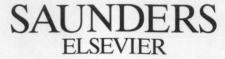

# SAUNDERS
## ELSEVIER

11830 Westline Industrial Drive
St. Louis, Missouri 63146

STUDY GUIDE
INTRODUCTION TO MEDICAL-SURGICAL NURSING 4/E

ISBN-13: 978-1-4160-9995-6
ISBN-10: 1-4160-9995-6

---

### Notice

Neither the Publisher nor the Authors assume any responsibility for any loss or injury and/or damage to persons or property arising out of or related to any use of the material contained in this book. It is the responsibility of the treating practitioner, relying on independent expertise and knowledge of the patient, to determine the best treatment and method of application for the patient.

The Publisher

---

ISBN-13: 978-1-4160-9995-6
ISBN-10: 1-4160-9995-6

*Acquisitions Editor:* Robin Richman
*Developmental Editor:* Ryan Creed
*Publishing Services Manager:* Deborah Vogel
*Project Manager:* Jodi Willard
*Design Direction:* Teresa McBryan

Printed in the United States of America
Last digit is the print number:   9   8   7   6   5   4   3   2

To my family:

*My husband, Jed*
*My children, Stephen, Maria, Elizabeth, Tom, Brian, Justine, Andrew and Clayton*
*My grandchildren, Allison, Sarah, Jessica, Erica, George, Ella, Emma, Colter and Hudson*

To my vocational nursing students:

*From whom I have learned so much about thinking, learning, dedication and commitment to nursing.*

# TO THE STUDENT

This study guide was created to assist you in achieving the objectives of each chapter in *Introduction to Medical-Surgical Nursing*, Fourth Edition, and establishing a solid base of knowledge in Medical-Surgical nursing. Completing the exercises in each chapter in this guide will help to reinforce the material studied in the textbook and learned in class. Such reinforcement also helps students to be successful on the NCLEX-PN®.

## STUDY HINTS FOR ALL STUDENTS

### Ask Questions!

There are no stupid questions. If you do not know something or are not sure, you need to find out. Other people may be wondering the same thing but may be too shy to ask. The answer could mean life or death to your patient. That is certainly more important than feeling embarrassed about asking a question.

### Chapter Objectives

At the beginning of each chapter in the textbook are objectives that you should have mastered when you finish studying that chapter. Write these objectives in your notebook, leaving a blank space after each. Fill in the answers as you find them while reading the chapter. Review to make sure your answers are correct and complete. Use these answers when you study for tests. This should also be done for separate course objectives that your instructor has listed in your class syllabus.

### Key Terms

At the beginning of each chapter in the textbook are key terms that you will encounter as you read the chapter. Text page number references are provided, for easy reference and review, and the key terms are in color the first time they appear in the chapter. Phonetic pronunciations are provided for terms that students might find difficult to pronounce. The terms that were assigned simple phonetic pronunciations were selected because they are either (1) difficult medical, nursing, or scientific terms or (2) other

words that may be difficult for students to pronounce. The goal is to help the student reader with limited proficiency in English to develop a greater command of the pronunciation of scientific and nonscientific English terminology. It is hoped that a more general competency in the understanding and use of medical and scientific language may result.

### Key Points

Use the Key Points at the end of each chapter in the textbook to help with review for exams.

### Reading Hints

When reading each chapter in the textbook, look at the subject headings to learn what each section is about. Read first for the general meaning. Then reread parts you did not understand. It may help to read those parts aloud. Carefully read the information given in each table and study each figure and its caption.

### Concepts

While studying, put difficult concepts into your own words to see if you understand them. Check this understanding with another student or the instructor. Write these in your notebook.

### Class Notes

When taking lecture notes in class, leave a large margin on the left side of each notebook page and write only on right-hand pages, leaving all left-hand pages blank. Look over your lecture notes soon after each class, while your memory is fresh. Fill in missing words, complete sentences and ideas, and underline key phrases, definitions, and concepts. At the top of each page, write the topic of that page. In the left margin, write the key word for that part of your notes. On the opposite left-hand page, write a summary or outline that combines material from both the textbook and the lecture. These can be your study notes for review.

## Study Groups

Form a study group with some other students so you can help one another. Practice speaking and reading aloud. Ask questions about material you are not sure about. Work together to find answers.

## References for Improving Study Skills

Good study skills are essential for achieving your goals in nursing. Time management, efficient use of study time, and a consistent approach to studying are all beneficial. There are various study methods for reading a textbook and for taking class notes. Some methods that have proven helpful can be found in *Saunders Student Nurse Planner: A Guide to Success in Nursing School.* This book contains helpful information on test taking and preparing for clinical experiences. It includes an example of a "time map" for planning study time and a blank form that the student can use to formulate a personal time map.

# ADDITIONAL STUDY HINTS FOR ENGLISH AS SECOND-LANGUAGE (ESL) STUDENTS

## Vocabulary

If you find a nontechnical word you do not know (e.g., *drowsy*), try to guess its meaning from the sentence (e.g., *With electrolyte imbalance, the patient may feel fatigued and drowsy*). If you are not sure of the meaning, or if it seems particularly important, look it up in the dictionary.

## Vocabulary Notebook

Keep a small alphabetized notebook or address book in your pocket or purse. Write down new nontechnical words you read or hear along with their meanings and pronunciations. Write each word under its initial letter so you can find it easily, as in a dictionary. For words you do not know or for words that have a different meaning in nursing, write down how they are used and sound. Look up their meanings in a dictionary or ask your instructor or first-language buddy. Then write the different meanings or usages that you have found in your book, including the nursing meaning. Continue to add new words as you discover them. For example:

*primary*
- of most importance; main: *the primary problem or disease*
- the first one; elementary: *primary school*

*secondary*
- of less importance; resulting from another problem or disease: *a secondary symptom*
- the second one: *secondary school (in the United States, high school)*

## First Language Buddy

ESL students should find a first-language buddy— another student who is a native speaker of English and who is willing to answer questions about word meanings, pronunciations, and culture. Maybe your buddy would like to learn about your language and culture as well. This could help in his or her nursing experience as well.

# Contents

# CHAPTER 1

# The Health Care System

---

## OBJECTIVES

1. Describe the organization of the health care system in the United States.

2. Describe the focus of public health services.

3. Define the three levels of prevention.

4. Discuss financing of health care in the United States, including Medicare and Medicaid programs.

5. Describe the components of the health care system that provide both outpatient and inpatient care and the types of service each provides.

6. Describe the impact of cost-containment measures on the delivery of care.

---

## LEARNING ACTIVITIES

**A. Prevention.** Match the example in the numbered column with the most appropriate term in the lettered column. Answers may be used more than once.

1. _____ Providing Pap smears at reduced cost *(3)*

2. _____ Educating people to wear seat belts *(3)*

3. _____ Teaching a person with diabetes proper diet and foot care *(3)*

4. _____ Offering reduced-cost screening mammograms *(3)*

5. _____ Use of physical therapy to prevent contractures in a stroke patient *(3)*

6. _____ Educational campaigns to prevent people from smoking *(3)*

7. _____ Exercise programs to increase strength and cardiovascular fitness *(3)*

A. Primary
B. Secondary
C. Tertiary

B. **Key Terms.** Match the definition in the numbered column with the most appropriate term in the lettered column.

1. _____ Branch of the Department of Health and Human Services (DHHS) of the U.S. government whose chief purpose is to provide better health services for the American people *(2)*

2. _____ Provision of comprehensive health care at a reasonable cost through enrollment in an HMO, PPO, or similar plan, with incentives to reduce costs *(1)*

3. _____ Law passed in 1965 to ensure that older adults have an adequate income and suitable housing, physical and mental health services, community services, and the opportunity to pursue meaningful activities *(9)*

4. _____ System of reimbursement standards for hospitals for care based on a fixed fee for a diagnostic category, regardless of cost *(4)*

5. _____ A level of residential care that includes medical, nursing, social, and rehabilitative services to individuals who cannot manage independently *(11)*

6. _____ Nursing home that provides care for people who are unable to care for themselves because of chronic illnesses and physical impairments *(11)*

7. _____ Steps taken to prevent disease recurrence or complications of diagnosed disease or injury *(3)*

8. _____ Steps taken to improve health and prevent disease and injury *(2)*

9. _____ Steps taken to detect disease early and begin treatment as soon as possible *(3)*

A. Public Health Service (USPHS)
B. Diagnosis-related group (DRG)
C. Managed health care
D. Older Americans Act
E. Skilled nursing facility
F. Long-term care facility
G. Primary prevention
H. Secondary prevention
I. Tertiary prevention

**C. Financing.** Match the definition in the numbered column with the most appropriate term in the lettered column.

1. _____ Accepting a fixed amount of money to pay for health care services to all health care plan members with no additional billing *(4)*

2. _____ An established fee set by physicians or health care providers for services or procedures actually provided *(3)*

3. _____ Program that provides health care services for needy, low-income, and disabled individuals with funds distributed at the state level *(5)*

4. _____ Health insurance program administered by the federal government that is funded by Social Security payments *(4)*

5. _____ Coverage that blends multiple options and enrollees select which option they want to use *(4)*

A. Medicare
B. Medicaid
C. Fee-for-service
D. Capitation
E. Point of service (POS)

**D. Health Care Facilities.** Match the description in the numbered column with the most appropriate term in the lettered column. Answers may be used more than once.

1. _____ Provide skilled care from a licensed nursing staff, including rehabilitative care *(11)*

2. _____ Nursing homes, skilled nursing facilities, and extended-care facilities *(11)*

3. _____ Provide care for people unable to care for themselves *(11)*

4. _____ Provide care for those who need observations during acute or unstable phase of illness *(11)*

5. _____ Permit a high degree of independence with limited access to nursing care *(11)*

6. _____ Residents' units have kitchens, but group meals are typically provided *(11)*

7. _____ Purpose is to care for and provide palliative care to dying people *(9)*

8. _____ Extended care for people who have the potential to regain function *(11)*

A. Long-term care facilities
B. Intermediate care facilities (extended care facilities)
C. Skilled nursing facilities
D. Assisted living centers
E. Hospices

E. **Medicare/Medicaid.** Match the description in the numbered column with the most appropriate term in the lettered column. Answers may be used more than once.

Funding

1. _____ Monthly premium from paycheck; funds matched by federal government *(4)*

2. _____ Federal, state, and local taxes *(4)*

Eligibility

3. _____ Needy, low-income, and disabled people and their dependent children younger than 65 years *(4)*

4. _____ All people older than 65 years plus disabled people younger than 65 who qualify for Social Security benefits *(4)*

How Administered

5. _____ Federal government *(4)*

6. _____ Both federal and state governments *(4)*

Benefits

7. _____ Includes nursing home care *(4)*

8. _____ Geared toward acute, short-term care *(4)*

9. _____ Offers prescription drug coverage option *(2)*

A. Medicare
B. Medicaid

## MULTIPLE-CHOICE QUESTIONS

F. Choose the most appropriate answer.

1. Which is an example of outpatient care? *(5)*
   1. Hospital operating room
   2. Acute care hospital
   3. Physician's office
   4. Long-term care facility

2. Managed care provides health care that includes: *(1)*
   1. incentives to save costs.
   2. increased treatment of acute diseases.
   3. increased hospital care.
   4. decreased cost sharing.

3. Which system groups patients according to the medical diagnosis so that hospitals receive a fixed payment based on the patient's diagnosis? *(4)*
   1. HMOs
   2. DRGs
   3. PPOs
   4. CQIs

4. Physicians are now discharging patients as early as possible to: *(10)*
   1. improve care, because the focus is on primary prevention.
   2. improve care, because hospice can take care of patients needing extended nursing services.
   3. reduce costs, because hospitals only receive a fixed amount of money as a result of DRGs.
   4. reduce costs, because hospitals can refer patients to home health and long-term care facilities.

5. Which of the following conditions is one of the five most frequent reasons for hospitalization? *(10)*
   1. Surgery for fractures
   2. Cardiovascular disease
   3. Trauma from accidents
   4. Osteoporosis

6. Which term describes the collection by physicians of a fixed amount of money each month for each member enrolled in the plan? *(4)*
   1. HMOs
   2. Capitation
   3. PPOs
   4. Fee-for-service

7. The demand for professional home health care services continues to increase for all age categories because: *(7)*
   1. ambulatory surgery center services are decreasing.
   2. health care costs are decreasing.
   3. managed health care is focused on acute care.
   4. hospitals are reducing the length of hospital stays.

8. What concerns do health insurance companies, HMOs, and PPOs have in common? *(3)*
   1. Health care service delivery for low-income people
   2. Delivery of health care services at a reasonable cost
   3. Establishment of ambulatory care centers
   4. Diagnosis-related groups (DRGs)

9. Which is an agency that carries out the activities of the Public Health Service? *(2)*
   1. Social Security Administration
   2. Centers for Medicare and Medicaid Services
   3. Food and Drug Administration
   4. Office of Human Development

10. In which setting is the number of patients decreasing? *(5)*
    1. Ambulatory care
    2. Home health
    3. Clinics
    4. Hospitals

11. A stroke patient who is aphasic will need the services of a(n): *(8)*
    1. occupational therapist.
    2. physical therapist.
    3. speech therapist.
    4. social worker.

12. Patients and their families needing assistance to manage chronic illness in the home will need the services of a(n): *(8)*
    1. speech therapist.
    2. social worker.
    3. occupational therapist.
    4. physical therapist.

13. The effects of managed care include: *(1)*
    1. increase in fee-for-service.
    2. decrease in home health care.
    3. decreased focus on wellness.
    4. increased focus on prevention.

14. In public health, the focus of attention is on: *(2)*
    1. emphasizing patients' rights.
    2. improving health of aggregates.
    3. increasing cost-sharing.
    4. decreasing home health care.

15. One aim of primary prevention is to: *(2)*
    1. promote health.
    2. detect disease early.
    3. treat disease to improve patient outcomes.
    4. prevent complications of disease.

16. *Cost-containment* refers to: *(3)*
    1. reducing costs.
    2. increasing fee-for-service plans.
    3. decreasing third-party reimburse-
       ments.
    4. controlling rates of increasing costs.

17. A strategy designed to control costs is: *(4)*
    1. capitation.
    2. fee-for-service.
    3. retrospective payment.
    4. voluntary enrollment.

18. The "revolving door syndrome" occurs
    when patients return to the hospital for
    care because: *(10)*
    1. hospice services were not available at
       home.
    2. high-technology services were needed.
    3. the emphasis was on preventive health
       care at home.
    4. they did not fully recover at home.

19. Which statement is true regarding the way
    DRGs have affected hospital finances? If the
    patient: *(4, 10)*
    1. gets better faster, the hospital loses
       money.
    2. gets better faster, the hospital makes
       money.
    3. requires a longer stay, the hospital
       makes money.
    4. requires a shorter stay, the hospital
       loses money.

20. Cost-effective health care methods began
    with DRGs. What method of health care
    delivery today is aimed at cost-effective
    health care delivery? *(1)*
    1. Primary prevention
    2. Long-term care
    3. Managed health care
    4. Extended care

21. The focus of hospice care is to: *(9)*
    1. extend life of the terminally ill.
    2. provide a better quality of life for dying
       patients and their families.
    3. provide assistance to families trying to
       manage chronic illness in the home.
    4. provide emergency care to dying pa-
       tients at home.

22. Assessment and intervention used by hos-
    pice nurses are centered around: *(9)*
    1. palliative care.
    2. treatment of disease.
    3. preservation of life.
    4. infection control.

23. Which type of prevention is the highest
    priority in preventing disease and injury?
    *(2)*
    1. Primary
    2. Secondary
    3. Health maintenance organization
       (HMO)
    4. Preferred provider organization (PPO)

24. A 66-year-old patient is admitted to the
    rehabilitation unit of a hospital following
    surgery for a fractured hip. Which type of
    preventive care is provided? *(3)*
    1. Primary
    2. Secondary
    3. Tertiary
    4. Comprehensive

25. Which type of medical insurance is ap-
    propriate to use for a 70-year-old patient
    recovering from a broken wrist? *(4)*
    1. Medicare
    2. Medicaid
    3. Private policy
    4. Social Security

26. The priority type of care for a 68-year-old
    patient who is on a rehabilitation unit fol-
    lowing a stroke is: *(11)*
    1. surgical care.
    2. acute care.
    3. palliative care.
    4. skilled nursing care.

27. Which patient is entitled to receive Medi-
    care insurance? *(4)*
    1. 25-year-old patient with asthma
    2. 72-year-old patient with hypertension
    3. 60-year-old patient with pneumonia
    4. 55-year-old patient with brain injury

28. Which low-income patient is most likely to be eligible for Medicaid funding? *(5)*
    1. 35-year-old patient with multiple sclerosis
    2. 65-year-old patient with a stroke
    3. 70-year-old patient with acute myocardial infarction
    4. 40-year-old patient with chronic allergies

## ALTERNATE FORMAT QUESTIONS

G. 1. Choose from the following activities the ones which represent tertiary care. Select all that apply. *(3)*
    1. Education about wearing seat belts
    2. Physical therapy to prevent contractures in patients who have had a stroke
    3. Use of screening mammograms in persons over the age of 50
    4. Exercise programs to increase strength and weight-bearing
    5. Teaching proper foot care to patients with diabetes

# Patient Care Settings

---

## OBJECTIVES

1.  Describe the role of the nurse in community and home health, rehabilitation, and long-term care settings.

2.  Differentiate community health and community-based nursing.

3.  Describe the types of specialty care that nurses may provide in home health care.

4.  Describe the principles of rehabilitation.

5.  List the four levels of disability.

6.  Discuss legislation passed to protect the rights of the disabled.

7.  Identify the goals of rehabilitation.

8.  Name the members of the rehabilitation team.

9.  List the types of extended care facilities.

10. Discuss the effects of institutionalization on the older adults.

11. Describe the principles of nursing home care.

---

## LEARNING ACTIVITIES

**A.  Key Terms.** Match the definition in the numbered column with the most appropriate term in the lettered column.

1. _____  Measurable loss of function, usually delineated to indicate a diminished capacity for work *(17)*

2. _____  Certain nursing procedures, such as dressing changes, Foley catheter insertions, and venipuncture *(17)*

3. _____  Physical or psychological disturbance in functioning *(18)*

4. _____  Inability to perform one or more normal daily activities because of mental or physical disability *(18)*

5. _____  Used to determine adequacy of home environment, knowledge level of the patient and family regarding care procedures and side effects of treatment, and family's level of comfort in performing specific procedures *(15)*

6. _____  Process of restoring individuals to best possible health and functioning following physical or mental impairment *(17)*

A.  Impairment
B.  Skilled observation and assessment
C.  Rehabilitation
D.  Handicap
E.  Skilled procedures
F.  Disability

**B.  Disability Levels.** Match the description of disability in the numbered column with the level of disability in the lettered column.

1. _____ Severe limitations in one or more ADLs; unable to work *(18)*

2. _____ Slight limitation in one or more ADLs; usually able to work *(18)*

3. _____ Total disability characterized by near complete dependence on others for assistance with ADLs; unable to work *(18)*

4. _____ Moderate limitation in one or more ADLs; able to work but workplace may need modifications *(18)*

A.  Level I
B.  Level II
C.  Level III
D.  Level IV

**C.  Health Care Workers.** Match the definition in the numbered column with the most appropriate term in the lettered column.

1. _____ Person who assists the patient in regaining swallowing or speaking functions *(20)*

2. _____ Person who assists patient with regaining fine motor skills necessary for dressing, eating, and grooming *(20)*

3. _____ Person who assists with coordinating resources for placement in the home or convalescent facility after discharge *(20)*

4. _____ Person who assists patient in all aspects of mobility *(20)*

A.  Physical therapist
B.  Occupational therapist
C.  Speech therapist
D.  Social worker

**D.  Rehabilitation.** Which of the following are goals of rehabilitation? Select all that apply.

1. _____ Improve health status of communities or groups of people through public education *(18)*

2. _____ Return disabled individuals to maximum state of functioning *(18)*

3. _____ Prevent further disabilities in patients *(18)*

**E. Home Health Care.** Check the following basic criteria for home health care that must be met to receive Medicare reimbursement. Select all that apply.

1. _____ Care must be continuous for 24 hours per day. *(14-15)*

2. _____ Care must be skilled. *(14-15)*

3. _____ Care must be reasonable and necessary. *(14-15)*

4. _____ The patient must be home-bound. *(14-15)*

5. _____ The physician must authorize a plan of care. *(14-15)*

6. _____ Visits must exceed 28 hours per week. *(14-15)*

7. _____ The patient must be bed-ridden. *(14-15)*

**F. Home Health IV Therapies.** Check five of the most common intravenous therapies that can be given at home.

1. _____ Hydration *(16)*

2. _____ Chemotherapy *(16)*

3. _____ Blood transfusions *(16)*

4. _____ Total parenteral nutrition (TPR) *(16)*

5. _____ Antibiotics *(16)*

6. _____ Platelets *(16)*

7. _____ Pain control *(16)*

**G. Institutional Care.** Match the descriptions in the numbered column with the five common effects of institutionalization in the lettered column.

1. _____ Patients are treated in light of their diagnosis or dysfunctional behavior patterns. *(22)*

2. _____ Behaviors considered normal at home are labeled abnormal or are unacceptable in the institution. *(23)*

3. _____ Family visits are few and include little discussion of the outside world. *(23)*

4. _____ A patient's physical, mental, and social abilities are lost because of disuse. *(23)*

5. _____ Residents of long-term care facilities are exposed unnecessarily when caregivers enter rooms without knocking. *(22)*

A. Depersonalization
B. Indignity
C. Redefinition of "normal"
D. Regression
E. Social withdrawal

**H. Long-Term Care.** Match the nursing interventions in the numbered column with the appropriate principle of long-term residential care in the lettered column.

1. _____ Place a urinal near the bed for immobile, incontinent patients. *(23)*

2. _____ Allow nursing home residents to assist in establishing care goals. *(24)*

3. _____ Give long-term care residents choices in activities. *(24)*

4. _____ Explore factors that may be responsible for the patient's incontinence. *(23)*

5. _____ Set specific goals for each resident that encourage independent functioning. *(23)*

A. Maintenance of function
B. Promotion of independence
C. Maintenance of autonomy

## MULTIPLE-CHOICE QUESTIONS

**I.** Choose the most appropriate answer.

1. The process of restoring an individual to the best possible health and functioning following a physical or mental impairment is called: *(17)*
   1. independent function.
   2. home health care.
   3. rehabilitation.
   4. autonomy.

2. A disturbance in functioning that may be either physical or psychological is called: *(17)*
   1. rehabilitation.
   2. impairment.
   3. restoration.
   4. independence.

3. People born without arms can perform ADLs by using their feet and assistive devices. These people are said to have: *(18)*
   1. a disability.
   2. a handicap.
   3. paralysis.
   4. return of function.

4. A measurable loss of function, usually indicating diminished capacity for work, is called: *(17)*
   1. impairment.
   2. alteration to integrity.
   3. compensation.
   4. disability.

5. An inability to perform daily activities is called: *(18)*
   1. impairment.
   2. disability.
   3. handicap.
   4. paralysis.

6. The ultimate goal of rehabilitation is to live with: *(18)*
   1. assistance.
   2. modification.
   3. independence.
   4. adaptation.

7. Which effect of institutionalization is diminished by not knocking before entering the room and not draping patients during care activities? *(22)*
   1. Redefinition of "normal"
   2. Social withdrawal
   3. Indignity
   4. Regression

8. The first comprehensive approach to problems experienced by people with disabilities was the: *(19)*
   1. Vocational Rehabilitation Act of 1920.
   2. Social Security Act of 1935.
   3. Medicare Act of 1965.
   4. Rehabilitation Act of 1973.

9. Which act began affirmative action programs to assist in the employment of disabled people and prohibited discrimination against them in programs receiving federal funds? *(19)*
   1. Vocational Rehabilitation Act of 1920
   2. Social Security Act of 1935
   3. Medicare Act of 1965
   4. Rehabilitation Act of 1973

10. The focus in rehabilitation is to: *(18)*
    1. promote self-esteem.
    2. assist with ADLs.
    3. restore maximal possible function.
    4. eliminate impairment.

11. An example of mental impairment is: *(17)*
    1. loss of memory.
    2. paralysis of an arm.
    3. brain hemorrhage.
    4. fractured neck.

12. Moderate limitation in one or more ADLs resulting in a person's being able to go to work, but requiring modifications in the workplace, is classified as: *(18)*
    1. Level I disability.
    2. Level II disability.
    3. Level III disability.
    4. Level IV disability.

13. Which of the following is an example of a skilled procedure? *(16)*
    1. Foley catheter insertion
    2. Enema administration
    3. Mouth care
    4. Ear drop administration

14. An individual with an injured back who has a diminished capacity for work is classified as: *(17)*
    1. handicapped.
    2. impaired.
    3. disabled.
    4. dependent.

15. Return of function and prevention of further disability are goals of: *(18)*
    1. community-based nursing.
    2. public health nursing.
    3. rehabilitation.
    4. long-term care.

16. Nursing homes and skilled nursing facilities are types of: *(20)*
    1. domiciliary care facilities.
    2. outpatient facilities.
    3. long-term facilities.
    4. health maintenance organizations.

17. By providing clear documentation of functional losses and goals for care, the nurse is meeting the Medicare criterion of: *(15)*
    1. skilled care.
    2. reasonable and necessary care.
    3. homebound patient care.
    4. intermittent care.

18. What percentage of people aged 65–74 live in nursing homes? *(21)*
    1. 1%
    2. 5%
    3. 10 %
    4. 20%

19. What percentage of people 85 and over reside in nursing homes? *(21)*
    1. 1%
    2. 6%
    3. 10%
    4. 20%

20. The best indicator of who will need nursing home placement is: *(21)*
    1. age.
    2. ADL dependency.
    3. presence of handicaps.
    4. severity of infectious disease process.

21. Which type of facility provides basic room, board, and supervision, where residents come and go as they please? *(21)*
    1. Domiciliary care facilities
    2. Sheltered housing
    3. Intermediate care
    4. Skilled care

22. Facilities that contain modifications to provide care for the frail elderly and usually provide community dining are called: *(21)*
    1. domiciliary care facilities.
    2. sheltered housing.
    3. intermediate care.
    4. skilled care.

23. Treating patients primarily in light of their diagnoses or dysfunctional behavior patterns is an example of: *(22)*
    1. indignity.
    2. regression.
    3. social withdrawal.
    4. depersonalization.

24. Being left in bed a great part of the day, finding it difficult to walk, and losing skills of conversation are examples of: *(23)*
    1. social withdrawal.
    2. indignity.
    3. regression.
    4. depersonalization.

25. Which is an example of the Medicare requirement for homebound care stating the care must be intermittent in nature? *(15)*
    1. Physician must sign off on all treatments prescribed.
    2. Patient must be bedridden.
    3. Care should not exceed 28 hours per week.
    4. Care must be skilled.

26. A patient rings the call bell. What is the first nursing action you should take to prevent the patient's feeling of indignity? *(23)*
    1. Knock on the patient's door before entering.
    2. Talk with the patient about events inside and outside the nursing home.
    3. Simplify language and activities for the patient, and avoid baby talk.
    4. Give the patient some flexibility and measure of control in the daily activities.

## ALTERNATE FORMAT QUESTIONS

J. 1. What types of care provided by home health nurses are considered skilled? Select all that apply. *(16)*
    1. Bathing the patient
    2. Weighing the patient
    3. Catheter insertion
    4. Dressing changes
    5. Mouth care
    6. Enema administration

2. Which are examples of secondary disabilities? Select all that apply. *(18)*
    1. Stroke
    2. Pneumonia
    3. Pressure ulcers
    4. Asthma
    5. Myocardial infarction
    6. Limb contractures

# Legal and Ethical Considerations

---

## OBJECTIVES

1. Define ethics, bioethics, values, morality, moral uncertainty, moral distress, moral outrage, and moral/ethical dilemma.

2. Explain the principles of ethics: autonomy, justice, fidelity, beneficence, and nonmaleficence.

3. Explain how values are formed.

4. Explain how values clarification is useful in nursing practice.

5. Discuss the relationship between culture and values.

6. Describe the following philosophical bases for ethics: deontology, utilitarianism, feminist ethics, and ethics of care.

7. Describe the steps in processing ethical dilemmas.

8. Describe the role of Institutional Ethics Committees.

9. Explain the role of the LVN/LPN in relation to informed consent.

---

## LEARNING ACTIVITIES

**A. Key Terms.** Match the definition in the numbered column with the most appropriate term in the lettered column.

1. _____ Principles or standards shared by members of a society that determine what is desirable or worthwhile *(28)*

2. _____ Shared ideas of what is right and good *(26)*

3. _____ Ethical questions related to health care *(26)*

4. _____ Belief that one's own culture is superior to others *(28)*

A. Ethnocentrism
B. Values
C. Bioethics
D. Morality

**B. Ethics Key Terms.** Match the basic concept of ethics on the left with the proper label in the lettered column.

1. _____ Do no harm *(27)*
2. _____ Obligation to do good *(27)*
3. _____ Obligation to be fair to everyone *(27)*
4. _____ Right to make one's own decisions *(27)*
5. _____ Obligation to be faithful to agreements *(27)*
6. _____ Telling the truth *(27)*

A. Veracity
B. Beneficence
C. Justice
D. Nonmaleficence
E. Fidelity
F. Autonomy

**C. Legal Terms.** Match the definition in the numbered column with the most appropriate term in the lettered column.

1. _____ Civil or criminal law *(29)*
2. _____ Result of judicial decisions made when individual cases are decided in the courts *(29)*
3. _____ Rules created by administrative bodies such as state boards of nursing *(29)*
4. _____ Civil wrong against a person or property *(29)*
5. _____ Conduct falling below the standard of care *(29)*
6. _____ Condition when injury was caused by the nurse's failure to carry out the duty *(30)*
7. _____ Spoken false information that could damage a person's reputation *(30)*
8. _____ Written false information that could damage a person's reputation *(30)*

A. Common law
B. Malpractice
C. Negligence
D. Regulatory law
E. Statutory law
F. Tort
G. Slander
H. Libel

D. **Negligence.** Which of the following are common negligence errors? Select all that apply.

1. _____ Failure to give complete report to oncoming shifts. *(30)*

2. _____ Restraining a patient against his wishes. *(30)*

3. _____ Failure to use aseptic technique when required. *(30)*

4. _____ Improper release of medical information. *(30)*

5. _____ Medicating a patient to keep him quiet. *(30)*

6. _____ Falls resulting in injury to a patient. *(30)*

7. _____ Failure to adequately monitor a patient's condition. *(30)*

E. **Autonomy.** Which of the following are related to the recognition of autonomy? Select all that apply.

1. _____ Reporting a coworker who is impaired *(27)*

2. _____ Advance directives *(27)*

3. _____ Patient's right to refuse treatment *(27)*

4. _____ Patient's right to expect that staff will not abandon him or her *(27)*

5. _____ Policies for fair distribution of scarce resources *(27)*

6. _____ Informed consent *(27)*

F. **Ethical Dilemmas.** List the seven steps for processing ethical dilemmas, in sequential order. *(29)*

1. _____

2. _____

3. _____

4. _____

5. _____

6. _____

7. _____

**G. Ethics Terms.** Match the definition in the numbered column with the most appropriate term in the lettered column.

1. _____   When the nurse senses that a situation is a moral problem but cannot define it clearly *(26)*

2. _____   When no one solution seems to be satisfactory because of conflicting morals *(26)*

3. _____   When another health care provider acts in a way the nurse believes is immoral and the nurse feels powerless to intervene *(26)*

4. _____   When the nurse feels powerless because moral beliefs cannot be followed due to institutional barriers *(26)*

A.   Moral distress
B.   Moral outrage
C.   Moral uncertainty
D.   Ethical dilemma

**H. Ethics Terms.** Match the definition in the numbered column with the most appropriate term in the lettered column.

1. _____   Defines right and wrong on the basis of whether an action meets the criteria of fidelity, veracity, autonomy, beneficence, and justice *(28)*

2. _____   Focuses on inequalities between people, particularly on the basis of gender, and places value on relationships *(28)*

3. _____   Theory that views care as a central activity of human behavior *(28)*

4. _____   The right action is that which produces the greatest good for the greatest number of people *(28)*

A.   Feminist ethics
B.   Ethics of care
C.   Utilitarianism
D.   Deontology

## MULTIPLE-CHOICE QUESTIONS

**I.** Choose the most appropriate answer.

1. A limitation of deontology occurs when: *(28)*
   1. an action produces the greatest good for the greatest number of people.
   2. the focus is on inequalities between people.
   3. an action represents conflicting values.
   4. the ethic of care emphasizes relationships.

2. What is the initial task when the nurse encounters an ethical dilemma? *(29)*
   1. State the ethical problem clearly so that everyone can agree on the problem.
   2. Decide whether the situation constitutes an ethical problem.
   3. Consider your own values in relation to the problem.
   4. Outline possible courses of action and consequences.

3. Where are the legal boundaries of nursing practice in a given state defined? *(29)*
   1. Hospital policy and procedures books
   2. Professional nursing organizations
   3. State legislatures
   4. Nurse practice acts

4. What group creates regulatory laws that address the conduct of nurses? *(29)*
   1. Professional nursing organizations
   2. State legislatures
   3. State boards of nursing
   4. State supreme courts

5. A threat of some contact without the patient's consent is called: *(30)*
   1. assault.
   2. battery.
   3. libel.
   4. slander.

6. The obligation to be fair to everyone is an ethical concept called: *(30)*
   1. fidelity.
   2. veracity.
   3. justice.
   4. beneficence.

7. What is the meaning of the ethical concept of autonomy? *(27)*
   1. Obligation to be fair
   2. The right to make one's own decisions
   3. Obligation to be faithful to agreements
   4. Telling the truth

8. The professional duty to help others is an example of: *(27)*
   1. veracity.
   2. beneficence.
   3. fidelity.
   4. autonomy.

9. A system or code of behavior related to what is right is known as: *(26)*
   1. ethics.
   2. empathy.
   3. caring.
   4. empowerment.

10. Which ethical concept is applied when the nurse provides quality care to patients, regardless of their socioeconomic status? *(27)*
    1. Justice
    2. Veracity
    3. Autonomy
    4. Fidelity

11. What is the ethical concept applied when the nurse reports substandard nursing practice? *(27)*
    1. Beneficence
    2. Veracity
    3. Fidelity
    4. Nonmaleficence

12. Which of the following people cannot give informed consent? *(32)*
    1. Patient having an appendectomy
    2. Patient receiving chemotherapy following a mastectomy
    3. Patient who just received a pre-operative sedative
    4. Patient having cataract surgery as day surgery

13. The nurse's best protection against negligence and malpractice is to follow: *(30)*
    1. hospital policies.
    2. scope of practice rules.
    3. standards of care.
    4. state nurse practice acts.

14. The law that went into effect in 2003 making health care providers acutely aware of the actions needed to protect patient confidentiality is the: *(32)*
    1. Nurse Practice Act.
    2. Social Security Act.
    3. Patient's Bill of Rights.
    4. HIPAA.

15. Which ethical concept refers to the patient's right to make his or her own decisions regarding treatment? *(27)*
    1. Beneficence
    2. Autonomy
    3. Fidelity
    4. Veracity

16. Which right do all patients have regarding informed consent? *(32)*
    1. Explanation of rehabilitation
    2. Have all questions answered
    3. The patient will not be abandoned
    4. Recommendation will be made indicating the best treatment

17. Who is responsible for obtaining informed consent? *(32)*
    1. Hospital
    2. Supervisory nurse
    3. Staff nurse
    4. Physician

18. The release of medical information or publication of patient photographs without the patient's consent constitutes: *(30)*
    1. defamation of character.
    2. slander.
    3. invasion of privacy.
    4. malpractice.

19. What action should the nurse take if the patient states that he does not understand the medical procedure for which he is scheduled, whien obtaining informed consent? *(32)*
    1. Explain the procedure to the patient.
    2. Ask the patient if he has any questions.
    3. Inform the patient that he may want to discuss this with his family members.
    4. Contact the physician.

## ALTERNATE FORMAT QUESTIONS

**J.**   1. Which topics must be discussed with patients to constitute sufficient information for the patient to give informed consent? Select all that apply. *(32)*
    1. Recommended treatment
    2. Risks
    3. Benefits
    4. Alternatives
    5. Consequences of refusing treatment
    6. Research data about treatment

2. What conditions must be met to be found liable for malpractice? Select all that apply. *(30)*
    1. The nurse owed a duty to the patient.
    2. The nurse communicated with other members of the health care team.
    3. The patient was injured.
    4. The nurse refused to work overtime.
    5. The nurse did not carry out the duty to the patient.
    6. Injury was caused by the nurse's failure to carry out the duty.

3. Which of the following are essential elements of informed consent? Select all that apply. *(32)*
    1. Mandatory agreement
    2. Patient decision-making capability
    3. Sufficient information
    4. Physician present when patient signs consent

4. Which of the following constitutes assault? Select all that apply. *(30)*
    1. Nurse touches the patient in offensive manner.
    2. Nurse threatens to restrain a patient against his wishes.
    3. Nurse gives false information that damages the patient's reputation.
    4. Nurse improperly releases information about the patient to a relative.
    5. Nurse threatens to medicate a patient against his wishes.

# The Leadership Role of the Licensed Practical Nurse

---

## OBJECTIVES

1. Differentiate leadership from management.

2. Describe leadership styles.

3. Discuss management theories.

4. List tips for effective management.

5. Describe the role of the licensed vocational nurse as a team leader.

---

## LEARNING ACTIVITIES

**A.  Leadership Styles and Management Theories.** Match the definition in the numbered column with the most appropriate term in the lettered column.

1.  _____   Authoritarian, directive, or bureaucratic types of leadership *(38)*

2.  _____   Mixture of autocratic and democratic leadership; feedback from group members is used by the leader to make a final decision *(39)*

3.  _____   Achievement of goals through participation by all group members *(38)*

4.  _____   Nondirective type of leadership *(38)*

5.  _____   Management by autocratic rule with little participation in decision-making by workers *(39)*

6.  _____   Democratic style of management with some participation in decision-making by workers *(40)*

7.  _____   Management with full participation in decision-making by workers *(40)*

8.  _____   All group members may assume leadership and follower roles in various circumstances based upon their unique skills and talents *(39)*

A.  Autocratic leadership
B.  Theory X
C.  Laissez-faire leadership
D.  Democratic leadership
E.  Participative leadership
F.  Transformational leadership
G.  Theory Y
H.  Theory Z

B. **Key Terms.** Match the definition in the numbered column with the most appropriate term in the lettered column.

1. _____ Turning over part of one person's responsibility to another person with that person's consent *(44)*

2. _____ Identification and delegation of specific tasks to a specific person who is hired and paid to perform these tasks *(44)*

3. _____ Guidance, or showing the way to others *(37)*

4. _____ Effective use of selected methods to achieve desired outcomes *(37)*

A. Leadership
B. Management
C. Assignment
D. Delegation

C. **Management Theory.** Following are characteristics of people in their work environments. Mark an "X" before the characteristic if it refers to the Theory X classical management theory, a "Y" if it refers to the Theory Y classical management theory, and a "Z" if it refers to the Theory Z classical management theory.

1. _____ Work together for the good of the company *(39-40)*

2. _____ Care about what they are doing *(39-40)*

3. _____ Find no pleasure in work *(39-40)*

4. _____ Constantly striving to grow *(39-40)*

5. _____ Naturally lazy and prefer to do nothing *(39-40)*

6. _____ Work mainly for the money *(39-40)*

7. _____ Do not want to think for themselves *(39-40)*

8. _____ Mature and responsible *(39-40)*

9. _____ Self-directed *(39-40)*

10. _____ Work only because they fear being fired *(39-40)*

11. _____ Child-like and like being told what to do *(39-40)*

12. _____ Work for rewards other than money *(39-40)*

13. _____ Active and enjoy setting their own goals *(39-40)*

14. _____ Not capable of making decisions for themselves *(39-40)*

15. _____ Based on mutual trust and loyalty *(39-40)*

16. _____ Dislike responsibility *(39-40)*

17. _____ Accept responsibility *(39-40)*

18. _____ Dynamic, flexible, and adaptive *(39-40)*

**D. Stages of Conflict.** Match the description of conflict in the numbered column with the related stages of conflict in the lettered column.

1. _____   The conflict leads to various behaviors that may or may not resolve the conflict. *(42)*

2. _____   Reformulation of goals that is acceptable to all parties. *(42)*

3. _____   People believe their goals are being blocked. *(42)*

4. _____   Each party formulates a view of the basis of conflict. *(42)*

A.  Frustration
B.  Conceptualization
C.  Action
D.  Outcomes

**E. Leadership Styles.** Match the characteristic of leadership style in the numbered column with the leadership style in the lettered column. The answers may be used more than once.

1. _____   Leader provides little or no directive leadership *(38)*

2. _____   Leader turns problems over to the group to manage *(38)*

3. _____   Leader leads by suggestion rather than domination *(38)*

4. _____   Opposite of autocratic *(38)*

5. _____   Cross between autocratic and democratic leaders *(38)*

6. _____   Authoritarian, directive, or bureaucratic *(38)*

7. _____   Leader analyzes feedback from the group and then makes all formal decisions *(39)*

8. _____   Leader presents personal views to group members who provide critique and comment *(39)*

9. _____   Leadership flows among members based on the task at hand and members' individual skills *(39)*

A.  Autocratic
B.  Democratic
C.  Laissez-faire
D.  Multicratic (situational)
E.  Transformational

F. **Conflict Resolution.** Match the positive outcomes and uses of conflict resolution modes in the numbered column with the related mode of conflict in the lettered column.

1. _____ Generates commitment to work together *(42)*

2. _____ Produces mutually accept-able solutions *(42)*

3. _____ Agreement is reached *(42)*

4. _____ Reflects strong stance to defend principles *(42)*

5. _____ Temporarily defuses highly charged emotional dis-agreement *(42)*

A. Accommodation
B. Collaboration
C. Compromise
D. Avoidance
E. Competition

G. **Management Tips.** Which of the following are tips for effective management? Select all that apply.

1. _____ Seek help and support from a variety of sources. *(42)*

2. _____ Keep confidential informa-tion confidential. *(42)*

3. _____ Stress the importance of documentation. *(42)*

4. _____ Collect data from each pa-tient upon admission. *(42)*

5. _____ Use an authoritarian ap-proach as a leader. *(42)*

6. _____ Use competition to avoid conflict. *(42)*

## MULTIPLE-CHOICE QUESTIONS

H. Choose the most appropriate answer.

1. Which of the following methods does the democratic leader use to make decisions? *(38)*
   1. Participation of all group members and group consensus
   2. Nondirective style, letting group mem-bers decide
   3. Makes decisions independently from group
   4. Presents personal views to group mem-bers for comments before making final decision

2. Four basic types of leadership are autocrat-ic, participative, democratic, and: *(38)*
   1. authoritarian.
   2. bureaucratic.
   3. directive.
   4. laissez-faire.

3. Individuals who achieve their goals by set-ting objectives and having them carried out without input or suggestions from others display what style of leadership? *(38)*
   1. Democratic
   2. Autocratic
   3. Laissez-faire
   4. Cooperative

4. Individuals who encourage people to provide input into problem-solving and come up with group consensus display what style of leadership? *(39)*
   1. Democratic
   2. Autocratic
   3. Laissez-faire
   4. Authoritarian

5. Individuals who lead by suggestion rather than by domination exhibit what style of leadership? *(39)*
   1. Autocratic
   2. Laissez-faire
   3. Authoritarian
   4. Democratic

6. A leadership style where individuals are allowed to do whatever they want is: *(38)*
   1. democratic.
   2. autocratic.
   3. authoritarian.
   4. laissez-faire.

7. Which style do leaders who use Theory Y of management usually have? *(38)*
   1. Autocratic
   2. Democratic
   3. Bureaucratic
   4. Laissez-faire

8. Which management step includes making assignments and explaining what needs to be done? *(41)*
   1. Coordinating
   2. Directing
   3. Planning
   4. Controlling

9. The process of selecting one course of action from alternatives is: *(40)*
   1. coordinating.
   2. decision-making.
   3. directing.
   4. evaluating.

10. Once the problem is identified, the next step in decision-making involves: *(40)*
    1. choosing the most desirable solution.
    2. evaluating the best response.
    3. coordinating the representative ideas.
    4. exploring all possible solutions.

11. The management step that helps eliminate overlap, duplication, and omissions is: *(41)*
    1. organizing.
    2. directing.
    3. coordinating.
    4. controlling.

12. The benefit of taking an active approach to planning is that the nurse is likely to: *(41)*
    1. emphasize the importance of documentation.
    2. avoid conflict before it occurs.
    3. make employees accountable for their actions.
    4. treat other employees with respect.

13. Which leadership style provides the quickest response? *(38)*
    1. Laissez-faire
    2. Democratic
    3. Participative
    4. Autocratic

14. Which leader is described as multicratic or situational? *(39)*
    1. Laissez-faire
    2. Democratic
    3. Participative
    4. Autocratic

15. In making assignments, an attempt should be made to match the skills of the assigned personnel with: *(41)*
    1. patient personalities.
    2. nursing needs.
    3. patient needs.
    4. institutional needs.

16. When making assignments for patient care, which approach encourages cooperation and tends to get more work done? *(41)*
    1. Directly ordering that a task be done
    2. Requesting that a task be done
    3. Delegating tasks to more than one person
    4. Asking to see the staffing plan

17. Which step of the management process involves developing objectives, policies, and procedures? *(41)*
    1. Directing
    2. Planning
    3. Organizing
    4. Coordinating

18. Controlling is basically a form of: *(42)*
    1. evaluation.
    2. assessment.
    3. planning.
    4. implementation.

19. Which should *not* be delegated to unlicensed personnel? *(44)*
    1. Making a bed
    2. Weighing a patient
    3. Writing a nursing care plan
    4. Feeding a patient

20. *Continuous quality improvement* (CQI) is a term frequently used in relation to: *(42)*
    1. organization.
    2. direction.
    3. coordination.
    4. control.

21. Which of the following is likely to occur when an autocratic leader hires an autocratic manager? *(38)*
    1. Group concerns
    2. Problem solving
    3. Power struggle
    4. Confusion

22. Which type of leadership style requires a highly motivated, focused group to work well? *(38)*
    1. Democratic
    2. Laissez-faire
    3. Autocratic
    4. Participative

23. Group members assist the participative leader with setting goals, achieving for themselves a sense of: *(39)*
    1. empowerment.
    2. structure.
    3. domination.
    4. creativity.

24. Characteristics of an effective team include: *(46)*
    1. continuous quality improvement (CQI).
    2. established standards.
    3. clear goals.
    4. active listening.

25. When the other person really does have a better idea than you, an effective mode of conflict resolution is: *(43)*
    1. accommodation.
    2. collaboration.
    3. compromise.
    4. competition.

26. A mode of conflict resolution that wastes time if used for resolution of trivial issues is: *(43)*
    1. accommodation.
    2. collaboration.
    3. compromise.
    4. competition.

27. Which leadership style provides a minimal leader activity level? *(38)*
    1. Democratic
    2. Authoritarian
    3. Multicratic
    4. Laissez-faire

28. Which leadership style provides the most creative output of the group? *(38)*
    1. Democratic
    2. Authoritarian
    3. Multicratic
    4. Laissez-faire

29. Which leadership theory places more emphasis on the followers than the leaders? *(39)*
    1. Trait
    2. Attitudinal
    3. Situational
    4. Contemporary

30. Which method of conflict resolution is used when you are wrong and the other person really does have a better idea? *(43)*
    1. Accommodation
    2. Collaboration
    3. Avoidance
    4. Competition

31. Which method of conflict resolution is used when time pressures require a quick solution and each party is finally committed to different views? *(43)*
    1. Collaboration
    2. Compromise
    3. Avoidance
    4. Competition

32. When delegating a task or making an assignment to unlicensed assistive personnel, the nurse has the duty to maintain: *(43)*
    1. patient safety.
    2. caring relationships.
    3. patient autonomy.
    4. autocraitc leadership.

33. Involving others and brainstorming is used in the decision-making process as part of: *(41)*
    1. identifying the problem.
    2. exploring possible solutions.
    3. choosing the most desirable action.
    4. planning evaluation.

34. Directing a patient to do something that creates a power struggle for resistance is an example of: *(54)*
    1. false reassurance.
    2. premature advice.
    3. communication cut-off.
    4. commanding.

## ALTERNATE FORMAT QUESTIONS

I.  1. Which characteristics describe the authoritarian leadership style? Select all that apply. *(38)*
       1. Little freedom
       2. No control
       3. Decision-making by the leader
       4. Shared responsibility
       5. High quantity output of the group
       6. Minimal leader activity

    2. Which of the following are major leadership theories? Select all that apply. *(39)*
       1. Multicratic
       2. Trait
       3. Attitudinal
       4. Situational
       5. Laissez-faire

    3. Which are characteristics of leaders and managers? Select all that apply. *(37)*
       1. Sets realistic goals
       2. Is easily self-satisfied
       3. Makes decisions not involving risks
       4. Answers questions of co-workers

J.  List in sequential order the steps in the decision-making process. The first step is 1 and the last step is 5. *(41)*

    A. _____ Implement action
    B. _____ Identify the problem
    C. _____ Plan evaluation
    D. _____ Choose the most desirable action
    E. _____ Explore possible solutions

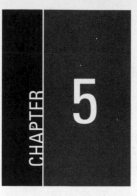
# The Nurse-Patient Relationship

---

## OBJECTIVES

1. Define holistic view of nursing.

2. Define the concept of *self*.

3. Discuss the use of self in the practice of nursing.

4. Compare the meaning of the terms *patient* and *client*.

5. List commonly held expectations of patients and families.

6. Describe the meaning of the Patient's Bill of Rights and the AHA Patient Care Partnership document.

7. Describe guidelines for nurse-patient relationships.

8. Describe basic components of communication.

---

## LEARNING ACTIVITIES

A. **Helper Roles.** What characteristics must a nurse must have to assume the helper role in a nurse-patient relationship? Select all that apply.

1. _____ Sense of responsibility to the patient *(48)*

2. _____ Ability to express feelings and attitudes with the patient *(48)*

3. _____ Ability to form a long-term relationship *(48)*

4. _____ Nonjudgmental attitude *(48)*

5. _____ Ability to keep secrets *(48)*

6. _____ Ability to form friendship or support relationships *(48)*

B. **Nonverbal Communication.** Which are examples of nonverbal communication? Select all that apply.

1. _____ Laughing *(52)*
2. _____ Facial expression *(52)*
3. _____ Explanation of patient care *(52)*
4. _____ Patient is a partner in care *(52)*
5. _____ Assertive communication *(52)*
6. _____ Body position *(52)*
7. _____ Making gestures *(52)*

C. **Communication.** Fill in the blank.

1. Observation is to nonverbal language as listening is to _____. *(52)*

D. **Helper Role.** Indicate by an X in the appropriate column whether the description refers to a helping person or a friend. *(52)*

| | Helping Person | Friend | |
|---|---|---|---|
| 1. | _____ | _____ | Shares personal information |
| 2. | _____ | _____ | Responsible to client |
| 3. | _____ | _____ | Sexual overtones or a sexual relationship may develop |
| 4. | _____ | _____ | Both individuals express feelings, attitudes, and opinions |
| 5. | _____ | _____ | Attitude is nonjudgmental |
| 6. | _____ | _____ | Relationship is goal-directed |
| 7. | _____ | _____ | Individuals meet each other's needs |
| 8. | _____ | _____ | Relationship is time-limited |
| 9. | _____ | _____ | Objective of relationship is to meet client's needs |
| 10. | _____ | _____ | Relationship may continue |
| 11. | _____ | _____ | No plan involved |
| 12. | _____ | _____ | Discourages any sexual overtones in relationship |
| 13. | _____ | _____ | Tries to influence each other in discussing issues |
| 14. | _____ | _____ | Does not keep secrets |
| 15. | _____ | _____ | Attempts to influence patient to his or her way of thinking |

**E.  Communication.** Match the example of communication technique in the numbered column with the proper label in the lettered column.

1. _____ Resisting the urge to fill quiet periods with conversation. *(54)*

2. _____ "Tell me your reactions to your new treatment." *(54)*

3. _____ "You say you're feeling better since your brother has returned?" *(54)*

4. _____ "So, you have decided to have surgery, but delay it until after Christmas." *(54)*

5. _____ "I hear you're concerned about your son." *(54)*

6. _____ "Do you mean 'sad' when you say 'upset'?" *(54)*

A.  Reflecting
B.  Clarifying
C.  Silence
D.  Restating
E.  Summarizing
F.  Open-ended statement

**F.  Communication.** Match the example of nontherapeutic communication technique in the numbered column with the proper label in the lettered column.

1. _____ "You shouldn't worry about the new treatment." *(54)*

2. _____ "Try to think positively." *(54)*

3. _____ "The first thing you need to do is to make your teenagers help you more." *(54)*

4. _____ "You must quit smoking immediately." *(54)*

5. _____ "It's incredible that your doctor did not tell you when to take this medication." *(54)*

A.  False reassurance
B.  Premature advice
C.  Commanding
D.  Communication cut-off
E.  Assuming truth of statements rather than checking them out

## MULTIPLE-CHOICE QUESTIONS

**G.  Choose the most appropriate answer.**

1.  The ability to be open and honest about one's feelings is characteristic of: *(52)*
    1.  self-image.
    2.  self-esteem.
    3.  self-disclosure.
    4.  self-trust.

2.  Exchanging ideas, beliefs, thoughts, and feelings between two or more people is: *(52)*
    1.  empathy.
    2.  caring.
    3.  self-disclosure.
    4.  communication.

3. An active process that involves trying to understand what is being said is: *(52)*
   1. listening.
   2. talking.
   3. explaining.
   4. self-awareness.

4. Understanding another's feelings and becoming immersed in the situation is: *(53)*
   1. empathy.
   2. helping.
   3. sympathy.
   4. apathy.

5. The main difference between a therapeutic relationship and a social relationship is that the therapeutic helping person: *(52)*
   1. has a spontaneous approach.
   2. discusses own beliefs.
   3. shares feelings and opinions.
   4. is responsible to the client.

6. A goal-directed focus on one patient is a description of: *(48)*
   1. self-disclosure.
   2. self-awareness.
   3. therapeutic relationship.
   4. reflection.

7. The ability to be honest and open about one's feelings relates to: *(52)*
   1. reflection.
   2. clarification.
   3. self-disclosure.
   4. nonjudgmental attitude.

8. Encouraging patients to be active participants in their own care is called: *(50)*
   1. empowerment.
   2. veracity.
   3. fidelity.
   4. empathy.

9. According to the Patient's Bill of Rights, a basic right of patients is the right to: *(50)*
   1. complete medical care regardless of the ability to pay.
   2. choose the best method of health care delivery.
   3. considerate and respectful care from all health care providers.
   4. determine treatment for medical care.

10. Protection of the patient's confidentiality is stated in the: *(50)*
    1. Joint Commission of Accreditation Act.
    2. Social Security Act.
    3. Patient's Bill of Rights.
    4. Right to Privacy Act.

## ALTERNATE FORMAT QUESTIONS

H. 1. Which of the following are patient rights described in the AHA patient care partnership? Select all that apply. *(50)*
   1. Discussion of the treatment plan
   2. Promotion of self-image
   3. Understanding of health goals
   4. Therapeutic communication
   5. Protection of privacy
   6. Telling the truth

# 6 Cultural Aspects of Nursing Care

---

## OBJECTIVES

1. Describe cultural concepts related to nursing and health care.

2. Identify traditional health habits and beliefs of major ethnic groups in the United States.

3. Explain cultural influences on the interactions of patients and families with the health care system.

4. Discuss cultural considerations in providing culturally sensitive nursing care.

5. Discuss ways in which planning and implementation of nursing interventions can be adapted to a patient's ethnicity.

---

## LEARNING ACTIVITIES

**A.  Key Terms.** Match the definition in the numbered column with the most appropriate term in the lettered column. Answers may be used more than once.

1. _____   A group of individuals within a culture whose members share different beliefs, values, and attitudes from those of the dominant culture *(57)*

2. _____   Replacing values and beliefs with those of another culture *(66)*

3. _____   The existence of many cultures in a society *(57)*

4. _____   Learned values, beliefs, and practices that are characteristic of a society and that guide individual behavior *(57)*

5. _____   Integration of cultural considerations into all aspects of nursing care *(57)*

6. _____   Group of individuals with a unique identity based on shared traditions and customs *(58)*

7. _____   The process of learning to be part of a culture *(57)*

A.  Cultural diversity
B.  Enculturation
C.  Subculture
D.  Culture
E.  Assimilation
F.  Ethnic group

**B.  Culture.** List the three basic characteristics of all cultures. *(57)*

1. _____

2. _____

3. _____

**C.  Ethnic Groups.** Match the healers in the numbered column with the ethnic group that may be likely to use them in the lettered column. Answers may be used more than once.

1. _____   Spiritualists *(67)*
2. _____   Curanderos *(67)*
3. _____   Root doctors *(67)*
4. _____   Medicine men *(67)*
5. _____   Herbalists *(67)*
6. _____   Acupuncturists *(67)*

A.  Asian
B.  Native American
C.  Latino
D.  African-American

**D. Culture Shock.** List in the proper sequence the three phases of culture shock associated with hospitalization. *(68)*

A. _____    Patient becomes disenchanted and frustrated.

B. _____    Patient adapts to new environment, maintaining a sense of humor.

C. _____    Patient asks questions about hospital routines and environment.

## MULTIPLE-CHOICE QUESTIONS

**E.** Choose the most appropriate answer.

1. The ideas, beliefs, values, and attitudes that a group of people possess represent: *(57)*
   1. race.
   2. religion.
   3. ethnicity.
   4. culture.

2. The effort of many immigrants to assimilate into society is known as: *(57)*
   1. salad bowl.
   2. melting pot.
   3. cultural diversity.
   4. true ethnicity.

3. The way in which new arrivals seek to maintain individual differences while acclimating to new surroundings is termed: *(57)*
   1. melting pot.
   2. salad bowl.
   3. cultural diversity.
   4. true ethnicity.

4. The Latinos are examples of a: *(57)*
   1. salad bowl.
   2. melting pot.
   3. subculture.
   4. democracy.

5. What percentage of households in the United States are single-parent families? *(58)*
   1. less than 1%
   2. 10%
   3. 20%
   4. 50%

6. People who claim that illness is a result of punishment for a sin that an individual has committed believe in: *(66)*
   1. divine punishment.
   2. corporal punishment.
   3. legal punishment.
   4. ethnic punishment.

7. People who believe that health and illness are influenced by four humors that regulate body function believe in: *(66)*
   1. divine punishment theory.
   2. cultural diversity theory.
   3. salad bowl theory.
   4. hot-and-cold theory.

8. Culture shock associated with hospitalization occurs in three stages. They include asking questions, being disenchanted, and: *(68)*
   1. generalization.
   2. denial.
   3. adaptation.
   4. bargaining.

9. The integration of cultural considerations into all aspects of nursing care is called: *(57)*
   1. cultural diversity.
   2. transcultural nursing.
   3. enculturation.
   4. subcultural nursing.

10. Kosher dietary laws which state that there is no mixing of milk and meat at a meal is a belief of which religious group? *(59)*
    1. Seventh-Day Adventist
    2. Eastern Orthodox
    3. Judaism
    4. Protestant

11. Which ethnic group values self-respect, respect for elders, and pride? *(67)*
    1. Whites
    2. African-Americans
    3. Latinos
    4. Asians

12. Which religious group believes that the body should not be left alone until buried? *(59)*
    1. Judaism
    2. Protestant
    3. Eastern Orthodox
    4. Mormon

13. Which religious group believes in reincarnation and calls in a priest at the time of death, who ties a thread around the neck of the dead person as a blessing? *(65)*
    1. Mormon
    2. Hinduism
    3. Eastern Orthodox
    4. Judaism

14. Which religious group believes that the body should be washed, prepared, and placed in a position facing Mecca following death? *(68)*
    1. Judaism
    2. Eastern Orthodox
    3. Catholic
    4. Muslim

15. Which ethnic group responds better to diuretics for hypertension? *(70)*
    1. African-Americans
    2. Latinos
    3. Native Americans
    4. Whites

16. A 24-year-old woman has been given an antidepressant for depression. Which ethnic group will respond better to a lower dose of antidepressants? *(70)*
    1. Whites
    2. African-Americans
    3. Europeans
    4. Asians

17. Why are antihypertensive drugs less effective in Japanese patients? *(69)*
    1. They metabolize the drug more quickly.
    2. They eat Kosher foods.
    3. Their diet is high in salt.
    4. They are at greater risk for drug toxicity.

18. Utilizing interpersonal skills to adapt nursing care to the cultural differences of your patients is called: *(67)*
    1. holistic care.
    2. complementary care.
    3. cultural competence.
    4. cultural diversity.

19. The integration of culture into all aspects of nursing is known as: *(57)*
    1. multicultural nursing.
    2. enculturation.
    3. transcultural nursing.
    4. assimilation.

# CHAPTER 7

# The Nurse and the Family

---

## OBJECTIVES

1. Describe the concept of *family* and its relationship to society.

2. Compare various family structures or lifestyles that characterize modern American families.

3. Discuss the family from a developmental perspective.

4. Describe roles and communication patterns within families.

5. Describe adaptive and maladaptive mechanisms used by families to cope with various stressors.

6. Describe the role of the nurse in dealing with families experiencing various stresses.

7. Identify community resources that may help to meet the family's needs.

---

## LEARNING ACTIVITIES

**A. Family Types.** Match the type of family in the numbered column with the most appropriate term in the lettered column.

1. _____ Nuclear family *(72)*
2. _____ Extended family *(72)*
3. _____ Step-parent *(72)*
4. _____ Nontraditional *(72)*

A. Cohabiting couples
B. Blended family
C. Relatives of either spouse who live with the nuclear family
D. Biologic or adoptive mother and father and their children

B. **Developmental Tasks.** Match the developmental task in the numbered column with the correct stage of the family life cycle in the lettered column.

1. _____   Establish mutually satisfy-     A.   Launching children and moving on
ing marriage; make deci-       B.   Families with adolescents
sions about parenthood         C.   Families with young children
*(74)*                                D.   Families in later life

2. _____   Set up young family as a     E.   Beginning families
stable unit; socialize chil-
dren *(74)*

3. _____   Balance freedom with
responsibility for children;
communicate openly be-
tween parents and children
*(74)*

4. _____   Expand family circle to
include new family mem-
bers acquired by marriage;
assist aging and ill parents
of husband or wife *(74)*

5. _____   Maintain a satisfying living
arrangement; adjust to
loss of spouse; maintain
intergenerational family
ties *(74)*

C. **Family Roles.** Match the family role in the numbered column with the type of role in the lettered column. Answers may be used more than once.

1. _____   Harmonizer *(74)*        A.   Informal role
2. _____   Encourager *(74)*        B.   Formal role
3. _____   Wife-mother *(74)*
4. _____   Family scapegoat *(74)*
5. _____   Husband-father *(74)*
6. _____   Son-brother *(74)*
7. _____   Family caretaker *(74)*
8. _____   Daughter-sister *(74)*

**D. Family Communication.** Match the characteristic of communication in the numbered column with the type of communication in the lettered column. Answers may be used more than once.

1. _____ Dynamic, two-way process *(75)*
2. _____ Acceptance of individual differences *(75)*
3. _____ Unclear transmission of a message *(75)*
4. _____ Verbal messages of caring *(75)*
5. _____ Inability to focus on one issue *(75)*
6. _____ Forbidden subjects for discussion *(75)*
7. _____ Mutual respect for each other's feelings *(75)*

A. Functional communication
B. Dysfunctional communication

## MULTIPLE-CHOICE QUESTIONS

**E.** Choose the most appropriate answer.

1. The most consistent family developmental task that must be met throughout the family life cycle is: *(74)*
   1. defining the roles of the family members.
   2. continuing education.
   3. maintaining the marital relationship.
   4. maintaining individual independence.

2. One of the most important influences on family interaction is: *(75)*
   1. self-esteem of each member.
   2. family income.
   3. family size.
   4. type of family configuration.

3. A negative strategy for adapting to family stress is: *(76)*
   1. problem-solving.
   2. mastery.
   3. coping behavior.
   4. defense mechanism.

4. Assessment of families and their coping strategies consists of all *except* which one of the following? *(76)*
   1. Determine stressors being experienced.
   2. Assess family communication patterns.
   3. Find out what kinds of coping strategies are used.
   4. Explore each family member's political views.

5. When assisting families to cope, it is most important to: *(77)*
   1. encourage all family members to be involved in the process.
   2. work with the most influential member of the family.
   3. make the family members use all new coping strategies.
   4. tell the family they are dysfunctional and need help.

6. When taking care of a patient in the hospital, it is important to: *(77)*
   1. keep the family members out of the room.
   2. ignore the family members because the patient is the focus of care.
   3. determine whether the family members are supportive or detrimental in the recovery process.
   4. provide information only to the patient because of confidentiality.

7. Which is an external family coping strategy? *(76)*
   1. Joint family problem-solving
   2. Maintaining active links with the community
   3. Normalizing family life
   4. Utilizing a sense of humor

8. Maintaining ties between aging parents and growing children is a developmental task of: *(73)*
   1. beginning families.
   2. families with young children.
   3. launching children and moving on.
   4. families in later life.

## ALTERNATE FORMAT QUESTIONS

F. 1. Which are internal family coping strategies? Select all that apply. *(76)*
   1. Family group reliance
   2. Role flexibility and changing roles
   3. Using support groups
   4. Obtaining spiritual support

## OBJECTIVES

1. Describe the health-illness continuum.

2. Discuss traditional and current views of health and illness.

3. List Maslow's five basic human needs, explaining why they constitute a hierarchy.

4. Explain the four levels of adaptability to stress.

5. Discuss concepts related to health promotion, disease prevention, and health maintenance.

6. Define acute and chronic illness.

7. Discuss illness behavior and the impact of illness on the family.

8. Describe nursing measures for health promotion, health maintenance, and illness.

9. Describe complementary and alternative therapies and the nurse's role in relation to both.

## LEARNING ACTIVITIES

**A.  Maslow's hierarchy.**  List the five levels of human needs in Maslow's hierarchy. *(80)*

1. _____

2. _____

3. _____

4. _____

5. _____

**B.  Maslow's hierarchy.** Match the need in the numbered column with the correct level in the lettered column.

1. _____   Oxygen, fluid, nutrition, temperature, elimination, shelter, rest, and sex *(80)*

2. _____   Security, protection from harm, freedom from anxiety and fear *(80)*

3. _____   Feeling loved by family and friends, and accepted by peers and community *(81)*

4. _____   Feeling good about oneself and feeling that others hold one in high regard *(81)*

5. _____   Self-fulfillment; able to problem-solve, accept criticism from others, and eager to acquire new knowledge; self-confidence; maturity *(81)*

A.  Self-esteem
B.  Safety and security
C.  Physiologic
D.  Self-actualization
E.  Love and belonging

**C. Adaptation.** List the three stages of the general adaptation syndrome. *(82)*

1. _____

2. _____

3. _____

**D. Maslow's hierarchy.** Match Henderson's 14 components of basic nursing care in the numbered column with Maslow's hierarchy of human needs in the lettered column. Answers may be used more than once.

1. _____ Learn, discover, or satisfy curiosity *(86)*

2. _____ Breathe normally *(86)*

3. _____ Worship according to one's faith *(86)*

4. _____ Eat and drink adequately *(86)*

5. _____ Eliminate body wastes *(86)*

6. _____ Play or participate in various forms of recreation *(86)*

7. _____ Move and maintain desirable posture *(86)*

8. _____ Sleep and rest *(86)*

9. _____ Select suitable clothing, dress and undress *(86)*

10. _____ Avoid dangers in the environment and avoid injuring others *(86)*

11. _____ Maintain body temperature within the normal range by adjusting clothing and modifying the environment *(86)*

12. _____ Communicate with others in expressing emotions, needs, fears, and opinions *(86)*

13. _____ Work in such a way that there is a sense of accomplishment *(86)*

14. _____ Keep the body clean and well-groomed and protect the integument *(86)*

A. Physiologic needs
B. Safety and security needs
C. Love and belonging needs
D. Self-esteem and self-actualization needs

E.  **Adaptation to Stress.** Match the statement in the numbered column with the correct method of increasing adaptability in the lettered column.

1. _____   "What is your worst possible stressor, and how does this present stress compare with the worst?" *(86)*

2. _____   "What ways have you coped with stress in the past that have been successful for you?" *(86)*

3. _____   "What kinds of things do you do when you are stressed? Do you eat more or less?" *(86)*

4. _____   "Whom do you turn to when you are feeling stressed?" *(86)*

A.  Collect data concerning past methods of coping with stress
B.  Collect data about internal coping strategies
C.  Determine external coping strategies
D.  Monitor the degree of stress

F.  **Views of Health.** Match the descriptions in the numbered column with traditional or current view in the lettered column. Answers may be used more than once.

1. _____   Emphasis is on maintenance of health and prevention of disease. *(79-80)*

2. _____   Health and illness are separate entities. *(79-80)*

3. _____   Focus is on curing disease or injury. *(79-80)*

4. _____   Health and illness are relative and ever-changing. *(79-80)*

A.  Traditional view
B.  Current view

G.  **Herbal-Drug Interactions.** Match the herbal-drug combination in the numbered column with the interaction in the lettered column. Answers may be used more than once.

1. _____   Echinacea and immunosuppressants *(89)*

2. _____   Aloe and diuretics *(89)*

3. _____   Garlic and anticoagulants *(89)*

4. _____   Ephedra and antihypertensives *(89)*

5. _____   Kava-kava and CNS depressants *(89)*

6. _____   Goldenseal and antihypertensives *(89)*

7. _____   Ginseng and aspirin *(89)*

8. _____   Hawthorne and cardiac glycosides *(89)*

A.  Inhibit immunosuppression
B.  Increased risk of bleeding
C.  Increased blood pressure
D.  Increased risk of digitalis toxicity
E.  Increased risk of hypokalemia
F.  Increased sedation

**H. Complementary Therapies.** Match the examples of complementary therapies in the numbered column with the type of therapy in the lettered column. Answers may be used more than once.

1. _____ Acupuncture *(88)*
2. _____ Meditation *(88)*
3. _____ Ginkgo biloba *(88)*
4. _____ Antioxidants *(88)*
5. _____ Herbal tea for a cold *(88)*
6. _____ Laser surgery *(88)*
7. _____ Chiropractic *(88)*
8. _____ High-dose vitamin therapy *(88)*
9. _____ St. John's wort *(88)*
10. _____ Prayer *(88)*

A. Alternative systems of medical practice
B. Mind-body interventions
C. Manual healing methods
D. Bioelectromagnetic applications
E. Herbal medicine
F. Pharmacologic and biologic treatments
G. Diet and nutrition changes

**I. Maslow's hierarchy.** Maslow's hierarchy: Indicate for each finding in the numbered column the appropriate level of needs to which it relates in Maslow's hierarchy in the lettered column. Answers may be used more than once.

Your patient is a 45-year-old male who has been admitted to the hospital with pneumonia. As you are conducting your admission interview, you find out the following:

1. _____ He has recently separated from his wife and three children. *(80-81)*
2. _____ He is afraid to jog due to crime in neighborhood. *(80-81)*
3. _____ He states that he feels like he will never amount to anything. *(80-81)*
4. _____ He eats "fast foods" and drinks a lot of coffee. *(80-81)*
5. _____ He states he does not feel very positive about himself right now. *(80-81)*
6. _____ His parents live 300 miles away; he has few close friends in town. *(80-81)*
7. _____ He states he fears he will lose his job if he is in the hospital too long. *(80-81)*
8. _____ He states he feels alone a lot. *(80-81)*
9. _____ He sleeps only 4–5 hours per night. *(80-81)*
10. _____ He lives in a poor section of town. *(80-81)*

A. Physiologic needs
B. Safety and security
C. Love and belonging
D. Self-esteem and self-actualization

## MULTIPLE-CHOICE QUESTIONS

**J.** Choose the most appropriate answer.

1. Which of the following is an internal stressor? *(81)*
   1. Loss of relationship
   2. Economic inadequacies
   3. Sensory deprivation
   4. Feelings of powerlessness

2. Which is an appropriate coping strategy for making plans? *(83)*
   1. Problem-solving
   2. Self-control
   3. Confrontation
   4. Faith

3. Which type of stress occurs when you feel angry while fearing the consequences of expressing it? *(81)*
   1. Internal, physical
   2. Internal, psychological
   3. External, interpersonal relations
   4. External, socioeconomic

4. Oxygen, food, and safety are examples of: *(80)*
   1. psychological needs.
   2. physiologic needs.
   3. emotional needs.
   4. affectional needs.

5. A patient's refusal of treatment is an example of which coping strategy? *(83)*
   1. Confrontation
   2. Denial
   3. Problem-solving
   4. Event review

6. What is one of the leading health indicators covered in the *Healthy People 2010* report? *(84)*
   1. Physical activity
   2. Vision and hearing
   3. Medical product safety
   4. Oral health

7. The highest level of Maslow's hierarchy is: *(80)*
   1. love and belonging.
   2. self-esteem.
   3. physiologic needs.
   4. self-actualization.

8. The most fundamental needs that sustain life are: *(80)*
   1. physiologic needs.
   2. safety needs.
   3. belonging needs.
   4. self-esteem needs.

9. Which is included as one of the top 10 major stressors? *(81)*
   1. Death of a close family member
   2. Marriage of a child
   3. Celebration of 25th wedding anniversary
   4. First employee evaluation

10. Areas in which most people seek control even while they are sick include their: *(82)*
    1. work environment.
    2. play environment.
    3. treatments and procedures.
    4. local adaptation syndrome.

11. Wound healing and inflammation are examples of: *(82)*
    1. general adaptation syndrome.
    2. local adaptation syndrome.
    3. negative feedback response.
    4. countercurrent response.

12. A physiologic response of the body to stress is: *(82)*
    1. bronchoconstriction.
    2. increased heart rate.
    3. decreased respirations.
    4. decreased blood pressure.

13. Increased hormone levels, heart rate, and oxygen intake are components of the: *(82)*
    1. resistance stage.
    2. exhaustion stage.
    3. alarm reaction.
    4. local adaptation stage.

14. Adaptation to a stressor occurs in the: *(83)*
    1. resistance stage.
    2. alarm stage.
    3. exhaustion stage.
    4. initial stage.

15. With a long-term stressor such as a chronic physical or mental illness, the individual enters the third stage of adaptation, or the: *(83)*
    1. alarm stage.
    2. exhaustion stage.
    3. resistance stage.
    4. local adaptation stage.

16. Cold hands and feet and tensed muscles are signs or symptoms of: *(83)*
    1. withdrawal.
    2. depression.
    3. adaptation.
    4. stress.

17. Slowed speech, inability to concentrate, and hesitant speech may be signs of: *(83)*
    1. stress.
    2. adaptation.
    3. depression.
    4. alarm.

18. Behavioral or cognitive activities used to deal with stress are: *(83)*
    1. feedback behaviors.
    2. coping behaviors.
    3. depressive behaviors.
    4. automatic behaviors.

19. Maintaining stability of the internal environment is a definition of: *(84)*
    1. adaptation.
    2. coping.
    3. resistance.
    4. homeostasis.

20. An illness or disease that has a relatively rapid onset and short duration is said to be: *(85)*
    1. chronic.
    2. acute.
    3. disabling.
    4. an emergency.

21. Permanent impairments or disabilities, requiring long-term rehabilitation and treatment, are said to be: *(85)*
    1. disabling.
    2. challenging.
    3. chronic.
    4. acute.

22. Nursing interventions to increase adaptability in older adults should be geared toward helping older clients to: *(83)*
    1. use past successful coping mechanisms to deal with new stressors.
    2. assess their strengths and weaknesses in dealing with new stressors.
    3. develop new coping mechanisms to deal with new stressors.
    4. learn new methods of dealing with stressors.

23. Biofeedback, meditation, and imagery are examples of measures that patients may use to help: *(86)*
    1. encourage exercise.
    2. increase appetite.
    3. relieve stress.
    4. promote bowel regularity.

24. Tasks for chronically ill individuals include: *(87)*
    1. ignoring disease.
    2. preventing and managing crises.
    3. curing disease.
    4. promoting social isolation.

25. Activities directed toward maintaining or enhancing well-being as a protection against illness are related to: *(84)*
    1. health adaptation.
    2. health promotion.
    3. prevention of illness.
    4. homeostasis measures.

26. Health and illness are: *(80)*
    1. absolute, unchanging states of being.
    2. unconditional states of being.
    3. relative, ever-changing states of being.
    4. homeostasis measures.

27. A leading health indicator for *Healthy People 2010* is: *(84)*
    1. infectious disease.
    2. cardiovascular disease.
    3. tobacco use.
    4. nutrition.

28. When garlic is taken by a patient who is also taking an anticoagulant, the patient is at risk for: *(89)*
    1. sedation.
    2. hypotension.
    3. bleeding.
    4. infection.

29. Immunosuppression may be inhibited when a patient who is taking immunosuppressant drugs also takes: *(89)*
    1. echinacea.
    2. ginseng.
    3. kava-kava.
    4. garlic.

30. Which is an example of a psychological internal stressor? *(81)*
    1. Unemployment
    2. Sensory deprivation
    3. Feeling of powerlessness
    4. Ethnic difference

31. The priority focus area of *Healthy People 2010* relates to: *(84)*
    1. food safety.
    2. access to quality health services.
    3. environmental health.
    4. chronic kidney disease.

32. When a patient discusses a situation that has occurred as a method of coping, this is an example of: *(83)*
    1. self-control.
    2. accepting responsibility.
    3. event review.
    4. positive reappraisal.

## ALTERNATE FORMAT QUESTIONS

K. 1. Which are examples of complementary and alternative therapies? Select all that apply. *(88)*
    1. Acupuncture
    2. Surgery
    3. Guided imagery
    4. Antioxidants
    5. Generic drugs
    6. Biofeedback

2. Which are focus areas of the *Healthy People 2010* document? Select all that apply. *(84)*
    1. Cancer
    2. Thyroid disorders
    3. Diabetes
    4. HIV
    5. Autoimmune disorders
    6. Sexually transmitted infections

3. Which are leading health indicators of *Healthy People 2010*? Select all that apply. *(84)*
    1. Substance abuse
    2. Occupational health
    3. Diabetes
    4. Physical activity
    5. Environmental quality

# CHAPTER 9

# Nutrition

---

## OBJECTIVES

1. Explain the role of the alimentary system in the digestion of food.

2. Describe how food is digested and absorbed.

3. List the functions of each of the six classes of essential nutrients.

4. List the functions of proteins, carbohydrates, and fats.

5. Identify the food sources of proteins, carbohydrates, and fats.

6. Identify the food sources of dietary fiber.

7. List the possible health benefits of dietary fiber.

8. Identify the food sources of each of the vitamins and minerals.

9. Describe the changes in nutrient needs as an individual ages.

10. Differentiate anorexia nervosa, bulimia, and binge eating disorder.

11. Discuss the different types of nutritional support.

12. Identify guidelines for the nutritional assessment.

---

## LEARNING ACTIVITIES

A. **Key Terms.** Match the definition in the numbered column with the most appropriate term in the lettered column.

1. _____ Lipid-wrapped proteins carried into the blood-stream; includes high-density and low-density lipoproteins, which carry cholesterol *(97)*

2. _____ Small amounts of metals (calcium, sodium, and potassium) and nonmetals (chloride, phosphate) that are essential to the body; can build up *(105)*

3. _____ Lipids composed of three fatty acid chains and a glycerol molecule *(96)*

4. _____ Combination of incomplete proteins that provide all nine essential amino acids when consumed together *(104)*

5. _____ Compounds that come chiefly from animal sources and are usually solid at room temperature; also coconut and palm oils *(96)*

6. _____ Large organic compounds made of various combinations of amino acids; found in meat, milk, fish, and eggs *(103)*

7. _____ Organic compounds supplied by food that the body requires for normal growth and development *(104)*

8. _____ A group of 22 substances that can be bonded in different ways to make a variety of proteins; the body can manufacture sufficient amounts of these, provided the nine essential amino acids are derived from the diet *(103)*

A. Saturated fatty acids
B. Incomplete protein
C. Triglycerides
D. Calorie
E. Vitamins
F. Lipids
G. Minerals
H. Basal metabolic rate
I. Amino acids
J. Complementary protein
K. Complete protein
L. Insoluble fiber
M. Lipoproteins
N. Resting metabolic rate
O. Proteins
P. Unsaturated fatty acids

9. _____ Indigestible roughage found in plant cells; aids in stool formation and elimination *(95)*

10. _____ Compounds that come from plants or fish and are generally liquid at room temperature; can be monounsaturated (olive, peanut, canola, and avocado oils) or polyunsaturated (corn, safflower, and sesame oils) *(96)*

11. _____ Energy expended in the resting state; measured in the morning with the body at complete mental and physical rest, but not asleep *(93)*

12. _____ Plant protein lacking one or more essential amino acids *(104)*

13. _____ Fats in solid or liquid form; store energy, carry fat-soluble vitamins, and maintain healthy skin and hair; supply essential fatty acids and promote a feeling of fullness (satiety) *(96)*

14. _____ Standard unit for measuring energy; the amount of heat needed to raise the temperature of 1 kg of water at a standard temperature by 1° Celsius *(94)*

15. _____ Measurement of energy expenditure taken at any time of the day and 3–4 hours after the last meal *(93)*

16. _____ Protein containing all nine essential amino acids; usually of animal origin (e.g., meat, eggs) *(103)*

B. **Macronutrients.** Which of the following are macronutrients? Select all that apply. *(92)*

1. _____ Minerals
2. _____ Vitamins
3. _____ Hormones
4. _____ Carbohydrates
5. _____ Lipids
6. _____ Amino acids
7. _____ Fluids
8. _____ Vegetables
9. _____ Proteins
10. _____ Fluids

C. **Basal Metabolic Rate (BMR).** Which are hormones that affect the basal metabolic rate (BMR)? Select all that apply. *(93-94)*

1. _____ Dopamine
2. _____ Insulin
3. _____ Estrogens
4. _____ Growth hormone
5. _____ Epinephrine
6. _____ Aldosterone
7. _____ Cortisol
8. _____ Thyroxine

D. **Basal Metabolic Rate (BMR).** Which are reasons why the BMR of a sleeping person is lower than that of an awake, alert person? Select all that apply. *(94)*

1. _____ Increased activity of the sympathetic nervous system
2. _____ Muscle relaxation
3. _____ Decreased thyroxine
4. _____ Increased body temperature

E. List the number of calories per gram provided by lipids, carbohydrates, and protein. *(102)*

   1. Lipids _____

   2. Carbohydrates _____

   3. Protein _____

F. How many calories are provided when a person consumes 2 grams of lipids, 4 grams of carbohydrates, and 4 grams of protein? *(102)*

G. **Complete Protein.** Which are sources of complete proteins in foods? Select all that apply. *(104)*

   1. _____ Fish             5. _____ Rice

   2. _____ Milk            6. _____ Meat

   3. _____ Dry beans      7. _____ Nuts

   4. _____ Eggs             8. _____ Cheese

H. **MyPyramid Guides.** Refer to MyPyramid Figure 9-1(B) on p. 111 and MyPyramid Figure 9-1(C) on p. 112 in your textbook and answer questions H1-H7.

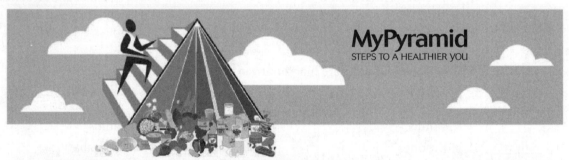

   1. What is the difference in amounts of vegetables, fruits, milk, and meat and beans between a person on an 1800-calorie diet and a 3000-calorie pattern? How much more will the 3000-calorie pattern require? List the differences in the chart above. *(111-112)*

2. What are the basic four food groups considered to be the standard food guide until 1992? *(109)*

3. In July 1992, what addition was made to the basic four food groups to form the Food Pyramid? *(109)*

4. What is the new, current, science-based food guidance system called, which incorporates the 2005 USDA Dietary Guidelines for Americans? *(110)*

5. What are the six foods represented by the six colored bands on MyPyramid? *(110)*

6. In addition to nutrition, what additional topic is included in MyPyramid? *(110)*

7. Refer to MyPyramid in the chart below and to Box 9-2 on p. 105 in your textbook. Which of the following foods provide protein content? Select all that apply. *(105)*

   _____ Fish                    _____ Meat

   _____ Potatoes                _____ Cheese

   _____ Nuts                    _____ Milk

   _____ Beans

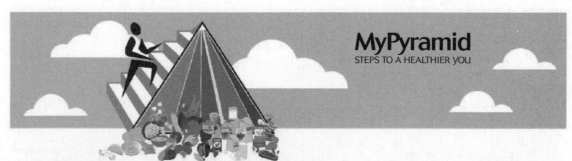

Based on the information you provided, this is your daily recommended amount from each food group.

| GRAINS | VEGETABLES | FRUITS | MILK | MEAT & BEANS |
|---|---|---|---|---|
| **Make half your grains whole** | **Vary your veggies**<br>Aim for these amounts each week:<br>**Dark green veggies**<br>**Orange veggies**<br>**Dry beans & peas**<br>**Starchy veggies**<br>**Other veggies** | **Focus on fruits**<br><br>Eat a variety of fruit<br>Go easy on fruit juices | **Get your calcium-rich foods**<br><br>Go low-fat or fat-free when you choose milk, yogurt, or cheese | **Go lean with protein**<br><br>Choose low-fat or lean meats and poultry<br><br>Vary your protein routine—choose more fish, beans, peas, nuts, and seeds |

**Find your balance between food and physical activity**          **Know your limits on fats, sugars, and sodium**

**Your results are based on a 3000 calorie pattern.**          **Name:** _____

This calorie level is only an estimate of your needs. Monitor your body weight to see if you need to adjust your calorie intake.

8. Based on an 1800-calorie pattern, how much of meats and beans should be included in the diet? Choose the best response. *(111)*

   1. _____    3 cups
   2. _____    5 cups
   3. _____    5 ounces
   4. _____    8 ounces

9. Which vegetable groups are recommended on a weekly basis? *(111)*

   _____    Dark green
   _____    Green grapes
   _____    Dry beans and peas
   _____    Red
   _____    Starchy vegetable
   _____    Orange

10. Label the feeding tubes in the figure below (Figure 9-4) using the following terms: *(119)*

   nasogastric
   nasoduodenal
   nasojejunal
   PEG

   A. _____

   B. _____

   C. _____

   D. _____

I.  **Nutrition Labels.** Refer to Figure 9-2 in the textbook. Read the nutrition label and fill in the blanks below. *(113)*

   1.  How many calories per serving are provided? _____

   2.  How many servings are in this container? _____

   3.  What is the size of one serving? _____

   4.  What percentage of vitamin A is provided in one serving? _____

   5.  How many calories are provided in one container? _____

   6.  Dietary guidelines recommend that people get no more than what percentage of their kilocalories from fat? _____

J.  **Skin Measurement.** Refer to Figure 9-3 in the textbook. *(116)*

   1.  What is the instrument shown in this picture? _____

   2.  What is being measured? _____

   3.  Measuring the thickness of subcutaneous fat tissue provides a measure of:
       1.  edema.
       2.  adiposity.
       3.  dehydration.
       4.  muscle mass.

K.  **Energy Requirement.** Refer to Table 9-9 in the textbook.

   1.  What are the energy requirements (number of kcal/day) for women with a BMI of 18.5 kg/in$^2$? *(102)*
       1.  1623 kcal
       2.  1762 kcal
       3.  1803 kcal
       4.  1956 kcal

   2.  What are the energy requirements for a very active man with a BMI of 24.99 kg/in$^2$? *(102)*
       1.  2490 kcal
       2.  2842 kcal
       3.  2880 kcal
       4.  3296 kcal

## MULTIPLE-CHOICE QUESTIONS

L.  Choose the most appropriate answer.

   1.  The stomach is normally emptied in: *(92)*
       1.  30–60 minutes.
       2.  1–4 hours.
       3.  5–8 hours.
       4.  10–12 hours.

   2.  What is one type of carbohydrate that cannot be digested and is excreted unchanged in the feces? *(92)*
       1.  Fiber
       2.  Glucose
       3.  Glycogen
       4.  Monosaccharide

3. What is the parasympathetic effect in the stomach carried by the vagus nerve in response to the sight or smell of food? *(92)*
   1. Increases the appetite
   2. Increases gastric acid secretions
   3. Increases the feeling of fullness
   4. Speeds the movement of food through the intestines

4. Which lipoprotein increases the risk of atherosclerosis by contributing to plaque buildup on the artery walls? *(97)*
   1. Triglycerides
   2. LDLs
   3. HDLs
   4. Phospholipids

5. Colonic bacteria are needed to help form vitamin: *(93)*
   1. C.
   2. D.
   3. K.
   4. A.

6. Which foods are the most easily digested? *(93)*
   1. Raw foods
   2. Cooked foods
   3. Fried foods
   4. Foods with additives

7. An endocrine hormone that regulates the metabolic rate is: *(93)*
   1. thyroxine.
   2. melatonin.
   3. aldosterone.
   4. estrogen.

8. For which body tissues are lipids NOT a source of energy? *(97)*
   1. Bladder
   2. Stomach
   3. Heart
   4. Brain

9. A calorie is the amount of heat energy required to raise the temperature of 1 gram of water at a standard initial temperature by: *(94)*
   1. 1° C.
   2. 10° C.
   3. 25° C.
   4. 50° C.

10. Carbohydrates are organic compounds that consist of carbon, hydrogen, and: *(94)*
    1. nitrogen.
    2. oxygen.
    3. iron.
    4. calcium.

11. For immediate use by the body's cells, carbohydrates are converted primarily to: *(94)*
    1. glycogen.
    2. glucose.
    3. sucrose.
    4. fructose.

12. What acts like a sponge to absorb many times its weight in water and helps provide a full feeling long after eating? *(95)*
    1. Soluble fiber
    2. Monosaccharides
    3. Insoluble fiber
    4. Glycerols

13. Diets without at least 50–100 grams of carbohydrates per day are likely to lead to: *(96)*
    1. ketosis.
    2. alkalosis.
    3. hyperglycemia.
    4. hypernatremia.

14. Which of the following nutrients releases the most energy? *(96)*
    1. Fiber
    2. Carbohydrates
    3. Protein
    4. Lipid

15. Which nutrient can be stored in the body compactly with little or no water? *(96)*
    1. Carbohydrate
    2. Lipid
    3. Protein
    4. Glucose

16. Neutral fats, the most common fats found in foods of both plant and animal origin, are called: *(96)*
    1. corticosteroids.
    2. insoluble fibers.
    3. soluble fibers.
    4. triglycerides.

17. Adipose cells can store up to 95% of their volume as: *(97)*
    1. glucose.
    2. glycogen.
    3. amino acids.
    4. triglycerides.

18. Most human adipose cells are in the form of white fat, which accumulates in: *(97)*
    1. subcutaneous tissue.
    2. epidermis.
    3. dermis.
    4. muscles.

19. Lipids are a major source of energy for: *(97)*
    1. subcutaneous tissue.
    2. epidermis tissue.
    3. muscle tissue.
    4. mucous membrane.

20. Where are most lipids carried to be converted to energy or used in the synthesis of new triglycerides? *(102)*
    1. Gallbladder
    2. Liver
    3. Heart
    4. Kidney

21. Most nutritionists recommend that the daily fat intake should be what percentage of the daily caloric intake? *(102)*
    1. 50% or less
    2. 30% or less
    3. 15% or less
    4. 10% or less

22. To minimize the risk of heart disease, people should eat more: *(102)*
    1. saturated fats.
    2. polyunsaturated fats.
    3. glycerol fats.
    4. unsaturated fats.

23. The main source of saturated fats in the American diet comes from: *(96)*
    1. vegetable oil.
    2. cottonseed oil.
    3. animal products.
    4. safflower oil.

24. When various incomplete proteins are consumed at the same time, the body can use them together to obtain a balance of the essential amino acids. Incomplete proteins consumed together are called: *(104)*
    1. plant proteins.
    2. complementary proteins.
    3. animal proteins.
    4. enzyme proteins.

25. The nine amino acids that must be obtained from the diet are called: *(103)*
    1. dietary amino acids.
    2. essential amino acids.
    3. incomplete amino acids.
    4. complementary amino acids.

26. Which of the following foods has the highest protein content? *(104)*
    1. Cereals
    2. Beans
    3. Poultry
    4. Lentils

27. Vitamins A, D, E, and K are: *(105)*
    1. fat-soluble.
    2. water-soluble.
    3. insoluble.
    4. complementary.

28. In addition to fat-soluble vitamins, which group of nutrients needs bile and pancreatic juices for absorption? *(96)*
    1. Carbohydrates
    2. Proteins
    3. Amino acids
    4. Lipids

29. The intake of water is controlled by: *(106)*
    1. exercise.
    2. thirst.
    3. metabolism.
    4. stress.

30. How much water should adults drink daily? *(107)*
    1. 500 ml
    2. 1000 ml
    3. 2500 ml
    4. 5000 ml

31. The diet for older adults should include:
    *(108)*
    1. low-fat foods.
    2. low-sodium foods.
    3. all the food groups.
    4. high-protein foods.

32. Older adults with chronic diseases have an
    increased risk for negative nitrogen balance
    and: *(109)*
    1. protein deficiency.
    2. vitamin deficiency.
    3. mineral deficiency.
    4. carbohydrate deficiency.

33. Guidelines for the amounts of nutrients
    that healthy people should consume daily
    are called: *(98)*
    1. basic four food groups.
    2. recommended daily allowances.
    3. food pyramid.
    4. minimum food requirements.

34. Overweight individuals are considered
    obese if their weight is what percent above
    the ideal body weight? *(113)*
    1. 5% or more
    2. 10% or more
    3. 20% or more
    4. 30% or more

35. Which nutrient must be eaten daily, as it
    cannot be stored in the body? *(104)*
    1. Carbohydrates
    2. Protein
    3. Lipids
    4. Minerals

36. A method of administering nutrients only
    if the gastrointestinal tract cannot be used
    is called: *(119)*
    1. enteral tube feeding.
    2. nasogastric tube feeding.
    3. duodenal tube feeding.
    4. total parenteral nutrition.

37. Total parenteral nutrition (TPN) feedings
    are used for patients who are usually debili-
    tated and malnourished with a weight loss
    of what percent of body weight? *(119)*
    1. 10% or more
    2. 20% or more
    3. 50% or more
    4. 75% or more

38. What type of solution is administered
    through a Hickman- or Broviac-type cath-
    eter? *(119)*
    1. Hypotonic
    2. Hypertonic
    3. Isotonic
    4. Glucose and sterile water

39. What is a complication of enteral tube
    feedings when viscous formulas and
    crushed medications are inadequately
    flushed? *(119)*
    1. Dumping syndrome
    2. Diarrhea
    3. GI bleeding
    4. Tube blockage

40. If patients who have been without food for
    an extended period of time are given food
    too quickly, they may develop: *(120)*
    1. hypernatremia.
    2. hypercalcemia.
    3. hypophosphatemia.
    4. hypoglycemia.

41. When moving from enteral to oral feed-
    ings, the patient may experience: *(120)*
    1. breathing difficulties.
    2. bleeding at the TPN site.
    3. heart palpitations.
    4. poor appetite.

42. Which grain product has the highest carbo-
    hydrate content? *(95)*
    1. Tapioca
    2. Popcorn
    3. Crackers
    4. Macaroni

43. Which of the following vegetables has the highest carbohydrate content? *(95)*
    1. Carrots
    2. Peas
    3. Tomatoes
    4. Cabbage

44. Which hormones increase the rate of glucose utilization? *(95)*
    1. Insulin
    2. Glucagon
    3. Epinephrine
    4. Growth hormone

45. Which of the following foods has the highest dietary fiber content? *(97)*
    1. Breads
    2. Vegetables
    3. Rice
    4. Pasta

46. Why is folate necessary for the human body? *(106)*
    1. Aids in removal of $CO_2$
    2. Acts in metabolism of carbohydrates and amino acids
    3. Essential for normal metabolism of red blood cells
    4. Important in immune responses

47. How is vitamin C helpful for the human body? *(106)*
    1. Enzyme development
    2. Wound healing
    3. Night vision
    4. Blood clotting

48. What nutrition-related metabolic change occurs in older adults? *(108)*
    1. Basal metabolic rate (BMR) decreases
    2. Lean body mass increases
    3. Plasma glucose levels decrease
    4. Tolerance to glucose increases

49. What nutrition-related change occurs in older adults? *(108)*
    1. Appetite increases
    2. Salivary secretions increase
    3. Acid secretion increases
    4. Absorption of vitamin $B_{12}$ decreases

50. What is the most common fluid and electrolyte disturbance in older adults? *(109)*
    1. Hyponatremia
    2. Hypokalemia
    3. Dehydration
    4. Edema

51. For a 2000-calorie diet, how many cups of orange vegetables are needed each week? *(111)*
    1. 2 cups/week
    2. 3 cups/week
    3. 4.5 cups/week
    4. 7 cups/week

52. Which of the following has over 25 grams of fat? *(103)*
    1. Bran muffin
    2. Hot dog
    3. Cheesecake
    4. Cheeseburger

53. Which as zero grams of fat? *(103)*
    1. Angel food cake
    2. Chicken noodle soup
    3. Yogurt
    4. Sunflower seeds

54. Which contains 7–8 grams of protein? *(105)*
    1. Canned corn
    2. Bran cereal
    3. Navy beans, cooked
    4. French fries

## ALTERNATE FORMAT QUESTIONS

M. 1. Which of the following are grain products? Select all that apply. *(95)*
    1. Oatmeal
    2. White bread
    3. Lima beans
    4. Saltine crackers
    5. Spaghetti

2. Which of the following foods contain high amounts of dietary fiber? Select all that apply. *(97)*
   1. Macaroni
   2. Bagel
   3. Raisin bran cereal
   4. Lima beans
   5. Dried peas

3. Intake of which nutrients should be kept as low as possible? Select all that apply. *(102)*
   1. Dietary cholesterol
   2. Dietary fiber
   3. Trans-fatty acids
   4. Saturated fatty acids

4. Which foods are high in calcium? Select all that apply. *(104)*
   1. Poultry
   2. Milk
   3. Sardines
   4. Whole-grain cereals

**N.** Ranking Questions

1. Rank in order (from 1 to 7) the following foods from those with the lowest amount of fat to those with the highest amount of fat. *(103)*
   A. _____ Hot dog
   B. _____ Tuna
   C. _____ Cup of whole milk
   D. _____ Fruits and vegetables
   E. _____ Chicken pot pie
   F. _____ Macaroni with cheese
   G. _____ Popcorn

2. Rank in order (from 1 to 6) the following foods from those with the lowest protein content to those with the highest protein content. *(102)*
   A. _____ Egg, one
   B. _____ Hamburger
   C. _____ Bread
   D. _____ Peanuts
   E. _____ Butter
   F. _____ Potatoes

# 10 Developmental Processes

---

## OBJECTIVES

1. List the developmental tasks for successful adulthood.

2. Identify the health problems specific to the adult age groups.

3. Discuss the health care needs of young, middle-aged, and older adults.

---

## LEARNING ACTIVITIES

**A. Key Terms.** Match the definition in the numbered column with the most appropriate term in the lettered column.

1. _____ Focus on the functional ca-
pabilities of various organ
systems in the body *(126)*

2. _____ Focus on the behavioral
capacity of a person to
adapt to changing environmental demands *(126)*

3. _____ Focus on the roles and
habits of a person in relation to other members of
society *(126)*

A. Social age
B. Biologic age
C. Psychological age

**B. Developmental Stages.** Match the definition in the numbered column with the most appropriate developmental stage in the lettered column. Answers may be used more than once.

1. _____    Focus on marriage, child-bearing, and work *(122)*

2. _____    45–65 years of age *(125)*

3. _____    Over the age of 65 *(126)*

4. _____    "Sandwich" generation *(125)*

5. _____    Redirection of energy and talents to new roles and activities *(126)*

6. _____    20–45 years of age *(122)*

A. Young adulthood
B. Middle adulthood
C. Older adulthood

**C. Developmental Stages.** Match the characteristic in the numbered column with the most appropriate developmental stage in the lettered column. Answers may be used more than once.

1. _____    Earn most of their money *(125)*

2. _____    Retirement *(126)*

3. _____    Marriage, childbearing, and work *(122)*

4. _____    Settling down to job and raising a family *(122)*

5. _____    Decreased short-term memory *(126)*

6. _____    Pay most of taxes *(125)*

7. _____    Establish career goals *(122)*

A. Young adulthood
B. Middle adulthood
C. Older adulthood

**D. Developmental Stages.** Match the developmental task in the numbered column with the developmental stage in the lettered column. Answers may be used more than once.

1. _____ Guidance of grown children *(125)*

2. _____ Home and time management *(122-123)*

3. _____ Learn to combine new dependency needs with the continuing need for independence *(126)*

4. _____ Help growing and grown children to become happy, responsible adults *(125)*

5. _____ Adjust to decreasing physical strength and health changes *(126)*

6. _____ Establish independence from parental home and financial aid *(122-123)*

7. _____ Accept role-reversal with aging parents *(125)*

8. _____ Adjust to loss of physical strength, illness, and one's own mortality *(126)*

9. _____ Accept self and stabilize self-concept *(122-123)*

10. _____ Become established in a vocation or profession *(122-123)*

11. _____ Balance work and other roles, preparing for retirement *(125)*

12. _____ Maintain emotional satisfaction in relationships with spouse, children, grandchildren, and other living relatives *(126)*

A. Young adulthood
B. Middle adulthood
C. Older adulthood

**E. Developmental Tasks.** Match the health developmental task in the numbered column with the developmental stage in the lettered column.

1. _____ Generativity versus stagnation *(123)*

2. _____ Intimacy versus isolation *(123)*

3. _____ Ego integrity versus despair *(123)*

A. Young adulthood
B. Middle adulthood
C. Older adulthood

F. **Health Problems.** Match the health problem in the numbered column with the most appropriate developmental stage in the lettered column. Answers may be used more than once.

1. _____ Benign or malignant prostate enlargement *(127)*
2. _____ Respiratory disease, causing absence from work among women *(125)*
3. _____ Bone mass begins to decline *(125)*
4. _____ Complications of pregnancy *(123)*
5. _____ Smoking; alcohol and drug abuse *(123)*
6. _____ Injuries, frequently causing absence from work among men *(125)*
7. _____ Chronic illness a major cause of death *(127)*
8. _____ Vehicular accidents and suicide *(123)*
9. _____ Breast cancer common in women *(124)*
10. _____ Stress related to managing a household *(123)*
11. _____ Perimenopausal period *(125)*
12. _____ Stress related to caregiving role of older parents *(125)*

A. Young adulthood
B. Middle adulthood
C. Older adulthood

G. **Age-Related Health Problems.** Match the health problem in the numbered column with the most appropriate developmental stage in the lettered column. Answers may be used more than once.

1. _____ Development of presbyopia *(125)*
2. _____ GI problems *(127)*
3. _____ Homicide and accidents *(123)*
4. _____ Arthritis *(127)*
5. _____ Obesity *(125)*
6. _____ Childbearing complications *(123)*
7. _____ Accidental falls *(127)*
8. _____ Emphysema *(127)*
9. _____ HIV infection *(123)*
10. _____ Alcoholism *(125)*

A. Young adulthood
B. Middle adulthood
C. Older adulthood

**H. Health Risks.** Match the harmful health practices in the numbered column with possible effects on health in the lettered column.

1. _____ Cigarette smoking *(124)*
2. _____ Alcohol abuse *(124)*
3. _____ Lack of physical activity *(124)*
4. _____ Obesity *(124)*

A. Osteoporosis
B. Degenerative joint disease
C. Cancer of the bladder
D. Malnutrition

## MULTIPLE-CHOICE QUESTIONS

**I.** Choose the most appropriate answer.

1. Establishing independence from parental home and financial aid is a developmental task of the: *(122)*
   1. middle-aged adult.
   2. older adult.
   3. young adult.
   4. adolescent.

2. Guidance of grown children and care of aging parents are developmental tasks of the: *(125)*
   1. young adult.
   2. middle-aged adult.
   3. older adult.
   4. retired adult.

3. Learning to combine new dependency needs with the need for independence are developmental tasks of the: *(127)*
   1. teenager.
   2. young adult.
   3. middle-aged adult.
   4. older adult.

4. Developmental tasks that focus on marriage, parenthood, and career choice are related to: *(122)*
   1. teenagers.
   2. young adults.
   3. middle-aged adults.
   4. older adults.

5. Stress and conflict related to balancing caring for children with caring for aging parents are related to: *(125)*
   1. teenagers.
   2. young adults.
   3. middle-aged adults.
   4. older adults.

6. If older adults cannot adjust to the physical, psychological, and sociologic changes that occur as they age, they are at risk for: *(123)*
   1. isolation.
   2. stagnation.
   3. generativity.
   4. despair.

7. To assess the developmental tasks of young adulthood, you ask: *(123)*
   1. whether the patient has meaningful, intimate relationships.
   2. what the patient does for leisure or recreation.
   3. what the patient does each day.
   4. what signs of depression the patient has.

8. A baseline mammogram is recommended for women during: *(123)*
   1. adolescence.
   2. older adulthood.
   3. young adulthood.
   4. middle adulthood.

9. Health promotion for people in their thirties includes: *(124)*
   1. effective parenting, stress management.
   2. yearly blood pressure screening.
   3. influenza vaccinations.
   4. yearly mammograms.

10. What is the average life expectancy of a child born in 2003? *(125)*
    1. 65.4 years
    2. 70.2 years
    3. 77.6 years
    4. 82.4 years

11. Asking the patient about meaningful relationships is a way of monitoring the developmental task of: *(123)*
    1. Generativity versus stagnation.
    2. Intimacy versus isolation.
    3. Ego integrity versus despair.
    4. Trust versus distrust.

2. Which preventive measures for improving health are included in *Healthy People 2010*? Select all that apply. *(124)*
    1. Reduce sedentary lifestyle
    2. Have annual Pap smears
    3. Maintain ideal weight
    4. Use stress-management programs
    5. Monitor blood pressure once a day

## ALTERNATE FORMAT QUESTIONS

J.  1. Which health screening tests should begin in young adulthood? Select all that apply. *(123-124)*
    1. Routine glucose testing
    2. Pelvic exams
    3. Pap smears
    4. Routine cholesterol
    5. Routine blood pressure screens
    6. Mammograms

# CHAPTER 11

# The Older Patient

---

## OBJECTIVES

1. Describe the roles of the gerontological nurse.

2. Determine the extent to which selected myths and stereotypes about older adults are factual.

3. Describe biologic and physiologic factors associated with aging.

4. Explain psychosocial factors associated with aging.

5. Describe modifications needed for activities of daily living.

6. Explain why drug dosage adjustments may be needed for older persons.

---

## LEARNING ACTIVITIES

A. **Drug Therapy.** Match the drug in the numbered column with the adverse drug reaction in older people in the lettered column. Answers may be used more than once.

1. _____ E    Analgesics (aspirin) *(140)*
2. _____ G & _____    Antibiotics (doxycycline) *(140)*
3. _____ E    Anticoagulants (warfarin) *(140)*
4. _____ B    Antidepressants (amitriptyline) *(140)*
5. _____ D    Antihypertensives (Verapamil) *(140)*
6. _____ H    Antiparkinsonians (levodopa) *(140)*
7. _____ C    Antipsychotics (Haloperidol) *(140)*
8. _____ A    Diuretics (chlorothiazide) *(140)*
9. _____ B    Sedative/hypnotics (flurazepam) *(140)*

A. Hypokalemia
B. Drowsiness or sedation
C. Confusion
D. Hypotension
E. Bleeding or hemorrhage
F. Uremia
G. Nephrotoxicity
H. Dystonia

B. **Age-Related Changes.** Match the change in the numbered column with the result in older people described in the lettered column. Answers may be used more than once.

1. ___C___ Pain, touch, and tactile sensation *(133)*

2. ___A___ Sense of smell *(133)*

3. ___A___ Conduction speed in CNS *(133)*

4. ___A___ Renal function *(134)*

5. ___A___ Pulmonary blood flow *(133)*

6. ___B___ Force of pulse *(133)*

7. ___C___ Intellectual capability *(132)*

8. ___C___ Sound judgment *(132)*

9. ___C___ Creativity *(132)*

10. ___B___ Exertional dyspnea *(133)*

11. ___A___ Cerebral blood flow *(133)*

12. ___B___ Loss of neurons (brain cells) *(132)*

13. ___C___ Functional ability of brain cells *(132)*

14. ___A___ Conduction speed associated with synaptic transmission *(133)*

15. ___C___ Intelligence *(132)*

16. ___C___ Heart size *(133)*

17. ___A___ Short-term memory *(132)*

18. ___A___ Vital capacity *(133)*

19. ___C___ Long-term memory *(132)*

20. ___B___ Chronic hypoxia of brain *(132)*

A. Decrease
B. Increase
C. No change

C. **Causes of Age-Related Changes.** Match the physiological assessment values in the numbered column with age-related causes in the lettered column.

1. ___B___   By the age of 70, BP is 150/90 *(133)*
2. ___D___   Resting cardiac output falls 30–40% *(134)*
3. ___C___   Difficulty remembering planned events for the day *(132)*
4. ___A___   Slow responses, impeded short-term memory *(132)*
5. ___J___   Problems with acid-base regulation *(134)*
6. ___I___   Increased residual urine and urinary tract infections *(134)*
7. ___K___   Increased BUN *(134)*
8. ___H___   Decreased ability to concentrate or dilute urine *(134)*
9. ___F___   Increased urge incontinence *(134)*
10. ___G___   Constipation *(135)*
11. ___E___   Heart murmurs *(133)*

A. Decreased neurons and conduction speed at synapses
B. Decreased baroreceptor reflexes and inelasticity of vessel walls
C. Chronic hypoxic state of the brain
D. Decreased heart rate and stroke volume
E. Increasing valvular rigidity and incomplete closure of the aortic and pulmonic valves
F. Bladder capacity reduced by half; delayed response to stretch receptors in the bladder
G. Decreased intestinal motility
H. Decreased secretion of ADH by the pituitary gland
I. Lax muscle tone and incomplete emptying of bladder
J. Decreases in filtration rate, plasma flow rate, and tubular reabsorption and secretion
K. Renal tubules are less able to eliminate excess hydrogen ions

D. **Drug Therapy.** Match the age-related changes in the numbered column with the drug effects in the lettered column.

1. ___B___   Increased body fat *(139)*
2. ___D___   Decreased body water *(139)*
3. ___F___   Decreased hepatic blood flow *(139)*
4. ___A___   Decreased lean muscle mass *(139)*
5. ___E___   Decreased renal function *(139)*
6. ___C___   Decreased serum albumin *(139)*

A. Increased drug tissue concentration
B. Increased drug storage
C. Increased free drug concentration
D. Increased drug/active concentration
E. Decreased drug elimination
F. Decreased drug clearance

## MULTIPLE-CHOICE QUESTIONS

E. Choose the most appropriate answer.

1. The study of aging is called: *(129)*
   1. geriatrics.
   2. ageism.
   3. gerontology.
   4. pulmonology.

2. A stressor, such as illness, may impair the older person's ability to compensate, resulting in: *(137)*
   1. disorientation.
   2. hypotension.
   3. loss of brain neurons.
   4. sedation.

3. Which system shows only slight decline with age? *(132)*
   1. Renal system
   2. Central nervous system
   3. Respiratory system
   4. Cardiovascular system

4. A frequent concern of older adults is: *(132)*
   1. long-term memory loss.
   2. creativity loss.
   3. short-term memory loss.
   4. judgment loss.

5. Neurologic features that show age-related changes include: *(133)*
   1. size of the brain, oxygenation function, and emotions.
   2. personality, cardiac output, and excretion of drugs.
   3. elasticity of cells, vision changes, and gastric secretions.
   4. temperature regulation, pain perception, and tactile sensation.

6. To compensate for neurologic changes, the aged individual may: *(133)*
   1. avoid temperature extremes and accomplish tasks at a slower pace.
   2. wear warm clothes and exert extra effort to get tasks accomplished.
   3. wear hats and concentrate for longer periods of time.
   4. check blood pressure frequently.

7. Kyphosis, vertebral loss of calcium, and calcification of costal cartilage result in: *(133)*
   1. increased vital capacity.
   2. decreased vital capacity.
   3. decreased anteroposterior chest diameter.
   4. contractures.

8. A frequent respiratory complaint of older adults is: *(133)*
   1. orthostatic hypotension.
   2. inability to breathe.
   3. increased respirations.
   4. exertional dyspnea.

9. Standard components of respiratory care for the older adult include: *(133)*
   1. coughing and deep-breathing exercises and range-of-motion exercises to facilitate lung expansion.
   2. frequent ambulation and auscultation of lungs.
   3. intake and output and postural drainage exercises.
   4. deep-breathing exercises and positioning to facilitate lung expansion and gas exchange.

10. In the absence of cardiovascular disease, heart size: *(133)*
    1. remains unchanged or slightly decreases.
    2. increases markedly.
    3. decreases markedly.
    4. remains unchanged or slightly increases.

11. With increasing age, a person's reduced tolerance for physical work may be due to the decreased: *(133)*
    1. size of the brain.
    2. capacity of heart cells to utilize oxygen.
    3. size of the heart.
    4. resistance to blood flow in many organs.

12. Which change occurs in aging kidneys? *(134)*
    1. Decreased filtration rate
    2. Increased extracellular fluid
    3. Increased cell mass
    4. Increased renal function

13. One of the first signs of aging of the skin is: *(134)*
    1. infection.
    2. thickening.
    3. elasticity.
    4. wrinkles.

14. An age change that occurs due to loss of oils in the skin is: *(134)*
    1. infection.
    2. itching.
    3. wrinkles.
    4. brown spots.

15. Which symptom is suggestive of possible gastrointestinal system illness? *(135)*
    1. Anorexia
    2. Dry mouth
    3. Constipation
    4. Unexplained weight loss

16. The leading cause of disability in old age is: *(135)*
    1. urinary tract infection.
    2. pelvic inflammatory disease.
    3. pressure ulcers.
    4. arthritis.

17. The curvature of the thoracic spine that causes a bent-over appearance in some older adults is: *(135)*
    1. kyphosis.
    2. arthritis.
    3. scoliosis.
    4. lordosis.

18. The term for hearing loss associated with age is: *(135)*
    1. tinnitus.
    2. ototoxicity.
    3. presbyopia.
    4. presbycusis.

19. What percentage of older adults are hearing-impaired? *(135)*
    1. 10%
    2. 50%
    3. 25%
    4. 75%

20. The type of hearing loss most easily treated is: *(135)*
    1. sensorineural.
    2. tinnitus.
    3. conduction.
    4. ototoxicity.

21. The type of hearing loss that results from exposure to loud noises, disease, and certain drugs is: *(135)*
    1. conduction.
    2. ototoxicity.
    3. infection.
    4. sensorineural.

22. The leading cause of new cases of blindness in older people is age-related: *(136)*
    1. glaucoma.
    2. cataracts.
    3. corneal abrasion.
    4. macular degeneration.

23. Which of the following is a normal aging change? *(135)*
    1. Decreased secretion of saliva
    2. Increased acidity of saliva
    3. Increased peristalsis
    4. Decreased gastric emptying

24. Presbyopia is corrected by: *(136)*
    1. laser surgery.
    2. reading eyeglasses.
    3. treatment with antibiotics.
    4. eye patches.

25. The leading cause of blindness in this country is: *(136)*
    1. glaucoma.
    2. presbyopia.
    3. cataract.
    4. conjunctivitis.

26. What percentage of older adults are able to function independently and sustain a sense of well-being? *(136)*
    1. 15%
    2. 25%
    3. 50%
    4. 85%

27. The developmental challenge in old age is to: *(137)*
    1. develop close relations with other people; to learn and experience love.
    2. find a vocation or hobby where the individual can help others or in some way contribute to society.
    3. establish trusting relationships with other people.
    4. review life and gain a feeling of accomplishment or fulfillment.

28. Two-thirds of the suicides among older people are due to depression resulting from: *(137)*
    1. loneliness.
    2. loss.
    3. medication.
    4. denial.

29. For effective gerontological care, the crucial denominator in deciding care needs is: *(138)*
    1. medical diagnosis.
    2. functional assessment.
    3. activities of daily living.
    4. community resources.

30. With aging, there is decreased body size and increased: *(139)*
    1. serum albumin.
    2. drug clearance.
    3. lean body mass.
    4. fat.

31. A highly fat-soluble drug such as diazepam (Valium) may result in: *(139-140)*
    1. shorter storage of drug before excretion.
    2. higher blood concentrations of the drug.
    3. lower blood concentrations of the drug.
    4. longer storage of drug before excretion.

32. Age-related changes of decreased liver size, reduced blood flow through the liver, and reduced liver enzyme activity affect the: *(140)*
    1. storage of drugs.
    2. tissue sensitivity of drugs.
    3. inactivation of drugs.
    4. absorption of drugs.

33. Which drug may counteract the effects of diuretics in the older adult? *(140)*
    1. Tylenol
    2. Nasal decongestant
    3. Sodium bicarbonate
    4. Aspirin

34. The developmental task associated with old age is: *(137)*
    1. generativity versus stagnation.
    2. intimacy versus isolation.
    3. autonomy versus dependence.
    4. ego-integrity versus despair.

35. Because older adults have a decreased number and sensitivity of sensory receptors and neurons, they should: *(133)*
    1. avoid temperature extremes and accomplish tasks at a slower pace.
    2. do deep-breathing exercises and positioning to facilitate lung expansion.
    3. use mnemonics and rehearsal memory training to improve memory performance.
    4. use assistive devices for walking and preventing falls.

36. Because of age-related changes in bone density in the spine, the thoracic spine curves, causing: *(135)*
    1. lordosis.
    2. scoliosis.
    3. kyphosis.
    4. arthritis.

37. Progressive slowing of responses and reflexes is due to: *(132)*
    1. decreased impulse conduction speed.
    2. loss of neurons in the brain.
    3. inadequate tissue oxygenation.
    4. atherosclerosis and decreased cellular respiration.

38. What is the effect on drugs an older patient is taking, related to renal function decreases in older adulthood? *(139-140)*
    1. Decreased body fat
    2. Decreased drug elimination
    3. Increased drug storage
    4. Increased drug tissue concentration

# CHAPTER 12

# The Nursing Process and Critical Thinking

---

## OBJECTIVES

1. Describe the five components of the nursing process.

2. Describe the formats for North American Nursing Diagnosis Association (NANDA) diagnoses, Nursing Interventions Classification (NIC) interventions, and Nursing Outcome Classification (NOC) outcomes.

3. Explain the role of the licensed practical nurse in the nursing process.

4. Describe the proper documentation of the nursing process using a problem-oriented medical record format, nurses' notes, and flow sheets.

5. Explain the relationship between the nursing process and critical thinking.

6. Describe the characteristics of a critical thinker.

7. Describe how critical thinking skills are used in clinical practice.

8. Describe principles of setting priorities for nursing care.

---

## LEARNING ACTIVITIES

A. **Key Terms.** Match the definition in the numbered column with the most appropriate term in the lettered column.

1. _____ A systematic, thorough way of obtaining objective data *(144)*

2. _____ Method of record-keeping that focuses on patient problems rather than on medical diagnoses *(143)*

3. _____ Systematic, problem-solving approach to providing nursing care in an organized, scientific manner *(146)*

4. _____ Tapping on the skin to assess the underlying tissues *(146)*

5. _____ Method of physical examination that uses the sense of touch to assess various parts of the body *(146)*

6. _____ Listening to sounds produced by the body, such as heart, lung, and intestinal sounds *(146)*

7. _____ Purposeful observation or scrutiny of the person as a whole and then of each body system *(146)*

8. _____ Actual or potential health problems derived from data gathered during the assessment of a patient or client *(148)*

9. _____ Information reported by patients or family members *(144)*

10. _____ Collection of data about the health status of a patient or client *(143)*

11. _____ Information about the patient collected by the nurse or other members of the health care team *(144)*

12. _____ Standard care plan with patient outcomes and timelines for specific interventions *(151)*

A. Auscultation
B. Objective data
C. Clinical pathway
D. Nursing diagnosis
E. Problem-oriented medical record
F. Subjective data
G. Nursing process
H. Percussion
I. Inspection
J. Assessment
K. Palpation
L. Physical assessment

B.  **Nursing Process.** Match the definition in the numbered column with the most appropriate component of the nursing process in the lettered column. Answers may be used more than once.

|   |   |   |   |
|---|---|---|---|
| 1. _____ | Putting the plan into action *(151)* | A. | Assessment |
| 2. _____ | Systematic collection of data relating to patients and their problems *(143)* | B. | Nursing diagnosis |
| 3. _____ | Assessing the achievement of patient goals *(151)* | C. | Planning |
| 4. _____ | Setting goals *(149-150)* | D. | Intervention |
| 5. _____ | Interpretation of the data for problem identification *(148-149)* | E. | Evaluation |

1.  _____ Putting the plan into action *(151)*
2.  _____ Systematic collection of data relating to patients and their problems *(143)*
3.  _____ Assessing the achievement of patient goals *(151)*
4.  _____ Setting goals *(149-150)*
5.  _____ Interpretation of the data for problem identification *(148-149)*
6.  _____ Identify health problems or potential health problems *(148-149)*
7.  _____ Determine priorities from the list of nursing diagnoses *(149-150)*
8.  _____ Collect data, including height, weight, and vital signs *(143-144)*
9.  _____ Obtain information through a health history by direct questioning *(143-144)*
10. _____ Measure the patient's progress toward meeting goals *(151)*
11. _____ Actual performance of nursing interventions identified in the care plan *(151)*
12. _____ Set short-term and long-term goals to determine outcomes of care *(149-150)*

A.  Assessment
B.  Nursing diagnosis
C.  Planning
D.  Intervention
E.  Evaluation

C.  **Objective Data.** Match the description in the numbered column (objective data) with the problem in the lettered column.

1.  _____ A patient's disheveled appearance based on sight *(144)*
2.  _____ A patient's noisy and labored breathing based on hearing *(144)*
3.  _____ A fruity mouth odor based on smell *(144)*
4.  _____ Cold, clammy skin based on touch *(144)*

A.  Possible respiratory problems
B.  Possible sign of diabetic acidosis
C.  May indicate that patient is in shock
D.  May indicate inability to carry out self-care activities at home

**D.  Charting Methods.** Match the description in the numbered column with the method of charting in the lettered column.

1. _____  Charting by different health care team members on the same page *(156)*

2. _____  Charting narrative notes only when there is a change in the patient's condition *(156-157)*

3. _____  Nursing notes recorded on computers *(157)*

4. _____  Using key words to organize charting, such as action or response *(156)*

5. _____  Charting on separate sheets for different health care workers *(156)*

6. _____  Recordkeeping that focuses on patient problems rather than on medical diagnoses *(157)*

7. _____  Charting that includes the problem, intervention, and evaluation *(157)*

A.  POMR
B.  Focus charting
C.  Source-oriented charting
D.  Multidisciplinary charting
E.  CBE
F.  CPR
G.  PIE

**E.  Critical Thinking.** Match the description of critical thinking tools in the numbered column with the corresponding critical thinking tool in the lettered column.

1. _____  Deriving alternatives and drawing conclusions *(158)*

2. _____  Clarifying the meaning of events and data *(158)*

3. _____  Reconsidering conclusions and recognizing the need to make changes *(158)*

4. _____  Presenting arguments for decisions and justifying *(158)*

5. _____  Examining ideas and breaking them down into components *(158)*

6. _____  Assessing possibilities, opinions, and usual practices *(158)*

A.  Interpretation
B.  Analysis
C.  Evaluation
D.  Inference
E.  Explanation
F.  Self-regulation

F. **Charting Methods.** Match the description in the numbered column with the correct component of SOAPE notes in the lettered column.

1. _____ Turn from side to side q 2 hr. Get out of bed at least twice a day. Begin ambulating as tolerated. *(157)*

2. _____ Turned q 2 hr. OOB twice a day; taking 6 small steps to and from bed. Pressure ulcer healing; now 1.5 cm. *(157)*

3. _____ Feels weak; "does not have the energy" to move around. *(157)*

4. _____ Pressure ulcer on sacrum related to immobility. *(157)*

5. _____ Does not turn self in bed; 2 cm, stage 2 pressure ulcer on sacrum. *(157)*

A. S
B. O
C. A
D. P
E. E

G. **Critical Thinking.** Match the description of critical thinking characteristics in the numbered column with the critical thinking characteristic in the lettered column. Answers may be used more than once.

1. _____ Willing to consider various alternatives *(159)*

2. _____ Examines parts and sees how they fit together *(159)*

3. _____ Recognizes that many variables are at work in patient situations *(159)*

4. _____ Seeks answers and reevaluates "common knowledge" *(159)*

5. _____ Uses an organized approach to problem solving *(159)*

6. _____ Sense of assurance that the problem-solving process produces a good plan *(159)*

7. _____ The desire, not just to know, but to understand how to apply the knowledge *(159)*

8. _____ Recognizes that sometimes the best plans do not work and goes back to the drawing board *(159)*

9. _____ Applies knowledge from various disciplines *(159)*

A. Systematic thinking
B. Analytical
C. Open-minded
D. Self-confident
E. Maturity
F. Truth-seeking
G. Curiosity

**H. Nursing Diagnosis.** List five new nursing diagnoses included in the 2005 NANDA list. *(149-150)*

1. _____

2. _____

3. _____

4. _____

5. _____

**I. Nursing Diagnosis.** Match the term in the numbered column with the type of diagnosis in the lettered column. Answers may be used more than once.

1. _____ Peptic ulcer *(148)*

2. _____ Pneumonia *(148)*

3. _____ Ineffective airway clearance *(148)*

4. _____ Myocardial infarction *(148)*

5. _____ Hiatal hernia *(148)*

6. _____ Impaired mobility *(148)*

7. _____ Wandering *(148)*

8. _____ Powerlessness *(148)*

9. _____ Fatigue *(148)*

10. _____ Risk for falls *(148)*

A. Nursing diagnosis

B. Medical diagnosis

**J. Data Collection.** Match the description in the numbered column with the type of data it represents in the lettered column. Answers may be used more than once.

1. _____ A shooting pain in my arm *(144-145)*

2. _____ Noisy, labored breathing *(144-145)*

3. _____ Fruity mouth odor *(144-145)*

4. _____ Cold, clammy skin *(144-145)*

5. _____ Blood pressure of 120/80 *(144-145)*

6. _____ Headache *(144-145)*

7. _____ Fear of surgery *(144-145)*

8. _____ Disheveled appearance *(144-145)*

A. Subjective data

B. Objective data

**K. Physical Assessment Techniques.** Match the condition to be assessed in the numbered column with the appropriate technique in the lettered column. Answers may be used more than once.

1. _____ Bowel sounds *(146)*
2. _____ Pitting edema *(146)*
3. _____ Mucous membranes *(146)*
4. _____ Jaundice *(146)*
5. _____ Blood pressure *(146)*
6. _____ Radial pulse *(146)*
7. _____ Lung sounds *(146)*
8. _____ Cyanosis *(146)*

A. Inspection
B. Percussion
C. Palpation
D. Auscultation

# MULTIPLE-CHOICE QUESTIONS

**L.** Choose the most appropriate answer.

1. The goal of the nursing process is to: *(143)*
   1. obtain information through observation, physical examination, or diagnostic testing.
   2. interview the patient or family in a goal-directed, orderly, and systematic way.
   3. record objective data, writing exactly what is observed.
   4. alleviate, minimize, or prevent real or potential health problems.

2. In the planning phase of the nursing process, which of the following actions occurs first? *(149)*
   1. Set short-term goals to determine outcomes of care.
   2. Set long-term goals to determine outcomes of care.
   3. Develop objectives to meet goals.
   4. Determine priorities from the list of nursing diagnoses.

3. The role of the LPN in relation to the planning phase of the nursing process is to: *(149)*
   1. perform a physical assessment.
   2. perform therapeutic nursing measures.
   3. assist with the development of nursing care plans.
   4. evaluate the nursing care given.

4. The role of the LPN in relation to the evaluation phase of the nursing process is to: *(144)*
   1. report observed outcomes and make necessary changes.
   2. carry out the established plan of care.
   3. collect data and take objective measurements of body functions.
   4. develop nursing care plans.

5. When admitting a patient with pneumonia, which step of the nursing process is done first? *(143)*
   1. Implementation
   2. Determine outcome criteria
   3. Set short-term goals
   4. Collect data

6. Which step of the nursing process do you use to determine whether outcome criteria have been met? *(143)*
   1. Assessment
   2. Planning
   3. Implementation
   4. Evaluation

7. An organization that requires systematic review of hospitals and other health care organizations is: *(151)*
   1. Joint Commission on Accreditation of Healthcare Organizations (JCAHO).
   2. Medicare.
   3. Medicaid.
   4. ANA Standards of Care.

8. Why is auscultation done before percussion and palpation when doing a physical assessment of the abdomen? *(146)*
   1. Auscultation aids in the palpation process.
   2. Palpation can alter auscultation findings.
   3. Auscultation can alter palpation findings.
   4. Auscultation findings determine where to perform percussion.

9. The POMR is a method of recordkeeping that focuses on: *(157)*
   1. medical diagnoses.
   2. patient problems.
   3. medical treatments.
   4. diagnostic tests.

10. If an error in charting is made, the entry should be: *(155)*
    1. erased, new entry entered, and initialed.
    2. erased, "error" or "mistaken entry" written in, and initialed.
    3. crossed out, "error" or "mistaken entry" written above, initialed.
    4. crossed out, new entry written above, and initialed.

11. Which of the following describes critical thinking? *(157)*
    1. Thinking based on learning many facts
    2. Reasonable thinking focused on deciding what to do
    3. Thinking based on the utilization of the nursing process
    4. Reflective thinking related to reading and gathering information

12. The statement, "Does not turn self in bed; 2 cm, stage 2 pressure ulcer on sacrum," refers to which component of SOAPIER charting? *(157)*
    1. Subjective information
    2. Assessment
    3. Plan
    4. Objective information

13. The statement, "Turn from side to side every 2 hours. Get out of bed at least twice a day. Begin ambulating as tolerated," refers to which component of SOAPE charting? *(157)*
    1. Plan
    2. Assessment
    3. Evaluation
    4. Objective information

14. Which would you chart under objective data? *(144)*
    1. Lumbar back pain
    2. Nausea
    3. No shortness of breath
    4. Pupils equal and reactive

15. Which is a correct recording of observational data? *(144)*
    1. The skin is cool and clammy.
    2. The skin looks good.
    3. The patient states, "My skin is cool and clammy."
    4. The patient's skin has improved.

16. Which is a nursing diagnosis? *(148)*
    1. Pneumonia
    2. Wandering
    3. Diabetes mellitus
    4. Urinary tract infection

17. Which is a medical diagnosis? *(148)*
    1. Altered tissue perfusion
    2. Impaired skin integrity
    3. Diabetes mellitus
    4. Fatigue

18. Which is a nursing diagnosis? *(148)*
    1. Fear
    2. Asthma
    3. Bronchitis
    4. Manic-depressive disorder

19. Auscultation is used to assess the: *(156)*
    1. skin.
    2. joints.
    3. lungs.
    4. head.

20. Which of the following observations about the patient is documented as subjective data? *(144)*
    1. Patient is 6' 3" tall and weighs 180 pounds.
    2. Patient's skin is jaundiced.
    3. Patient has pain associated with taking deep breaths.
    4. Patient's blood pressure is 130/80.

21. Which of the following is the best method for obtaining objective data? *(144)*
    1. Asking the patient about his pain
    2. Observing the patient to see if he is afraid
    3. Watching the patient for signs of fatigue
    4. Inspecting the color of the patient's skin

22. A new patient is admitted to the hospital with the following nursing diagnoses: Fatigue, Nausea, Ineffective individual coping, and Ineffective breathing pattern. Which diagnosis requires immediate attention? *(149)*
    1. Fatigue
    2. Nausea
    3. Ineffective individual coping
    4. Ineffective breathing pattern

23. Which of the following short-term goals is incomplete? *(150)*
    1. The patient will drink 1500 mL by 8:00 AM on 3/22.
    2. The patient will ambulate in the hall twice a day on 3/22.
    3. The patient will have less pain by 8:00 AM on 3/22.
    4. The patient will cough and deep breathe every 4 hours on 3/22.

24. A patient states, "I hope I can leave the hospital soon and return to my neighborhood association meetings. I am the president." According to Maslow's hierarchy of needs, which level does this indicate? *(150)*
    1. Physiological need
    2. Safety and security
    3. Love and belonging
    4. Self-esteem

25. Which critical thinking tool is associated with collection of data and focused assessment? *(158)*
    1. Inference
    2. Evaluation
    3. Interpretation
    4. Self-regulation

26. What is the critical thinking step that involves recognizing the need to make changes and reconsider conclusions? *(158)*
    1. Inference
    2. Self-regulation
    3. Interpretation
    4. Analysis

27. Which critical thinking tool is utilized when you think about the possible outcomes of each nursing action and you choose one intervention? *(158)*
    1. Interpretation: identifying data
    2. Evaluation: assessing possibilities
    3. Inference: drawing conclusions
    4. Self-regulation: reconsidering conclusions

28. The care plan states that you are supposed to give your patient a bath. The patient states that he feels "wobbly" when he stands up. You check his blood pressure, which is 90/60 mm Hg and his pulse is 120 and weak. What is the best nursing action? *(158)*
    1. Try again to get him up
    2. Give him a bed bath
    3. Let him rest and see how he feels later
    4. Exercise his legs before letting him stand

29. A benefit of clinical pathways for nurses and health team members is that it provides: *(151)*
    1. decreased length of stay.
    2. standardized, organized care.
    3. increased patient satisfaction.
    4. mutual goal setting.

30. Refer to Box 12-4 in the textbook, Clinical Pathway for Hepatic Cirrhosis. On what day is fluid restriction to 1500 mL/day started? *(155)*
    1. Day 1
    2. Day 2
    3. Day 3
    4. Day 4

31. Refer to Box 12-4 in the textbook. On what day can the patient with hepatic cirrhosis walk in the room with supervision? *(155)*
    1. Day 1
    2. Day 2
    3. Day 3
    4. Day 4

32. Refer to Box 12-4 in the textbook. What type of diet is the patient with hepatic cirrhosis following? *(154)*
    1. High protein, high carbohydrate
    2. Low protein, low carbohydrate
    3. High protein, high fat
    4. High carbohydrate, low fat

**M.** Nursing Care Plan Questions

1. Refer to Nursing Care Plan, Plan of Care for Mrs. C., on p. 152 in the textbook to answer M1 and M2. Into what level of Maslow's hierarchy does the nursing diagnosis of disturbed body image fall? *(152)*
   1. Physiological
   2. Safety
   3. Love and belonging
   4. Self-esteem

2. What is the priority initial nursing intervention for this patient, Mrs. C.? *(152)*
   1. Assist Mrs. C. to discuss changes caused by illness and surgery
   2. Monitor frequency of Mrs. C.'s statements of self-criticism
   3. Determine patient's and family's perception of Mrs. C.'s alteration in body image vs. reality
   4. Identify support groups available to Mrs. C.

# Inflammation, Infection, and Immunity

## OBJECTIVES

1. Describe physical and chemical barriers.

2. Describe how inflammatory changes act as bodily defense mechanisms.

3. Identify the signs and symptoms of inflammation.

4. Discuss the process of repair and healing.

5. Differentiate infection from inflammation.

6. Discuss the actions of commonly found infectious agents.

7. Describe the ways that infections are transmitted.

8. Identify the signs and symptoms of infection.

9. Compare community-acquired and nosocomial infections.

10. Discuss the nursing care of patients with infections.

11. Describe the Centers for Disease Control standard precautions guidelines for infection control.

12. Describe the Centers for Disease Control isolation guidelines for airborne, droplet, and contact (transmission-based) precautions.

13. Describe the immune response.

14. Identify organs involved in immunity.

15. Compare natural and acquired immunity.

16. Differentiate between humoral (antibody-mediated) and cell-mediated immunity.

17. Describe the nursing care of patients with immunodeficiency and of those with allergies.

18. Describe the process of autoimmunity.

## LEARNING ACTIVITIES

A. **Key Terms.** Match the definition in the numbered column with the most appropriate term in the lettered column. Some terms may be used more than once and some terms may not be used.

1. _____ An antigen that causes a hypersensitive reaction *(177)*

2. _____ A protein that is created in response to a specific antigen *(174)*

3. _____ Limiting the spread of microorganisms; often called *clean technique* *(169)*

4. _____ Elimination of microorganisms from any object that comes in contact with the patient; often called *sterile technique* *(170)*

5. _____ Nonspecific immune response that occurs in response to bodily injury; condition in which the body is invaded by infectious organisms that multiply, causing injury and inflammatory response *(162)*

6. _____ Hospital-acquired infections (infections that were not present at the time of admission) *(168)*

7. _____ Presence of an infectious organism on a body surface or an object *(166)*

8. _____ Vegetable-like organisms that feed on organic matter and are capable of producing disease *(165)*

9. _____ A substance, usually a protein, that is capable of stimulating a response from the immune system *(174)*

10. _____ A condition in which the body is invaded by infectious organisms that multiply, causing injury *(164)*

A. Allergen
B. Antibody
C. Antigen
D. Autoimmunity
E. Bacteria
F. Communicable disease
G. Contamination
H. Fungi
I. Immunity
J. Immunodeficiency
K. Infection
L. Inflammation
M. Medical asepsis
N. Nosocomial infections
O. Surgical asepsis
P. Viruses

11. _____ One-celled organisms capable of multiplying rapidly and causing illness *(164)*

12. _____ A condition in which the body is unable to distinguish self from nonself, causing the immune system to react and destroy its own tissues *(178)*

13. _____ Illness caused by infectious organisms or their toxins that can be transmitted, either directly or indirectly, from one person to another *(167)*

14. _____ Condition in which the immune system is unable to defend the body against organisms *(176)*

15. _____ Infectious microorganisms that can live and reproduce only within living cells; capable of causing illness, inflammation, and cell destruction *(165)*

16. _____ Resistance to or protection from a disease *(173)*

**B. Infectious Agents.** Match the definition in the numbered column with the most appropriate term in the lettered column. Some answers may be used more than once, and some may not be used.

1. _____ One-celled organisms capable of producing disease, which is usually spread by contaminated food and water *(165)*

2. _____ Vegetable-like organisms that exist by feeding on organic matter and that are capable of producing disease *(165)*

3. _____ Worms that are parasites found in the soil and water and are transmitted to humans from hand to mouth *(165)*

4. _____ Microorganisms that cause illness by stimulating an antigen-antibody response in the tissues, producing inflammation and cell destruction *(165)*

5. _____ Microorganisms that are usually transmitted to humans through flea and tick bites *(165)*

6. _____ Gram-negative organisms usually causing infections in the respiratory tract *(166)*

A. Helminths
B. Rickettsiae
C. Protozoa
D. Fungi
E. Mycoplasmas
F. Viruses

C.  **Signs of Infection.** Which of the following are observable signs (objective data) of infection? Select all that apply. *(166)*

1. _____  Redness
2. _____  Pus
3. _____  Pain
4. _____  Swelling

5. _____  Discoloration
6. _____  Heat
7. _____  Decreased skin turgor

D.  **Characteristics of Pain.** Match the definition in the numbered column with the most appropriate term in the lettered column.

1. _____  Tumor *(162)*
2. _____  Dolor *(162)*
3. _____  Calor *(162)*
4. _____  Rubor *(162)*

A.  Heat
B.  Swelling
C.  Redness
D.  Pain

E.  **Age-Related Changes.** What reasons explain why the healing process can be delayed in older adults? Select all that apply. *(164)*

1. _____  Decreased tissue elasticity
2. _____  Decreased lean muscle mass

3. _____  Decreased blood supply to tissues
4. _____  Decreased renal function

F.  **Bacteria.** Match the definition or description in the numbered column with the most appropriate term in the lettered column.

1. _____  Round bacteria that cluster in groups of two *(165)*
2. _____  Rod-shaped organisms that form spirals *(165)*
3. _____  Chains of round bacteria *(165)*
4. _____  One-celled microorganisms that retain a violet-colored stain *(165)*
5. _____  Bacteria that do not grow in the presence of oxygen *(165)*
6. _____  Clusters of round bacteria *(165)*
7. _____  Rod-shaped organisms *(165)*
8. _____  Bacteria that grow in the presence of oxygen *(165)*
9. _____  Round bacteria *(165)*
10. _____  Rod-shaped organisms with tapered ends *(165)*
11. _____  One-celled microorganisms that can be decolorized and counterstained pink *(164-165)*
12. _____  One-celled microorganisms capable of multiplying rapidly within a susceptible host *(164)*

A.  Anaerobes
B.  Gram-positive bacteria
C.  Bacilli
D.  Aerobes
E.  Spirochetes
F.  Diplococci
G.  Streptococci
H.  Bacteria
I.  Staphylococci
J.  Fusiform bacilli
K.  Gram-negative bacteria
L.  Cocci

G. **Infectious Agents.** Match each disease or infection in the numbered column with the most appropriate causative agent in the lettered column. Some agents may be used more than once and some agents may not be used.

1. _____ Malaria *(165)*
2. _____ Hookworm infection *(166)*
3. _____ Pneumocystis pneumonia *(165)*
4. _____ Primary atypical pneumonia *(166)*
5. _____ Measles *(165)*
6. _____ Typhus *(165)*
7. _____ Common cold *(165)*
8. _____ Rocky Mountain spotted fever *(165)*
9. _____ Tapeworm infection *(165)*
10. _____ Ringworm *(165)*

A. Fungi
B. Protozoa
C. Mycoplasmas
D. Viruses
E. Helminths
F. Rickettsiae

H. **Chain of Infection.** Place the six factors of the chain of infection in sequence: portal of entry, reservoir, susceptible host, mode of transmission, portal of exit, and causation agent. *(166)*

1. _____
2. _____
3. _____
4. _____
5. _____
6. _____

I. **Portals of Entry.** What are common portals of entry? Select all that apply. *(166)*

1. _____ Urethra
2. _____ Eyes
3. _____ Drains
4. _____ Ears
5. _____ Intravenous access devices
6. _____ Nervous system

**J.  Types of Infection.** Indicate which of the diseases below are (A) community-acquired and which are (B) hospital-acquired. *(167-169)*

1. _____   Urinary tract infections
2. _____   Food-borne illness
3. _____   Hepatitis B
4. _____   Nosocomial infection
5. _____   Superinfection
6. _____   Syphilis
7. _____   Gonorrhea

8. _____   Iatrogenic infection
9. _____   Tuberculosis
10. _____   Hepatitis A
11. _____   VRE
12. _____   AIDS
13. _____   Anthrax

**K.  Allergies.** Match each common allergic reaction in the numbered column with the most appropriate causative agent in the lettered column.

1. _____   Asthma *(177)*
2. _____   Anaphylaxis *(177)*
3. _____   Urticaria (hives) *(177)*
4. _____   Atopic dermatitis (eczema) *(177)*
5. _____   Allergic contact dermatitis *(177)*

A.  Food
B.  Latex gloves, plants (poison ivy)
C.  Pollens, dust
D.  Soaps
E.  Insect venom, antibiotics

**L.  VRE Infection.** Which of the following are CDC-recommended guidelines for limiting patient-to-patient transmission of VRE infection? Select all that apply. *(168)*

1. _____   Disinfect all patient care equipment used with VRE-infected patients.
2. _____   Wear a gown while in the room.
3. _____   Place VRE-infected patients in a single room or in a room with other VRE patients.
4. _____   Wear a mask while in the room.
5. _____   Use separate thermometers and stethoscopes.
6. _____   Remove gloves after leaving the patient's room.

**M.  Resistance.** Which of the following are reasons for the development of resistant bacterial strains? Select all that apply. *(168)*

1. _____   Bacterial cells develop mutations.
2. _____   Overuse of antibiotics.
3. _____   Introduction of allergens.
4. _____   Exposure to cigarette smoke.

**N.  Nosocomial Infection.** What are common sites for nosocomial infections in hospitalized patients? Select all that apply. *(169)*

1. _____   Respiratory tract
2. _____   Conjunctiva of the eye
3. _____   Surgical wounds
4. _____   Auditory canal of the ear
5. _____   Urinary tract

**O. Medical Asepsis.** What are examples of clean technique (medical asepsis) that help prevent infection in hospitalized patients? Select all that apply. *(169)*

1. _____ Changing bed linen
2. _____ Sterile wound dressing changes
3. _____ Washing hands frequently
4. _____ Insertion of Foley catheter
5. _____ Sanitizing bedpans
6. _____ Using individual medication cups
7. _____ Starting an IV infusion

**P. Standard Precautions.** Contact with which substances require the use of standard precautions when you are performing procedures? Select all that apply. *(170)*

1. _____ Patient's blood
2. _____ Sweat and perspiration
3. _____ Mucous membranes
4. _____ Intact skin
5. _____ Body fluids

**Q. Standard Precautions.** What are types of transmission-based precautions? Select all that apply. *(171)*

1. _____ Airborne
2. _____ Intact skin
3. _____ Droplet
4. _____ Contact
5. _____ Nosocomial

**R. Standard Precautions.** For each disease or condition in the numbered column, indicate all of the types of precautions in the lettered column that are appropriate.

1. _____ Mumps *(171)*
2. _____ Scabies *(171)*
3. _____ Influenza *(171)*
4. _____ Impetigo *(171)*
5. _____ Rubeola (measles) *(171)*
6. _____ Respiratory syncytial virus (RSV) *(171)*
7. _____ Varicella (chickenpox) *(171)*
8. _____ Rubella *(171)*
9. _____ Tuberculosis *(171)*
10. _____ Diphtheria (pharyngeal) *(171)*

A. Airborne precautions
B. Droplet precautions
C. Contact precautions

S.  **Lab Tests.** Which of the following are laboratory tests used to screen patients for infection? Select all that apply. *(173)*

1. _____        White blood cell differentiated count
2. _____        Liver function
3. _____        Electrolytes
4. _____        Blood cultures
5. _____        Platelet count

T.  **Hyperbaric Oxygen Therapy.** Which of the following are complications for which you monitor the patient during hyperbaric oxygen therapy? *(173)*

1. _____        Ear pain
2. _____        Eye pain
3. _____        Seizures
4. _____        Bradycardia
5. _____        Chest pain
6. _____        Allergic reaction

U.  Fill in the blank. *(173)*

The body's resistance to invading organisms and its ability to fight off invaders once they have gained access to the body is called _____.

V.  **Immune System.** Which of the following are factors that can compromise the immune system? Select all that apply. *(174)*

1. _____        Aging
2. _____        Disease
3. _____        Stress
4. _____        Use of antihypertensives
5. _____        Use of steroids

W.  **Antigens.** Which of the following are antigens? Select all that apply. *(174)*

1. _____        Microorganisms
2. _____        White blood cells
3. _____        Environmental substances
4. _____        Platelets
5. _____        Dust

X.  **Immune System Organs.** Which body organs are involved in immunity? Select all that apply. *(175)*

1. _____        Bone marrow
2. _____        Heart
3. _____        Lungs
4. _____        Lymph nodes
5. _____        Spleen
6. _____        Thyroid gland

Y.  **Drug Therapy.** Which classifications of medications often place patients at risk for infection? Select all that apply. *(168)*

1.  _____    Antibiotics
2.  _____    Antihypertensives
3.  _____    Steroids
4.  _____    Antineoplastics
5.  _____    Diuretics
6.  _____    Cholesterol lowering drugs

Z.  What is the primary nursing responsibility in cases of patients with immunodeficiencies? *(176)*

AA. **Antigens.** Match the example of antigen in the numbered column with the appropriate classification in the lettered column. Some classifications may be used more than once and some classifications may not be used.

1.  _____    Food *(174)*
2.  _____    Fungi *(174)*
3.  _____    Parasites *(174)*
4.  _____    Organ transplant cells *(174)*
5.  _____    Penicillin *(174)*
6.  _____    Bacteria *(174)*
7.  _____    Insect venoms *(174)*
8.  _____    Pollens *(174)*
9.  _____    Viruses *(174)*
10. _____    Blood transfusion cells *(174)*

A.  Environmental substances
B.  Drugs
C.  Microorganisms
D.  Transplanted cells

BB. **Allergens.** Which of the following are common allergens? Select all that apply. *(177)*

1.  _____    Animal dander
2.  _____    Molds
3.  _____    Foods
4.  _____    Viruses
5.  _____    Bacteria
6.  _____    Pollens
7.  _____    Cigarette smoke
8.  _____    Fungi
9.  _____    Latex gloves
10. _____    Pus

**CC. Anaphylaxis.** Which of the following are effects of histamine on the body when it is released during anaphylaxis? Select all that apply. *(177)*

1. _____    Shock from hypervolemia
2. _____    Decreased vascular permeability
3. _____    Edema
4. _____    Bronchospasm
5. _____    Vasoconstriction

**DD. Inflammatory Response.** Indicate the stages of the anti-inflammatory response following tissue injury outlined in the figure using the letters A–D.

1. _____    Release of chemical mediators *(163)*

2. _____    Ingestion and destruction of foreign agents *(163)*

3. _____    Repair and regeneration *(163)*

4. _____    Cellular injury *(163)*

5. _____    Movement of proteins, water, and white blood cells out of capillaries into injured tissues *(163)*

6. _____    Exudate formation *(163)*

7. _____    Normal tissue *(163)*

8. _____    Phagocytic lymphocytes enter area of injury *(163)*

9. _____    Dilated blood vessels and increased capillary permeability *(163)*

A.    Normal tissue
B.    Stage I
C.    Stage 2
D.    Stage 3

**EE. Immune System Organs.** Using the figure below, label organs involved in immunity (A–G). *(175)*

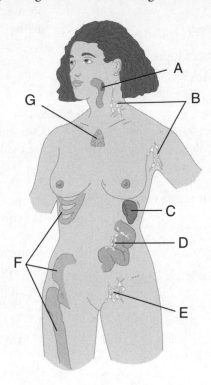

A. _____

B. _____

C. _____

D. _____

E. _____

F. _____

G. _____

**FF. Autoimmune Disorders.** Match the autoimmune disorders in the numbered column with the most appropriate targets in the lettered column.

1. _____ Diabetes mellitus type 1 *(179)*
2. _____ Addison's disease *(179)*
3. _____ Multiple sclerosis *(179)*
4. _____ Myasthenia gravis *(179)*
5. _____ Rheumatic fever *(179)*
6. _____ Ulcerative colitis *(179)*
7. _____ Crohn's disease *(179)*
8. _____ Rheumatoid arthritis *(179)*
9. _____ Autoimmune thrombocytopenia purpura *(179)*

A. Colon
B. Adrenal gland
C. Ileum
D. Joints
E. Brain and spinal cord
F. Pancreas
G. Neuromuscular junction
H. Heart
I. Platelets

## MULTIPLE-CHOICE QUESTIONS

**GG.** Choose the most appropriate answer.

1. Which types of leukocytes are especially involved with fighting infection? *(162)*
   1. Erythrocytes and neutrophils
   2. Neutrophils and monocytes
   3. Monocytes and thrombocytes
   4. Eosinophils and neutrophils

2. Which gram-positive bacteria clusters cause pneumonia, cellulitis, peritonitis, and toxic shock? *(165)*
   1. Staphylococcus
   2. Streptococcus
   3. Pneumococcus
   4. Enterococcus

3. The literal meaning of inflammation is: *(162)*
   1. red flame.
   2. great fire.
   3. inner infection.
   4. fire within.

4. What are small intracellular parasites that only live inside cells? *(165)*
   1. Gram-negative bacteria
   2. Gram-positive bacteria
   3. Viruses
   4. Fungi

5. The increase in blood flow to an inflamed area is due to: *(162)*
   1. increased permeability.
   2. chemical mediators.
   3. hemodynamic changes.
   4. hormonal factors.

6. The process by which the increased blood flow brings leukocytes to line the small blood vessel walls near the inflamed site is called: *(162)*
   1. phagocytosis.
   2. leukocytosis.
   3. pavementing.
   4. vasodilation.

7. The hemodynamic changes and vascular permeability in inflammation occur with the help of: *(162)*
   1. hormonal factors.
   2. chemical mediators.
   3. erythrocytes.
   4. thrombocytes.

8. Prostaglandins, histamine, and leukotrienes are examples of: *(162)*
   1. hormonal factors.
   2. chemical mediators.
   3. erythrocytes.
   4. thrombocytes.

9. A hormone produced by the adrenal cortex that is antiinflammatory is: *(162)*
   1. epinephrine.
   2. cortisol.
   3. aldosterone.
   4. thyroxine.

10. Cells that are produced to clean up inflammatory debris are called: *(162)*
    1. fibroblasts.
    2. platelets.
    3. neutrophils.
    4. macrophages.

11. Which of the following is a sign of local infection? *(162)*
    1. Fever
    2. Chills
    3. Warm skin
    4. Pale skin

12. One-celled microorganisms capable of multiplying rapidly within a susceptible host are called: *(164)*
    1. fungi.
    2. protozoa.
    3. bacteria.
    4. mycoplasmas.

13. Many childhood illnesses such as measles and chickenpox and some forms of hepatitis are caused by: *(165)*
    1. viruses.
    2. bacteria.
    3. protozoa.
    4. fungi.

14. The best way to fight viral illness is: *(165)*
    1. antibiotics.
    2. prevention.
    3. drug therapy.
    4. vitamin therapy.

15. It is seldom possible to kill viruses because: *(165)*
    1. replication of the virus occurs within the host cell.
    2. the cell wall can be destroyed with drugs.
    3. the cell wall requires oxygen for functions.
    4. the host cell is separate from the virus.

16. Vegetable-like organisms that exist by feeding on organic matter are called: *(165)*
    1. bacteria.
    2. viruses.
    3. protozoa.
    4. fungi.

17. Ringworm (tinea corporis) and athlete's foot (tinea pedis) are examples of disease caused by: *(165)*
    1. bacteria.
    2. viruses.
    3. fungi.
    4. protozoa.

18. One-celled organisms that produce diseases such as malaria and amoebic dysentery are called: *(165)*
    1. fungi.
    2. protozoa.
    3. viruses.
    4. helminths.

19. Microorganisms between the size of bacteria and viruses that are transmitted to humans through the bites of fleas and ticks are called: *(165)*
    1. rickettsiae.
    2. protozoa.
    3. helminths.
    4. mycoplasmas.

20. Parasites that are found in soil and water and are generally transmitted from hand to mouth are called: *(165)*
    1. rickettsiae.
    2. protozoa.
    3. helminths.
    4. mycoplasmas.

21. Gram-negative multishaped organisms without cell walls, also known as *pleuro-pneumonia-like organisms*, are called: *(165)*
    1. helminths.
    2. protozoa.
    3. mycoplasmas.
    4. viruses.

22. Microorganisms present in sufficient number and virulence to damage human tissue are called: *(166)*
    1. reservoirs.
    2. causative agents.
    3. portals of exit.
    4. portals of entrance.

23. The route by which the infectious agent leaves one host and travels to another is called: *(166)*
    1. portal of entry.
    2. mode of transfer.
    3. host.
    4. portal of exit.

24. Two groups of patients who are most susceptible to hospital-acquired infections include patients with: *(169)*
    1. pneumonia and patients requiring insulin.
    2. myocardial infarction and patients with tachycardia.
    3. AIDS and cancer patients receiving chemotherapy.
    4. emphysema and patients with bronchitis.

25. The type of infection resulting from giving immunosuppressive drugs to prevent rejection of a transplanted organ is: *(169)*
    1. sexually transmitted infection.
    2. superinfection.
    3. iatrogenic infection.
    4. fungal infection.

26. The overgrowth of a second microorganism that can cause illness following antibiotic therapy for one microorganism is called: *(169)*
    1. thrombophlebitis.
    2. superinfection.
    3. sexually transmitted infection.
    4. scpticemia.

27. The most basic and most effective method of preventing cross-contamination is: *(169)*
    1. handwashing.
    2. antibiotics.
    3. isolation.
    4. use of gown and gloves.

28. The primary cause of nosocomial infections is: *(169)*
    1. soiled hands.
    2. faulty equipment.
    3. airborne droplets.
    4. open wounds.

29. The elimination of microorganisms from any object that comes in contact with the patient is called: *(170)*
    1. medical asepsis.
    2. clean technique.
    3. isolation technique.
    4. surgical asepsis.

30. How much fluid is required by patients with infection? *(173)*
    1. 1 liter/day
    2. 2 liters/day
    3. 5 liters/day
    4. 10 liters/day

31. Patient teaching for people undergoing hyperbaric oxygen therapy includes: *(173)*
    1. do not take aspirin one week before.
    2. do not wear watches.
    3. swallow first to prevent pressure buildup.
    4. wear everyday clothes.

32. A CNS complication of oxygen toxicity that may occur during hyperbaric oxygen therapy is: *(173)*
    1. respiratory problems.
    2. sinus pain.
    3. bradycardia.
    4. seizures.

33. An advantage of home health care for infected patients is that the patient is: *(173)*
    1. exposed to fewer nosocomial infections.
    2. capable of spreading infections to others.
    3. susceptible to poorly prepared food.
    4. vulnerable to poor hygiene.

34. Which type of precaution is used to treat methicillin-resistant *Staphylococcus aureus* infections? *(171)*
    1. Airborne
    2. Droplet
    3. Respiratory
    4. Contact

35. Precautions developed to reduce the risk of airborne, droplet, and contact transmission in hospitals are known as: *(170)*
    1. reverse isolation.
    2. compromised host precautions.
    3. enteric precautions.
    4. transmission-based precautions.

36. Which precautions are used with patients who have MRSA? *(171)*
    1. Contact precautions
    2. Airborne precautions
    3. Droplet precautions
    4. Compromised host precautions

37. People with generalized infections become dehydrated because of: *(173)*
    1. poor skin turgor and dry mouth.
    2. dry mucous membranes and decreased metabolism.
    3. inflammation and pain.
    4. fever and anorexia.

38. A diet recommended for patients with
infection is: *(173)*
    1. low sodium.
    2. high fiber.
    3. high protein.
    4. low potassium.

39. Which guidelines are used for limiting
patient-to-patient transmission in order to
prevent VRE infection? *(168)*
    1. Check air conditioning system for
infected water
    2. Use separate thermometers and stetho-
scopes for VRE patients
    3. Change bed linen frequently
    4. Use sterile technique when caring for
VRE patients

40. Decreased bone mass due to the administration of cortisone is an example of a(n):
*(169)*
    1. VRE infection.
    2. MRSA infection.
    3. nosocomial infection.
    4. iatrogenic infection.

41. A common side effect of broad-spectrum
antibiotics is: *(169)*
    1. superinfection.
    2. hemorrhage.
    3. hypotension.
    4. hypokalemia.

42. Isolation precautions and disease-specific
precautions are now classified under standard precautions as: *(171)*
    1. universal precautions.
    2. enteric precautions.
    3. transmission-based precautions.
    4. compromised host precautions.

43. Food-borne illness is a common community-acquired infectious disease often caused
by: *(167)*
    1. pseudomonas.
    2. diphtheria.
    3. tuberculosis.
    4. *Salmonella.*

44. Antibody-mediated immunity is: *(175)*
    1. immediate.
    2. delayed.
    3. cell-mediated.
    4. altered.

45. A delayed response to injury or infection is
called: *(176)*
    1. humoral immunity.
    2. interferon immunity.
    3. cell-mediated immunity.
    4. pyrogen immunity.

46. What percentage of the U.S. population
suffers from allergies of some sort? *(177)*
    1. 20–25%
    2. Under 5%
    3. 40–45%
    4. 50–75%

47. Someone who is prone to allergies may be
referred to as: *(177)*
    1. infectious.
    2. immunocompromised.
    3. atopic.
    4. symptomatic.

48. Antigens that cause hypersensitivity reactions are called: *(177)*
    1. antibodies.
    2. complement.
    3. allergens.
    4. interferon.

49. Allergy testing is performed by injecting
small amounts of allergen: *(177)*
    1. intradermally.
    2. intramuscularly.
    3. intravenously.
    4. interstitially.

50. In anaphylaxis, what causes bronchospasm,
vasodilation, and increased vascular permeability? *(178)*
    1. Interferon
    2. Pyrogen
    3. Phagocytosis
    4. Histamine

51. Drugs used in the treatment of anaphylaxis include diphenhydramine, corticosteroids, epinephrine, and: *(178)*
    1. atropine.
    2. morphine.
    3. propranolol.
    4. aminophylline.

52. The body's ability to determine self from nonself is called: *(178)*
    1. tolerance.
    2. phagocytosis.
    3. immunity.
    4. inflammation.

53. Autoimmunity can involve any tissue or organ system. In multiple sclerosis, what is (are) affected? *(178)*
    1. Heart and kidney tissue
    2. White matter of brain and spinal cord
    3. Lung tissue and liver cells
    4. Spleen tissue and thymus gland

54. Two central nervous system autoimmune disorders are: *(179)*
    1. ulcerative colitis and Crohn's disease.
    2. rheumatoid arthritis and SLE.
    3. hyperthyroidism and Addison's disease.
    4. multiple sclerosis and myasthenia gravis.

55. Barriers to providing immunizations to large groups of the population include: *(168)*
    1. using fixed sites such as health departments.
    2. sliding fee schedules.
    3. educating people on benefits.
    4. increased infectious diseases caused by new organisms.

56. Control of vectors aimed at interrupting the transmission of infectious agents is: *(168)*
    1. spraying for mosquitoes.
    2. using antibiotics to prevent traveler's diarrhea.
    3. prompt treatment of strep throat.
    4. cooking meat, egg, and poultry until well-done.

57. Two measures to prevent the spread of VRE are: *(168)*
    1. careful use of antibiotics and infection control.
    2. proper hygiene and cooking meats until well-done.
    3. sanitation of water and antidiarrheal agents.
    4. screening and education of blood handlers.

58. Flu and cold viruses often enter the body through the mucous membranes of the nose and mouth; the nose and mouth areas are: *(166)*
    1. susceptible hosts.
    2. portals of exit.
    3. portals of entry.
    4. causative agents.

59. Malaise, anorexia, and prostration are symptoms of: *(167)*
    1. generalized infection.
    2. localized infection.
    3. community-acquired infection.
    4. nosocomial infection.

60. It is now necessary to give two or more drugs to tuberculosis patients because: *(167)*
    1. they prolong the effects of each drug.
    2. they potentiate the effect of each drug.
    3. strains of bacteria resistant to drugs have developed.
    4. more people are susceptible to tuberculosis.

61. A common protozoal infection that occurs as an opportunistic infection in HIV-positive people is: *(165)*
    1. *Pneumocystis carinii.*
    2. Rocky Mountain spotted fever.
    3. hookworms.
    4. conjunctivitis.

62. Gram-negative organisms without cell walls that are responsible for primary atypical pneumonia are: *(166)*
    1. viruses.
    2. rickettsia.
    3. helminths.
    4. mycoplasmas.

63. A life-threatening allergic reaction that can quickly deteriorate into shock, coma, and death is called: *(178)*
    1. resistance.
    2. septicemia.
    3. anaphylaxis.
    4. pneumonia.

64. Any items that have been touched or cross-contaminated by the host, such as bed linens or side rails, are: *(168)*
    1. vectors.
    2. common vehicles.
    3. pathogens.
    4. fomites.

65. The condition when the body's self defenses against foreign invasion fail to function normally is: *(176)*
    1. infection.
    2. inflammation.
    3. immunodeficiency.
    4. allergy.

## ALTERNATE FORMAT QUESTIONS

**HH.** 1. Which of the following are considered to be autoimmune disorders? Select all that apply. *(179)*
    1. Pneumonia
    2. Graves' disease (hyperthyroid disease)
    3. Crohn's disease
    4. Tuberculosis
    5. Hypertension
    6. Multiple sclerosis

2. Which of the following are common reportable diseases? Select all that apply. *(167)*
    1. Syphilis
    2. Crohn's disease
    3. Hypertension
    4. Encephalitis
    5. Diabetes mellitus
    6. Gonorrhea
    7. Hepatitis
    8. AIDS
    9. Pneumonia

3. Which of the following illnesses require the use of airborne precautions? See Box 13-3, p. 171. Select all that apply. in the textbook. *(171)*
    1. Pneumonia
    2. Measles
    3. Tuberculosis
    4. Pertussis
    5. Meningitis
    6. Varicella

4. Refer to Box 13-3, p. 171 in the textbook. Which of the following require contact precautions? Select all that apply. *(171)*
    1. Tuberculosis
    2. Influenza
    3. Impetigo
    4. Wound infection
    5. Viral conjunctivitis

# Fluids and Electrolytes

---

## OBJECTIVES

1. Describe the extracellular and intracellular fluid compartments.

2. Describe the composition of the extracellular and intracellular body fluid compartments.

3. Discuss the mechanisms of fluid transport and fluid balance.

4. Identify the causes, signs and symptoms, and treatment of fluid imbalances.

5. Describe the major functions of the major electrolytes—sodium, potassium, calcium, and magnesium.

6. Identify the causes, signs and symptoms, and treatment of electrolyte imbalances.

7. List data to be collected in assessing the fluid and electrolyte status.

8. Discuss the medical treatment and nursing management of people with fluid and electrolyte imbalances.

9. Explain why older adults are at increased risk for fluid and electrolyte imbalances.

10. List the four types of acid-base imbalances.

11. Identify the major causes of each acid-base imbalance.

12. Explain the management of acid-base imbalances.

---

## LEARNING ACTIVITIES

A. **Body Water.** Select the correct word to complete each sentence.

1. With increasing age, body water (increases/decreases). *(183)*

2. Fat cells contain (more/less) water than other cells. *(183)*

3. Females have (higher/lower) body water percentages than males. *(183)*

4. An obese person has a (higher/lower) percentage of body water than a thin person. *(183)*

B.  **Electrolytes.** Indicate for each substance whether it is an electrolyte (A) or a nonelectrolyte (B).

1.  _B_  Bilirubin *(184)*
2.  _B_  Urea *(184)*
3.  _A_  Magnesium *(183)*
4.  _A_  Phosphate *(183)*
5.  _B_  Creatinine *(184)*
6.  _A_  Bicarbonate *(183)*

7.  _A_  Potassium *(183)*
8.  _B_  Protein *(183)*
9.  _A_  Chloride *(183)*
10. _A_  Calcium *(183)*
11. _A_  Sodium *(183)*

C.  **Fluid Balance.** Which of the following conditions have great potential for altering fluid balance? Select all that apply. *(191)*

1.  _✓_  Burns
2.  ____  Multiple sclerosis
3.  _✓_  Ulcerative colitis
4.  ____  Dyspnea
5.  _✓_  Vomiting
6.  _✓_  Kidney disease
7.  ____  Tachycardia
8.  ____  Hypothermia
9.  _✓_  Diarrhea
10. ____  Congestive heart failure

D.  **Skin Turgor.** What are locations where skin turgor is best measured? Select all that apply. *(186)*

1.  ____  Wrist
2.  _✓_  Sternum
3.  ____  Inner aspects of thighs
4.  ____  Cheeks
5.  _✓_  Forehead
6.  ____  Fingertips

E.  **Edema Measurement.** What are common parts of the body against which skin is pressed to test for edema? Select all that apply. *(188)*

1.  _✓_  Radius
2.  _✓_  Ankle
3.  _✓_  Tibia
4.  _✓_  Fibula
5.  ____  Femur
6.  _✓_  Sternum
7.  _✓_  Sacrum

F.  **Age-Related Changes.** Which of the following are reasons older people are at high risk for fluid and electrolyte imbalance? Select all that apply. *(186)*

1.  _____✓_____  Decreased renal response
2.  _____  Decreased lean muscle mass
3.  _____✓_____  Decreased sense of thirst
4.  _____  Increased total body water

G.  What is the most serious effect of hyperkalemia? *(196)*  Dysrhythmias (Brady→Tachy→ cardiac Arrest)

H.  **Fluid Balance.** Indicate whether the statements are related to fluid volume excess (hypervolemia) (A) or fluid volume deficit (hypovolemia) (B).

1.  ____B____  Stimulates thirst *(191)*
2.  ____A____  Dilute urine *(191)*
3.  ____B____  Decreased urination *(191)*
4.  ____A____  Stimulates aldosterone *(191)*
5.  ____B____  Inhibits ADH *(191)*

I.  **Regulation of body fluid volume.** Match the condition in the numbered column with the most appropriate effect in the lettered column. Answers may be used more than once or not at all.

1.  _____  Hyperkalemia *(196)*
2.  _____  Increased plasma osmolality *(195)*
3.  _____  Hyponatremia *(192-193)*
4.  _____  Decreased plasma osmolality *(185)*

A.  Stimulates ADH release
B.  Inhibits ADH release
C.  Stimulates aldosterone release
D.  Inhibits aldosterone release

J.  **Fluid and Electrolyte Changes.** Match the vital sign change (assessment) finding in the numbered column with the most appropriate condition in the lettered column. More than one condition may be appropriate for each vital sign change. Not all choices may be used.

1.  _____  Bounding pulse *(188)*
2.  _____  Weak, irregular, and rapid pulse *(188)*
3.  _____  Increased pulse *(188)*
4.  _____  Decreased pulse *(188)*
5.  _____  Increased blood pressure *(188)*
6.  _____  Deep, fast respirations *(188)*
7.  _____  Slow, shallow respirations with intermittent periods of apnea *(188)*
8.  _____  Fall in systolic blood pressure >20 mm Hg from lying to standing *(188)*
9.  _____  Fever *(188)*
10.  _____  Increased respiratory rate *(188)*
11.  _____  Subnormal body temperature *(188)*
12.  _____  Hypotension *(188)*

A.  Hyponatremia
B.  Increased metabolism, with fluid loss
C.  Metabolic acidosis
D.  Hypernatremia
E.  Hyperkalemia
F.  Hypermagnesemia
G.  Metabolic alkalosis
H.  Hypomagnesemia
I.  Fluid volume excess
J.  Fluid volume deficit

**K.  Blood Gas Values.** Refer to Table 14-7 in the textbook. Add arrows ($\uparrow$, $\downarrow$) or Normal in the table below. *(198)*

### Arterial Blood Gas Values with Uncompensated Respiratory and Metabolic Acidosis and Alkalosis

| CONDITION | CAUSE | pH | HCO₃ | PaCO₂ |
|-----------|-------|-----|------|-------|
| Respiratory acidosis | Hypoventilation | | | |
| Respiratory alkalosis | Hyperventilation | | | |
| Metabolic acidosis | Diabetic ketoacidosis | | | |
| | Lactic acidosis | | | |
| | Diarrhea | | | |
| | Renal insufficiency | | | |
| Metabolic alkalosis | Vomiting | | | |
| | HCO₃ retention | | | |
| | Volume depletion | | | |
| | K⁺ depletion | | | |

**L.  Lab Values.** Refer to Table 14-4 in the textbook. Fill in the blanks with the normal values. *(190)*

1.  Normal urine pH: _____

2.  Urine specific gravity (SG): _____

3.  Arterial blood pH: _____

**M.  Fluid and Electrolyte Imbalances.** What respiratory changes occur with the following conditions? Fill in the blanks.

1.  Metabolic alkalosis: _____ *(199)*

2.  Metabolic acidosis: _____ *(199)*

3.  Fluid volume excess: _____ *(193)*

**MULTIPLE-CHOICE QUESTIONS**

**N.** Choose the most appropriate answer.

1. The major electrolytes in extracellular fluid are: *(183)*
   1. sodium and chloride.
   2. potassium and phosphate.
   3. calcium and bicarbonate.
   4. magnesium and phosphate.

2. Sodium, potassium, calcium, and magnesium are examples of: *(183)*
   1. anions.
   2. cations.
   3. filtrates.
   4. enzymes.

3. Chloride, bicarbonate, and phosphate are examples of: *(183)*
   1. cations.
   2. anions.
   3. filtrates.
   4. enzymes.

4. The concentration of electrolytes in a solution or body fluid compartment is measured in: *(183)*
   1. milligrams (mg).
   2. grams (g).
   3. milliliters (ml).
   4. milliequivalents (mEq).

5. What stimulates osmoreceptors in the hypothalamus to give the sensation of thirst? *(185)*
   1. Increased plasma osmolality
   2. Decreased plasma osmolality
   3. Less concentrated urine
   4. Decreased urine volume

6. Water loss via the skin and lungs increases in a: *(186)*
   1. hot, moist environment.
   2. hot, dry environment.
   3. cool, dry environment.
   4. cool, moist environment.

7. A measurement of the concentration of electrolytes in body water is called: *(184)*
   1. osmosis.
   2. diffusion.
   3. osmolality.
   4. filtration.

8. What percentage of the plasma is filtered by the glomerulus? *(185)*
   1. 5%
   2. 20%
   3. 50%
   4. 80%

9. Because the retention of sodium causes water retention, aldosterone acts as a regulator of: *(185)*
   1. acid balance.
   2. base balance.
   3. blood pH.
   4. blood volume.

10. One way the body tries to compensate for fluid volume deficits is to: *(191)*
    1. increase heart rate.
    2. decrease heart rate.
    3. increase blood pressure.
    4. decrease ADH.

11. ADH is decreased in response to: *(187)*
    1. fluid volume deficit.
    2. fluid volume excess.
    3. decreased urination.
    4. concentrated urine.

12. The body tries to compensate for fluid volume excess by: *(187)*
    1. inhibiting aldosterone.
    2. stimulating ADH.
    3. inhibiting epinephrine.
    4. stimulating thirst.

13. The two electrolytes that cause a majority of health problems when there is an imbalance are sodium and: *(192)*
    1. potassium.
    2. chloride.
    3. magnesium.
    4. bicarbonate.

14. The major cation involved in the structure of bones and teeth is: *(183)*
    1. sodium.
    2. chloride.
    3. calcium.
    4. potassium.

15. When your body goes without fluid intake, which hormone increases water reabsorption? *(185)*
    1. Thyroxine
    2. Epinephrine
    3. ADH
    4. Aldosterone

16. Low levels of serum potassium can result in serious disturbances of neuromuscular function and: *(194)*
    1. metabolic function.
    2. cardiac function.
    3. bone structure.
    4. acid-base balance.

17. An extracellular anion that is usually bound with other ions, especially sodium or potassium, is: *(183)*
    1. chloride.
    2. magnesium.
    3. calcium.
    4. iron.

18. Which of the following drugs cause hypokalemia? *(194)*
    1. Narcotics and salicylates
    2. Anticholinergics and antihistamines
    3. Calcium channel blockers and beta blockers
    4. Diuretics and corticosteroids

19. Ninety-nine percent of the body's calcium is concentrated in the: *(183)*
    1. blood and muscles.
    2. liver and brain.
    3. bones and teeth.
    4. kidneys and adrenal glands.

20. If more calcium is needed in the bones, it is taken from the blood as well as reabsorbed through the: *(183)*
    1. lungs.
    2. kidneys.
    3. heart.
    4. liver.

21. Next to potassium, the most abundant cation in the intracellular fluid is: *(183)*
    1. calcium.
    2. sodium.
    3. chloride.
    4. magnesium.

22. Hard, edematous tissue, called *brawny edema*, occurs commonly after: *(189)*
    1. hysterectomy.
    2. appendectomy.
    3. tonsillectomy.
    4. radical mastectomy.

23. One liter of fluid retention equals a weight gain of: *(187)*
    1. 1 pound.
    2. 2.2 pounds.
    3. 5.4 pounds.
    4. 10 pounds.

24. Puffy eyelids and fuller cheeks suggest: *(188)*
    1. fluid volume excess.
    2. fluid volume deficit.
    3. potassium excess.
    4. potassium deficit.

25. Which assessment finding is the *least* reliable indicator of fluid status in an 80-year-old person? *(188)*
    1. Pitting peripheral edema
    2. Poor tissue turgor
    3. Intake and output
    4. Mucous membrane moisture

26. If a depression remains in the tissue after pressure is applied with a fingertip, the edema is described as: *(188)*
    1. excessive.
    2. pitting.
    3. depressed.
    4. minimal.

27. A deep and persistent pit that is approximately 1 inch deep is described as: *(188)*
    1. 1+.
    2. 2+.
    3. 3+.
    4. 4+.

28. When the edema is so severe that pitting is not possible and the tissue feels hard, the edema is described as: *(189)*
    1. 10+.
    2. 5+.
    3. tenacious.
    4. brawny.

29. A red, swollen tongue suggests an excess of: *(189)*
    1. potassium.
    2. calcium.
    3. sodium.
    4. magnesium.

30. A dry mouth may be the result of: *(189)*
    1. fluid volume excess.
    2. fluid volume deficit.
    3. hypochloremia.
    4. hyperchloremia.

31. Distention of the jugular neck vein can indicate: *(189)*
    1. fluid volume excess.
    2. fluid volume deficit.
    3. hypocalcemia.
    4. hypercalcemia.

32. If the veins take longer than 3 to 5 seconds to fill when placed in a dependent position, the patient may have: *(189)*
    1. hypokalemia.
    2. hyperkalemia.
    3. hypovolemia.
    4. hypervolemia.

33. Weakness and muscle cramps are symptoms of: *(195)*
    1. hyponatremia.
    2. hypokalemia.
    3. fluid volume deficit.
    4. respiratory acidosis.

34. The normal range for urine pH is: *(189)*
    1. 2.0–7.0.
    2. 4.0–12.0.
    3. 4.6–8.0.
    4. 7.8–12.0.

35. A urine specimen that is not tested within 4 hours of collection may become: *(189)*
    1. alkaline.
    2. acidic.
    3. more concentrated.
    4. less concentrated.

36. A measure of the kidneys' ability to dilute or concentrate urine is called: *(190)*
    1. pH.
    2. urine potassium.
    3. creatinine clearance.
    4. specific gravity.

37. In most instances, normal urine specific gravity is between: *(190)*
    1. 1.010 and 1.025.
    2. 2.001 and 4.035.
    3. 4.001 and 6.035.
    4. 5.0 and 7.0.

38. A good indicator of fluid balance is urine: *(190)*
    1. sodium.
    2. creatinine clearance.
    3. specific gravity.
    4. potassium.

39. A more precise measurement of the kidneys' ability to concentrate urine than the specific gravity is: *(190)*
    1. urine sodium.
    2. urine pH.
    3. urine osmolality.
    4. urine potassium.

40. A 24-hour urine specimen is required for: *(190)*
    1. creatinine clearance.
    2. pH.
    3. specific gravity.
    4. osmolality.

41. When the blood is more concentrated in a patient with fluid volume deficit, which blood study result is expected? *(191)*
    1. Increased blood urea nitrogen (BUN)
    2. Increased creatine
    3. Increased hematocrit
    4. Decreased hemoglobin

42. BUN provides a measure of: *(191)*
    1. blood volume.
    2. renal function.
    3. cardiac function.
    4. liver function.

43. In a patient with fluid volume excess, which blood study result would you expect? *(191)*
    1. Increased albumin
    2. Decreased osmolality
    3. Decreased magnesium
    4. Increased potassium

44. What one of the following is a symptom of hyponatremia? *(193)*
    1. palpitations
    2. hypertension
    3. confusion
    4. insomnia

45. What amount of fluid per day is needed by the average person for adequate hydration? *(186)*
    1. 500–700 ml/day
    2. 800–1000 ml/day
    3. 1500–2000 ml/day
    4. 3500–5000 ml/day

46. When breathing problems occur in a patient with fluid volume excess, the patient should: *(193)*
    1. lie flat in bed.
    2. have head of bed elevated 30 degrees.
    3. ambulate frequently.
    4. be in side-lying position.

47. If pitting edema is present in patients with fluid volume excess, patients should: *(193)*
    1. be turned every 2 hours.
    2. cough every 2 hours.
    3. ambulate every 2 hours.
    4. have blood pressure checked every 2 hours.

48. To prevent hyponatremia in patients with feeding tubes, what should be used for irrigation? *(194)*
    1. Sterile water
    2. Normal glucose
    3. Normal saline
    4. Sterile dextrose

49. The heart rate of patients on digitalis should be closely watched because hypokalemia can contribute to: *(195)*
    1. congestive heart failure.
    2. pericarditis.
    3. digitalis toxicity.
    4. diuresis.

50. In order to prevent gastrointestinal irritation, oral potassium supplements should be given with: *(195)*
    1. meals.
    2. a full glass of water or fruit juice.
    3. a full glass of milk.
    4. a teaspoon of water.

51. Which must be checked before starting an intravenous infusion of potassium? *(195)*
    1. Blood pressure
    2. Temperature
    3. Weight
    4. Urine output

52. Decreased renal function can cause: *(196)*
    1. hyperkalemia.
    2. hypokalemia.
    3. hypercalcemia.
    4. hypocalcemia.

53. The homeostasis of the hydrogen ion concentration in the body fluids is: *(196)*
    1. acid-base balance.
    2. active transport.
    3. adaptation.
    4. osmosis.

54. The respiratory system regulates the pH by removing: *(197)*
    1. oxygen from the blood.
    2. carbon dioxide from the blood.
    3. sodium from the blood.
    4. chloride from the blood.

55. When the respiratory system fails to eliminate the appropriate amount of carbon dioxide to maintain the normal acid-base balance, what occurs? *(197)*
    1. Respiratory alkalosis
    2. Respiratory acidosis
    3. Metabolic acidosis
    4. Metabolic alkalosis

56. Nursing care for patients with hypokalemia includes monitoring serum potassium levels and: *(195)*
    1. EKG.
    2. EEG.
    3. arterial blood gas results.
    4. intake and output.

57. The most common cause of respiratory alkalosis is: *(198)*
    1. hypoventilation.
    2. hyperventilation.
    3. drowning.
    4. obesity.

58. Patients may develop high levels of magnesium in their blood if they are taking: *(196)*
    1. diuretics.
    2. antihypertensives.
    3. antacids.
    4. salicylates.

59. Hyperventilation is treated by having the patient: *(198)*
    1. breathe slowly.
    2. increase fluid intake.
    3. receive oxygen.
    4. elevate legs.

60. When patients with respiratory alkalosis are hyperventilating, they should be encouraged to breathe: *(198)*
    1. rapidly into a paper bag.
    2. shallow breaths.
    3. panting breaths.
    4. slowly into a paper bag.

61. When the body retains too many hydrogen ions or loses too many bicarbonate ions, what occurs? *(199)*
    1. Respiratory acidosis
    2. Respiratory alkalosis
    3. Metabolic acidosis
    4. Metabolic alkalosis

62. With too many acids and too few bases present in metabolic acidosis, the blood: *(199)*
    1. $PaCO_2$ increases.
    2. pH remains the same.
    3. pH rises.
    4. pH drops.

63. When cells are damaged because of an injury, which cation is released? *(196)*
    1. Calcium
    2. Chloride
    3. Potassium
    4. Sodium

64. Metabolic acidosis may be treated with intravenous infusion of: *(199)*
    1. potassium chloride.
    2. normal saline.
    3. calcium salts.
    4. sodium bicarbonate.

65. An increase in bicarbonate levels or a loss of hydrogen ions results in: *(199)*
    1. metabolic acidosis.
    2. metabolic alkalosis.
    3. respiratory alkalosis.
    4. respiratory acidosis.

66. Potassium is a critical factor for the transmission of nerve impulses, because it is necessary for: *(183)*
    1. muscular activity.
    2. acid-base balance.
    3. fluid balance.
    4. membrane excitability.

67. In addition to its role in regulating fluid balance, sodium is also necessary for: *(183)*
    1. nerve impulse conduction.
    2. bone structure.
    3. protein structure.
    4. breakdown of glycogen.

68. Symptoms of hyponatremia include: *(193)*
    1. headache, rapid breathing, nervousness.
    2. confusion, abdominal cramps.
    3. vomiting, diarrhea, shallow respirations.
    4. irritability, edema, convulsions.

69. The most common cause of hypocalcemia is related to problems with which hormone? *(196)*
    1. ADH
    2. Aldosterone
    3. Thyroxine
    4. PTH

70. Refer to Table 14-1 in the textbook. What is the percentage of total body fluids in a female? *(183)*
    1. 18%
    2. 36%
    3. 54%
    4. 60%

71. Refer to Table 14-1 in the textbook. What is the percentage of total intracellular fluid (ICF) in a male? *(183)*
    1. 20%
    2. 36%
    3. 40%
    4. 54%

72. How are most fluids lost from the body? *(185)*
    1. Kidneys
    2. Lungs
    3. Skin
    4. Intestine

73. What is the normal total daily intake of body fluids? *(186)*
    1. 1000 mL
    2. 1200 mL
    3. 1500 mL
    4. 2500 mL

74. What is the best position for the patient who is experiencing dyspnea? *(193)*
    1. Keep the bed flat
    2. Elevate the head of the bed 30 degrees
    3. Elevate the head of the bed 60 degrees
    4. Elevate the head of the bed 90 degrees

75. What does a weak, irregular, rapid pulse suggest? *(196)*
    1. Severe calcium excess
    2. Severe potassium excess
    3. Severe sodium excess
    4. Severe magnesium excess

76. A bounding pulse occurs in patients with: *(193)*
    1. dehydration.
    2. hypovolemia.
    3. circulatory overload.
    4. hyperthermia.

77. A subnormal temperature often occurs with: *(188)*
    1. hypotension.
    2. hypovolemia.
    3. dehydration.
    4. fluid volume excess.

78. A fall in systolic pressure of more than 20 mm Hg when the patient changes from a lying to standing position usually indicates: *(188)*
    1. fluid volume deficit.
    2. fluid volume excess.
    3. circulatory overload.
    4. hypoventilation.

79. What is the best way to decrease the incidence of serious fluid and electrolyte imbalances? *(188)*
    1. Monitor blood pressure carefully
    2. Monitor temperature carefully
    3. Monitor rate and rhythm of the pulse carefully
    4. Monitor records of fluid intake and output carefully

80. What is the patient at risk for when the total intake is substantially less than the total output? *(191)*
    1. Fluid volume excess
    2. Fluid volume deficit
    3. Hypoventilation
    4. Hyperventilation

81. What is the normal hourly adult urine output? *(188)*
    1. 30–40 mL/hour
    2. 40–80 mL/hour
    3. 50–60 mL/hour
    4. 100 mL/hour

82. A rapid weight gain of 8% is considered to be: *(188)*
    1. minimal.
    2. mild.
    3. moderate.
    4. severe.

83. If the patient has a rapid weight loss of 2 kilograms, what is the equivalent loss of fluid? *(188)*
    1. 1 liter
    2. 2 liters
    3. 4 liters
    4. 6 liters

## ALTERNATE FORMAT QUESTIONS

O. 1. Which electrolytes are present in greater amounts in the extracellular fluid (ECF) than in the intracellular fluid (ICF)? Select all that apply. *(184)*
    1. Sodium (Na)
    2. Potassium (K)
    3. Chloride (Cl)
    4. Bicarbonate (HCO$_3$)
    5. Calcium (Ca$^{++}$)
    6. Magnesium (Mg)
    7. Phosphate (HPO4)

2. Refer to Table 14-9 in the textbook. Which factors are related to causes of hypovolemia? Select all that apply. *(192)*
    1. Decreased oral fluid intake
    2. Vomiting
    3. Decreased ADH production
    4. High fever
    5. Diarrhea
    6. Excessive sweating

3. Which of the following are indicators of dehydration? Select all that apply. *(192)*
    1. Hypotension
    2. Decreased pulse
    3. Decreased respirations
    4. Increased temperature
    5. Weight loss
    6. Decreased hematocrit (Hct) and hemoglobin (Hgb)

4. Refer to Table 14-6 in the textbook. What are signs of fluid excess in a patient being treated for dehydration who receives excessive fluid replacement? Select all that apply. *(192)*
    1. Increased pulse
    2. Decreased blood pressure
    3. Dyspnea
    4. Decreased respirations

5. What are indicators of fluid volume excess? Select all that apply. *(188)*
    1. Increased blood pressure
    2. Bounding pulse
    3. Decreased respirations
    4. Weight loss
    5. Irritability

6. What is the treatment for fluid volume excess? Select all that apply. *(193)*
    1. Restrict sodium intake
    2. Increase water intake
    3. Give diuretics
    4. Give antiemetics

7. Which of the following are nursing interventions for the patient with fluid volume excess? Select all that apply. *(193)*
    1. Offer ice chips
    2. Offer clear liquids
    3. Use small fluid containers
    4. Turn every 2 hours
    5. Inspect skin for breakdown
    6. Check temperature

8. Refer to Box 14-1 in the textbook. With which conditions does increased pulse occur? Select all that apply. *(188)*
    1. Fluid volume excess
    2. Sodium excess
    3. Magnesium deficit
    4. Potassium deficit

9. Refer to Box 14-7 in the textbook. Which aspects of the health and physical exam are important in determining the fluid and electrolyte status of a patient? Select all that apply. *(197)*
   1. Numbness
   2. Seizures
   3. Vomiting
   4. Use of diuretics
   5. Use of salicylates
   6. Dyspnea
   7. Skin turgor

10. Refer to Box 14-5 (GB 14-5) in the textbook. Which foods are high in sodium? Select all that apply. *(194)*
    1. Natural cheese
    2. Sausage
    3. Cooked oatmeal
    4. Fresh chicken
    5. Pizza
    6. Frozen peas

11. Which foods are high in potassium? Refer to Box 14-6 (GB 14-6) in the textbook. Select all that apply. *(195)*
    1. Lima beans
    2. Fresh apricots
    3. Broccoli
    4. Banana
    5. Ginger ale
    6. Fresh apple
    7. Corn
    8. Watermelon

12. Which of the following are manifestations of acid-base imbalance? Select all that apply. *(197)*
    1. Dyspnea
    2. Confusion
    3. Vomiting
    4. Muscle weakness
    5. Numbness
    6. Decreased skin turgor

# Pain Management

---

## OBJECTIVES

1. Define pain.

2. Explain the physiologic basis for pain.

3. Identify situations in which patients are likely to experience pain.

4. Explain the relationships among past pain experiences, anticipation, culture, anxiety, or activity and a patient's response to pain.

5. Identify differences in the duration of pain and patient responses to acute and chronic pain.

6. Explain the special needs of older adult patients with pain.

7. List the data to be collected in assessing pain.

8. Describe interventions used in the management of pain.

9. Describe the nursing care of patients receiving opioid and nonopioid analgesics for pain.

10. List the factors that should be considered when pain is not relieved with analgesic medications.

---

## LEARNING ACTIVITIES

A.  **Key Terms.** Match the definition in the numbered column with the most appropriate term in the lettered column.

1. _____  Process of pain transmission *(203)*

2. _____  Unpleasant sensory and emotional experience associated with actual or potential tissue damage, existing whenever the person says it does *(202)*

3. _____  Drug that acts on the nervous system to relieve or reduce the suffering or intensity of pain *(202)*

4. _____  A physiologic result of repeated doses of an opioid where the same dose is no longer effective in achieving the same analgesic effect *(204)*

5. _____  Behavioral pattern of compulsive drug use characterized by craving for an opioid and obtaining and using the drug for effects other than pain relief *(217)*

6. _____  Physiologic adaptation of the body to an opioid so that a person exhibits withdrawal symptoms when the opioid is stopped abruptly after repeated administration *(217)*

7. _____  Amount of pain a person is willing to endure before taking action to relieve pain *(204)*

8. _____  Pain that lasts longer than 6 months *(205)*

9. _____  Point at which a stimulus causes the sensation of pain *(204)*

10. _____  Pain that occurs after injury to tissues from surgery, trauma, or disease *(205)*

A.  Pain
B.  Addiction
C.  Acute pain
D.  Pain tolerance
E.  Nociception
F.  Physical dependence
G.  Tolerance
H.  Chronic pain
I.  Pain threshold
J.  Analgesic

B. **Gate Control Theory.** Indicate for each statement in the numbered column whether it (A) opens the gate or (B) closes the gate according to gate-control theory. Answers may be used more than once.

1. _____ Distraction *(203)*

2. _____ Tissue damage *(203)*

3. _____ Massage *(203)*

4. _____ Heat application *(203)*

5. _____ Position change *(203)*

6. _____ Fear of pain *(203)*

7. _____ Guided imagery *(203)*

8. _____ Monotonous environment *(203)*

9. _____ Cold application *(203)*

10. _____ Preparatory information *(203)*

C. **Pain Response.** Match the description in the numbered column with the most appropriate factor affecting pain response in the lettered column.

1. _____ A patient who has received nitrous oxide during surgery and who says he does not have pain postoperatively *(204)*

2. _____ An older person who is stoic and does not want to bother the nurse *(204)*

3. _____ Pain associated with childbirth is usually short-lived, whereas cancer pain may be chronic *(205)*

4. _____ Anger, fatigue, insomnia, depression *(204)*

5. _____ A patient who prays and believes that divine intervention will help him to endure pain *(205)*

A. Situational factors
B. Pain threshold
C. Religious beliefs
D. Age, culture
E. Anesthetic

D. **Patient Situation.** A 42-year-old male with multiple fractures in the right arm used the numeric scale from 1 to 10 for rating pain. The patient complained of throbbing in his right arm and a backache. He rated the intensity of both pains at 7 on the scale at 8:00 PM. The nurse applied heat to the lower back as ordered, massaged his back, and administered 10 mg of morphine intramuscularly. At 9:00 PM, the patient rated intensity of both pains at 2 and stated that the pain was slowly going away. *(209)*

1. Were the interventions effective in relieving the pain?

2. What evidence do you have that the pain was or was not relieved?

**E. Pain Nursing Diagnoses.** List seven possible nursing diagnoses for patients who have pain. *(210-211)*

1. _____

2. _____

3. _____

4. _____

5. _____

6. _____

7. _____

**F. Pain Key Terms.** Match the characteristic in the numbered column with the most appropriate term in the lettered column. Answers may be used more than once.

1. _____    Physiologic changes that occur from repeated doses of opioids *(217)*

2. _____    Compulsive obtaining and use of drug for psychic effects *(217)*

3. _____    Withdrawal symptoms may occur if the opioid is stopped abruptly (e.g., irritability, chills, sweating, nausea) *(217)*

4. _____    Psychological dependence characterized by continued craving for opioid for other than pain relief *(217)*

5. _____    The need for higher doses to achieve pain relief *(217)*

A.   Addiction
B.   Tolerance
C.   Physical dependence

**G. Pain Response.** Which of the following are physical factors that influence response to pain? Select all that apply. *(204)*

1. _____    Age

2. _____    Type of surgery

3. _____    Pain tolerance

4. _____    Endocrine system activity

5. _____    Body temperature

6. _____    Physical activity

7. _____    Blood pressure

## MULTIPLE-CHOICE QUESTIONS

**H.** Choose the most appropriate answer.

1. One difference between acute and chronic pain is that a patient with acute pain: *(205)*
   1. often becomes depressed.
   2. shows little facial expression.
   3. feels isolated.
   4. has a fast heart rate.

2. Pathways that carry messages to the brain where the messages are interpreted are: *(203)*
   1. internal.
   2. external.
   3. afferent.
   4. efferent.

3. Factors influencing the response to pain include pain threshold, pain tolerance, age, physical activity, and the type of surgery. These factors are examples of: *(204)*
   1. psychosocial factors.
   2. emotional factors.
   3. sociological factors.
   4. physical factors.

4. The point at which a stimulus causes the sensation or feeling of pain is the pain: *(204)*
   1. duration.
   2. peak.
   3. threshold.
   4. tolerance.

5. When the pain threshold is lowered, the person experiences pain: *(204)*
   1. less easily.
   2. more easily.
   3. as excruciating.
   4. as mild.

6. Which age group tends to report their pain as much less severe than it really is? *(204)*
   1. Older patients
   2. Middle-aged patients
   3. Adolescent patients
   4. Children

7. Surgery in which area is reported to be the most painful for patients? *(204)*
   1. Skull region
   2. Thoracic region
   3. Upper abdominal region
   4. Lower abdominal region

8. Dilated pupils, perspiration, and pallor are results of which nervous system response to pain? *(205)*
   1. Voluntary
   2. Somatic
   3. Parasympathetic
   4. Sympathetic

9. Postoperative pain and pain in childbirth are examples of: *(205)*
   1. chronic pain.
   2. permanent pain.
   3. acute pain.
   4. nonmalignant pain.

10. An example of acute pain with recurrent episodes is pain associated with: *(206)*
    1. low back pain.
    2. migraine headaches.
    3. rheumatoid arthritis.
    4. cancer pain.

11. A pain that cannot be explained or that persists after healing has taken place is: *(206)*
    1. acute benign pain.
    2. acute metastatic pain.
    3. chronic benign pain.
    4. chronic metastatic pain.

12. The first step in pain management is: *(207)*
    1. assessment.
    2. planning.
    3. intervention.
    4. evaluation.

13. When possible, the information about pain should obtained from the: *(207)*
    1. nurse.
    2. patient.
    3. doctor.
    4. patient's family.

14. Factors that make the pain worse are called: *(209)*
    1. benign factors.
    2. stoic factors.
    3. psychological factors.
    4. aggravating factors.

15. The application of heat or cold, massage, and TENS are examples of: *(212)*
    1. physical comfort measures.
    2. cutaneous stimulation.
    3. environmental control.
    4. psychological comfort measures.

16. The longest time a cold application can be used without tissue injury would be: *(212)*
    1. 3 minutes.
    2. 15 minutes.
    3. 30 minutes.
    4. 60 minutes.

17. The application of cold is contraindicated in patients with: *(212)*
    1. hip fracture.
    2. muscle sprain.
    3. allergic reaction.
    4. peripheral vascular disease.

18. Fentanyl (Duragesic) transdermal patches are used to treat chronic pain by delivering: *(218)*
    1. NSAIDs.
    2. salicylates.
    3. opioids.
    4. steroids.

19. Which is the most expensive and least available pain treatment? *(212)*
    1. Cold
    2. Heat
    3. Massage
    4. TENS

20. Focusing on stimuli other than pain is called: *(213)*
    1. massage.
    2. stimulation.
    3. distraction.
    4. acupuncture.

21. Relaxation is most effective for: *(213)*
    1. delusional pain.
    2. mild to moderate pain.
    3. moderate to severe pain.
    4. severe pain.

22. Using a person's imagination to help control pain is called: *(214)*
    1. environmental control.
    2. stimulation.
    3. imagery.
    4. relaxation.

23. When pain is unpredictable, analgesics are more effective when given: *(214)*
    1. once a day.
    2. twice a day.
    3. around the clock.
    4. prn.

24. The initial treatment choice for mild pain is: *(215)*
    1. opioid analgesics.
    2. nonopioid analgesics.
    3. narcotics.
    4. anesthetics.

25. Aspirin, acetaminophen, and NSAIDs are examples of: *(215)*
    1. opioid analgesics.
    2. nonopioid analgesics.
    3. narcotics.
    4. anesthetics.

26. Ketorolac tromethamine (Toradol) is generally used for the short-term management of: *(215)*
    1. cancer pain.
    2. congestive heart failure.
    3. urinary tract infection.
    4. postoperative pain.

27. Drugs, such as nonopioids, that do not improve analgesia beyond a certain dosage are said to have a: *(215)*
    1. peak effect.
    2. duration effect.
    3. ceiling effect.
    4. onset effect.

28. Some nonopioids should be used cautiously in patients with congestive heart failure or hypertension because of the side effect of: *(215)*
    1. decreased circulation.
    2. depressed respiration.
    3. tachycardia.
    4. fluid retention.

29. Nonopioids tend to block pain transmission: *(215)*
    1. at the central nervous system.
    2. during cell wall synthesis.
    3. at the myocardium.
    4. on the peripheral nervous system.

30. Nalbuphine (Nubain), butorphanol (Stadol), and pentazocine (Talwin) are examples of: *(216)*
    1. nonopioid analgesics.
    2. anticholinergics.
    3. opioid agonist-antagonists.
    4. opioid agonists.

31. A patient receiving 10 mg morphine IM for pain will be given what dose PO to receive an equianalgesic dose? *(217)*
    1. 10 mg
    2. 30 mg
    3. 60 mg
    4. 80 mg

32. If the patient is nauseated or has difficulty swallowing, which route is useful for administering opioids? *(218)*
    1. Oral
    2. Rectal
    3. Topical
    4. Intradermal

33. To evaluate the patient for constipation, the nurse must assess the patient for: *(218)*
    1. black, tarry stools and anorexia.
    2. decreased blood pressure, itching, and respiratory distress.
    3. abdominal distention, cramping, and abdominal pain.
    4. intake and output, nausea and vomiting.

34. Which effect of opioids is not potentiated by the use of promethazine (Phenergan)? *(218)*
    1. Sedation
    2. Respiratory depression
    3. Hypotension
    4. Analgesia

35. A drug classification that is effective in treating neuropathic pain is: *(219)*
    1. muscle relaxants.
    2. benzodiazepines.
    3. antidepressants.
    4. corticosteroids.

36. A patient who has had back surgery complains of muscle spasms. Which drug may be most effective in relieving his pain? *(219)*
    1. Muscle relaxant
    2. Opioid
    3. NSAID
    4. Aspirin

37. Which nonpharmacologic pain intervention increases the pain threshold and reduces muscle spasm? *(211)*
    1. Jaw relaxation
    2. Simple imagery
    3. Music
    4. TENS

38. When observing sedation in a patient, which stage would you consider to be an emergency situation? *(219)*
    1. Sleeping, but arouses when called
    2. Drowsy, but easily aroused
    3. Frequently drowsy to drifting off to sleep during conversations
    4. Minimal response to physical stimulation

39. When a pain order states 10–20 mg IM prn for pain, what will you do when you have given 10 mg and it is not effective? *(221)*
    1. Adjust the dose up as ordered until pain is relieved with minimal or no side effects.
    2. Give an additional 10 mg as soon as possible.
    3. Wait 4 hours, and give 20 mg the next time.
    4. Determine if the patient has developed pain tolerance.

40. What is an advantage of using slow, rhythmic breathing to reduce pain? *(214)*
    1. It involves simple imagery.
    2. It increases the pain threshold and reduces muscle spasms.
    3. It decreases congestion in the injured area.
    4. It may be used for only a few seconds or up to 20 minutes.

## ALTERNATE FORMAT QUESTIONS

I.  1. Which of the following are characteristics of chronic pain? Refer to Table 15-1 in the textbook. Select all that apply. *(206)*
       1. Lasts 3–6 months
       2. Responds to analgesics
       3. Pain is a sign of tissue injury
       4. Normal heart rate and blood pressure
       5. Oral route is preferred route
       6. Minimal facial expression
       7. Restlessness
       8. Grimacing

    2. Which of the following are examples of conditions that cause acute pain? Select all that apply. *(206)*
       1. Low back pain
       2. Rheumatoid arthritis
       3. Neuralgia (herpes zoster)
       4. Sickle cell crisis
       5. Phantom limb pain
       6. Migraine headaches

    3. Which of the following are adjuvant analgesics and medications for the treatment of pain? Refer to Table 15-6 in the textbook. Select all that apply. *(219)*
       1. Antidepressants
       2. Muscle relaxants
       3. Anticonvulsants
       4. Antipsychotics
       5. Diuretics

    4. Which of the following are parasympathetic responses to pain? Select all that apply. *(205)*
       1. Constipation
       2. Increased blood pressure
       3. Dilated pupils
       4. Urinary retention
       5. Perspiration

    5. Refer to Box 15-4 in the textbook. What are common pain behaviors in cognitively impaired older adults? Select all that apply. *(211)*
       1. Grimacing
       2. Crying
       3. Aggressive behaviors
       4. Increased appetite
       5. Noisy breathing

# 16 First Aid, Emergency Care, and Disaster Management

---

## OBJECTIVES

1. List the principles of emergency and first aid care.

2. List the steps of the initial assessment and interventions for the person requiring emergency care.

3. Describe the components of the nursing assessment of the person requiring emergency care.

4. Outline the steps of the nursing process for emergency or first aid treatment of victims of cardiopulmonary arrest, choking, shock, hemorrhage, traumatic injury, burns, heat or cold exposure, poisoning, bites, and stings.

5. Explain the legal implications of administering first aid in emergency situations.

---

## LEARNING ACTIVITIES

**A.  Key Terms.** Match the definition in the numbered column with the most appropriate term in the lettered column.

1. _____  Tearing away of tissue *(232)*

2. _____  Presence of air in the pleural cavity that causes the lung on the affected side to collapse *(232)*

3. _____  Loss of a large amount of blood *(229)*

4. _____  An injury to muscle tissue or the tendons that attach them to bones, or both *(231)*

5. _____  A severe, potentially fatal, allergic reaction characterized by hypotension and bronchial constriction *(239)*

6. _____  Presence of blood in the pleural cavity causing the lung on the affected side to collapse *(232)*

7. _____  Elevation of body core temperature above 99° F *(235)*

8. _____  Blood in the pericardial sac that causes decreased cardiac output *(232)*

9. _____  Nosebleed *(230)*

10. _____  Decrease in body core temperature below 95° F *(235)*

11. _____  An injury to a ligament *(231)*

12. _____  Any substance that, in small quantities, is capable of causing illness or harm following ingestion, inhalation, injection, or contact with the skin *(237)*

13. _____  Absence of breathing *(225)*

14. _____  Protrusion of internal organs through a wound *(233)*

15. _____  Absence of heartbeat and breathing *(225)*

A.  Shock
B.  Hypothermia
C.  Cardiopulmonary arrest
D.  Hemothorax
E.  Flail chest
F.  Sprain
G.  Evisceration
H.  Avulsion
I.  Hemorrhage
J.  Hyperthermia
K.  Strain
L.  Poison
M.  Respiratory arrest
N.  Pneumothorax
O.  Anaphylactic shock
P.  Cardiac tamponade
Q.  Epistaxis

16. _____ Loss of support of chest wall where several adjacent ribs are broken in more than one place *(232)*

17. _____ Acute circulatory failure that can lead to death *(229)*

B. **Emergency Care.** List, in sequence, the five steps in the initial assessment and immediate intervention in emergency care. *(224)*

1. _____ Look for uncontrolled breathing
2. _____ Initiate CPR or rescue breathing
3. _____ Look for medical alert tag
4. _____ Assess the ABCs: airway, breathing, and circulation
5. _____ Assess for injuries

C. **First Aid.** What are general guidelines for first aid treatment of emergency patients? Select all that apply. *(225)*

1. _____ Splint injured parts in the position they are found.
2. _____ Prevent chilling, and do not add excessive heat.
3. _____ Remove any penetrating objects.
4. _____ Give the unconscious person sips of water.
5. _____ Stay with the injured person until help arrives.

D. **Cardiopulmonary Arrest.** Which of the following are nursing diagnoses for patients in cardiopulmonary arrest? Select all that apply. *(226)*

1. _____ Ineffective airway clearance
2. _____ Ineffective (cerebral, cardiopulmonary) tissue perfusion
3. _____ Increased cardiac output
4. _____ Ineffective breathing pattern
5. _____ Risk for suffocation

E. **CPR.** Complete the table for adult basic life support for adult lay rescuers maneuvers. Refer to Table 16-1 on p. 228 in the textbook. *(228)*

1. Compression rate: _____
2. Compression/ventilation ratio for adult lay rescuers: _____
3. Compression/ventilation ratio for two rescuer health care providers: _____
4. Defibrillation AED for sudden collapse: _____
5. Defibrillation AED out of hospital: _____

F. **Burns.** Refer to Table 16-4 in the textbook. Match the type of burn on the left in the numbered column with the emergency intervention on the right in the lettered column.

1. _____ Superficial, minor burn *(235)*
2. _____ Sunburn *(235)*
3. _____ Extensive burns *(235)*
4. _____ Chemical burns *(235)*

A. Cover burns with a clean, dry dressing or cloth.
B. Immerse the injured body part in cool water for 2–5 minutes.
C. Remove contaminated clothing and then flush skin with water for 30 minutes.
D. Apply topical preparations with benzocaine.

**G.  Bites.** Refer to Table 16-7 in the textbook. Match the intervention on the left with the type of bite on the right. Answers may be used more than once.

1. _____    Immobilize the body part with the bite and keep it at or below the heart, to minimize absorption of venom. *(239)*

2. _____    Clean thoroughly and apply a dressing. Seek medical attention for antibiotic therapy. *(239)*

3. _____    Clean the wound thoroughly and apply a bulky dressing. *(239)*

4. _____    Calamine lotion or a paste of baking soda or meat tenderizer is soothing. *(239)*

5. _____    The patient with severe allergies may be given epinephrine, Benadryl, aminophylline, or hydrocortisone. *(239)*

6. _____    Try to keep the patient still. *(239)*

7. _____    Advise the patient to have a tetanus booster if immunizations are not current. *(239)*

8. _____    Remove the stinger with a scraping motion. *(239)*

A.  Snake bite
B.  Insect bite or sting
C.  Animal bite
D.  Human bite

## MULTIPLE-CHOICE QUESTIONS

**H.**  Choose the most appropriate answer.

1. General guidelines for first aid treatment of emergency patients include: *(225)*
   1. cover with wool blanket to prevent chills.
   2. remove penetrating objects.
   3. splint injured parts in the position they are found.
   4. give orange juice with sugar if unconscious.

2. The first assessment priorities must be: *(225)*
   1. observation of uncontrolled bleeding or shock.
   2. systematic head-to-toe assessment.
   3. airway, breathing, and circulation.
   4. palpation of carotid and peripheral pulses.

3. The systematic assessment begins with inspection of the: *(225)*
   1. head.
   2. chest.
   3. abdomen.
   4. lungs.

4. When the heart stops beating, a person is in: *(225)*
   1. pulmonary arrest.
   2. anaphylactic shock.
   3. cardiac arrest.
   4. cardiopulmonary arrest.

5. When respirations cease, the person is in: *(225)*
   1. cardiac arrest.
   2. anaphylactic shock.
   3. cardiopulmonary arrest.
   4. pulmonary arrest.

6. In most cases, the brain begins to die after 4 minutes without oxygen due to susceptibility to hypoxia of: *(225)*
   1. heart tissue.
   2. nerve tissue.
   3. lung tissue.
   4. blood vessels.

7. Prompt recognition and treatment of cardiopulmonary arrest are so important due to the need to maintain the oxygen supply to the: *(225-226)*
   1. heart.
   2. brain.
   3. lungs.
   4. blood vessels.

8. The goal of CPR is to maintain: *(226)*
   1. the heartbeat until respirations are restored.
   2. respirations until the heartbeat is restored.
   3. circulation until the heartbeat and respirations are restored.
   4. oxygenation until the heartbeat and respirations are restored.

9. When cardiopulmonary arrest is suspected, the first step is to: *(226)*
   1. tap the victim urgently and ask "Are you okay?".
   2. place the victim supine on a firm, flat surface.
   3. put your ear near the victim's nose and mouth to listen for breathing.
   4. give two full breaths.

10. Check for cardiac arrest in the adult by palpating the: *(226)*
    1. brachial artery.
    2. femoral artery.
    3. carotid artery.
    4. coronary artery.

11. Airway obstruction caused by a foreign body that enters the airway is: *(228)*
    1. cardiac arrest.
    2. respiratory arrest.
    3. choking.
    4. cardiopulmonary arrest.

12. Grabbing the throat with one or both hands is the universal sign for: *(228)*
    1. heart attack.
    2. choking.
    3. danger.
    4. loss of consciousness.

13. If the choking victim is conscious, the rescuer performs: *(228)*
    1. the Heimlich maneuver.
    2. CPR.
    3. 15 chest compressions.
    4. assessment of breathing.

14. If a choking victim loses consciousness, the rescuer does a finger sweep, attempts to ventilate, straddles the victim's thighs, and gives: *(229)*
    1. 5 chest compressions.
    2. 15 chest compressions.
    3. 5 abdominal thrusts.
    4. 10 abdominal thrusts.

15. Choking deaths can be prevented by: *(229)*
    1. not talking while chewing.
    2. lowering blood pressure.
    3. decreasing weight.
    4. increasing exercise.

16. In an adult, what amount of blood loss may result in hypovolemic shock? *(229)*
    1. 30 ml or more
    2. 1 pint or more
    3. 1 liter or more
    4. 10 liters or more

17. Immediate treatment for external bleeding is: *(229)*
    1. application of ice.
    2. elevate the site of bleeding.
    3. direct, continuous pressure.
    4. check vital signs.

18. If direct wound pressure and elevation fail to control bleeding, pressure is applied to the: *(230)*
    1. coronary heart vessels.
    2. cerebral blood vessels.
    3. main artery that supplies the area.
    4. main vein that supplies the area.

19. A fracture that does not break the skin is: *(230)*
    1. compound.
    2. open.
    3. simple.
    4. complete.

20. A fracture in which the ends of the broken bone protrude through the skin is: *(230)*
    1. compound.
    2. simple.
    3. closed.
    4. incomplete.

21. A fracture in which the broken ends are separated is: *(230)*
    1. compound.
    2. simple.
    3. complete.
    4. incomplete.

22. A fracture in which the bone ends are not separated is: *(230)*
    1. complete.
    2. incomplete.
    3. compound.
    4. simple.

23. The primary symptom of fracture is: *(230)*
    1. numbness.
    2. tingling.
    3. pain.
    4  hemorrhage.

24. The key to emergency management of fractures is: *(231)*
    1. application of cold.
    2. elevation of injury.
    3. immobilization.
    4. application of heat.

25. Injuries to muscles and/or the tendons are called: *(231)*
    1. dislocations.
    2. strains.
    3. sprains.
    4. fractures.

26. Emergency treatment for sprains and strains include: *(231)*
    1. direct wound pressure.
    2. immobilization.
    3. application of heat.
    4. application of splint.

27. Nursing diagnoses that might apply to the patient with a head injury during the emergency phase of treatment include: *(231)*
    1. Decreased cardiac output related to hypovolemia and fear related to possible impending death.
    2. Altered cerebral tissue perfusion related to hypovolemia and anxiety related to panic.
    3. Ineffective breathing pattern related to neurologic trauma and risk for injury related to increasing intracranial pressure.
    4. Risk for trauma related to improper movements of the spine.

28. Altered mental function and unequal pupils are signs of: *(231)*
    1. anaphylactic shock.
    2. altered breathing.
    3. increased intracranial pressure.
    4. spinal cord injury.

29. When there is a neck or spinal injury, you first assess: *(231)*
    1. blood loss and level of consciousness.
    2. breathing and circulation.
    3. movement of extremities.
    4. sensation in extremities.

30. After a diving injury, while removing the victim from the water, efforts are made to: *(231)*
    1. immobilize the extremities.
    2. immobilize the neck and back.
    3. turn the victim in a prone position.
    4. turn the victim in a supine position.

31. The priority goal for the patient with a neck or spinal injury is to: *(232)*
    1. provide adequate ventilation.
    2. increase cardiac output.
    3. reduce fear.
    4. decrease risk of additional injury.

32. Outcome criteria for the patient with a neck or spinal injury is based on: *(232)*
    1. continuous monitoring for signs of increased intracranial pressure and oxygenation.
    2. continuous immobilization of the back and spine and transport for medical care.
    3. prevention of aspiration and maintenance of circulation.
    4. prevention of skin breakdown and shock.

33. The primary nursing diagnosis for the patient with an eye injury is: *(232)*
    1. Impaired self-image related to change in physical capacity.
    2. Impaired coping related to change in vision.
    3. Risk for impaired skin integrity related to immobility.
    4. Risk for injury related to foreign body in eye.

34. When chemicals come in contact with the eye, the nurse should: *(233)*
    1. cover the eye with a loose dressing.
    2. flush with water to irrigate the eye for 30 minutes.
    3. apply pressure with a sterile cloth.
    4. place patient in shower under cold water.

35. If bleeding is under control, the priority nursing diagnosis for a traumatic injury to the auricle is: *(232)*
    1. Impaired body image related to injury.
    2. Anemia related to blood loss.
    3. Impaired tissue integrity related to trauma.
    4. Decreased cardiac output related to blood loss.

36. The most critical chest injuries include: *(232)*
    1. tension pneumothorax, ulcer, and abdominal injuries.
    2. pericarditis, lung contusion, and flail chest.
    3. open pneumothorax, flail chest, and cardiac tamponade.
    4. lung concussion and closed pneumothorax.

37. Any chest injury at or below the nipple may cause both chest injuries and: *(232)*
    1. head injuries.
    2. neck injuries.
    3. shoulder injuries.
    4. abdominal injuries.

38. Signs and symptoms of chest injuries that impair respirations are: *(232)*
    1. unequal pupils and hypotension.
    2. dyspnea and tachycardia.
    3. shallow respirations and lethargy.
    4. bradycardia and cyanosis.

39. Open chest wounds that penetrate the pleural cavity allowing air to enter are referred to as: *(234)*
    1. pneumothorax.
    2. cardiac tamponade.
    3. flail chest.
    4. hemothorax.

40. The pneumothorax wound should be covered with which type of dressing? *(234)*
    1. Saline
    2. Occlusive
    3. Vented
    4. Porous

41. The term used when several adjacent ribs are broken in more than one place is: *(234)*
    1. pneumothorax.
    2. cardiac tamponade.
    3. flail chest.
    4. hemothorax.

42. The abnormal chest wall movement in flail chest would be described as what sort of motion? *(234)*
    1. Sawing
    2. Paradoxical
    3. Pulsating
    4. Sucking

43. The abnormal chest wall action in flail chest causes: *(234)*
    1. altered tissue perfusion.
    2. increased cardiac output.
    3. increased pulse strength.
    4. impaired gas exchange.

44. The accumulation of blood in the pleural cavity that causes the lung to collapse is: *(234)*
    1. pneumothorax.
    2. cardiac tamponade.
    3. flail chest.
    4. hemothorax.

45. Outcome criteria for evaluating emergency nursing care of the patient with an abdominal wound includes: *(234)*
    1. protection of injured tissue.
    2. control of bleeding.
    3. restoration of a strong pulse.
    4. reduction in fear.

46. First aid for minor superficial burns is to: *(235)*
    1. apply butter to the burn.
    2. apply petroleum jelly to the burn.
    3. cover the burn with a cloth.
    4. immerse the injured body part in cool water.

47. When a large body surface area is burned or any area is severely burned, the nurse should: *(235)*
    1. apply medications to the burn.
    2. cover the burn with a clean dry dressing or cloth.
    3. cover the burn with a cool wet dressing or cloth.
    4. apply ice to the burn.

48. Outcome criteria for emergency care of the burn victim are based on finding: *(235)*
    1. immobility, as well as circulatory and respiratory status maintained.
    2. absence of symptoms of shock, burned areas covered, and coping supported.
    3. improved gas exchange, skin surfaces free from burning materials, and pain reduced.
    4. no symptoms of ileus and monitoring in place for signs of gastrointestinal bleeding and circulation.

49. Heat exhaustion is treated by: *(236)*
    1. pushing fluids with caffeine.
    2. ambulating the victim.
    3. cooling and hydrating the victim.
    4. placing victim in ice.

50. Patients with heat exhaustion would be considered stable when they exhibit: *(236)*
    1. urine output of at least 10 ml/hr and pulse rate of 100 bpm or more.
    2. ability to take a regular diet without nausea.
    3. below-normal body temperature and tachycardia.
    4. lowered body temperature and intake and retention of fluids.

51. The skin is red, hot, and dry and perspiration is absent in: *(236)*
    1. heatstroke.
    2. heat exhaustion.
    3. hyperthermia.
    4. hypothermia.

52. Mild tissue damage caused by cold is called: *(236)*
    1. frostbite.
    2. frostnip.
    3. hypothermia.
    4. cyanosis.

53. The priority nursing diagnosis for the victim of frostbite is: *(236)*
    1. Sensory/perceptual alterations related to decreased circulation.
    2. Risk for impaired skin integrity related to vascular changes caused by extreme cold exposure.
    3. Risk for infection related to tissue damage.
    4. Risk for disuse syndrome related to vascular changes.

54. The immediate treatment of mild cold injury is: *(236)*
    1. rapid rewarming.
    2. massaging to increase circulation.
    3. covering with dressing.
    4. immersing in tepid water.

55. Any substance that in small quantities is capable of causing illness or harm following ingestion is a(n): *(237)*
    1. antitoxin.
    2. emetic.
    3. poison.
    4. antiemetic.

56. Carbon monoxide poisoning occurs because carbon monoxide: *(237)*
    1. is blown off too rapidly during exhalation.
    2. binds to hemoglobin and occupies sites needed to transport oxygen to the cells.
    3. binds to white blood cells and causes infection.
    4. is retained and prevents oxygen from being inhaled in adequate amounts.

57. The primary nursing diagnosis for the victim of carbon monoxide poisoning is: *(237)*
    1. Impaired gas exchange.
    2. Ineffective breathing pattern.
    3. Risk for aspiration.
    4. Anxiety related to ineffective breathing pattern.

58. The primary nursing diagnosis for the victim of drug or chemical poisoning is: *(237)*
    1. Altered thought processes.
    2. Risk for infection.
    3. Risk for injury.
    4. Risk for suffocation.

59. Flu-like symptoms following a tick bite may be symptoms of: *(240)*
    1. poisoning.
    2. Lyme disease.
    3. staph infection.
    4. hypersensitivity.

60. Which drugs increase the risk of heatstroke by affecting the body's heat-reducing mechanisms? *(237)*
    1. Adrenergics and bronchodilators
    2. Diuretics and anticholinergics
    3. Steroids and salicylates
    4. Anticoagulants and antihistamines

61. Local effects of venom on blood and blood vessels include: *(239)*
    1. skin breakdown, petechiae, and clubbing of nails.
    2. coolness of extremities, shiny skin, and blood clots.
    3. discoloration, pain, and edema.
    4. brittle nails, hair loss, and cellulitis.

62. After a bite, epinephrine may be given to prevent: *(239)*
    1. hypotension.
    2. aspiration.
    3. blood clots.
    4. anaphylaxis.

63. A victim of a bite would be considered improved when: *(238)*
    1. wound has only clear or white drainage, pulse is 100 bpm or fewer, and respiratory rate is increased.
    2. patient is sleepy but able to be aroused, wound has only slight drainage, and only slight toxic effects are noted.
    3. patient is alert, respiratory rate is 30 or more, and blood pressure is normal.
    4. wound is free from debris, patient is alert without dyspnea, and specific toxic effects are absent.

64. For a minor superficial burn, what is the immediate nursing care? *(235)*
    1. Apply butter to the injured body part.
    2. Apply topical preparations with benzocaine.
    3. Immerse the injured body part in cool water for 3–5 minutes.
    4. Cover the burn with a clean, dry dressing or cloth.

65. What is the danger of too rapid rewarming as the treatment for a patient with severe hypothermia? *(236)*
    1. Cardiac dysrhythmias
    2. Heatstroke
    3. Tingling and numbness of extremities
    4. Muscle cramps

66. What is the danger of too rapid rewarming as the treatment for a patient with severe hypothermia? *(236)*
    1. Decreased heart and respiratory rates
    2. Lactic acid and cold blood may be sent to the heart
    3. Irregular heartbeat and breathing patterns
    4. Numbness and tingling of the extremities.

67. What is the first nursing action for any chemical eye injury? *(233)*
    1. Gently touch the eye with the corner of a clean cloth.
    2. Flush the eye for 30 minutes.
    3. Tape an inverted paper cup over the eye.
    4. Apply a loose dressing to the eye.

68. Which of the following is a significant nursing diagnosis for a patient with an insect bite? *(238)*
    1. Decreased cardiac output
    2. Ineffective breathing patterns
    3. Impaired gas exchange
    4. Risk for infection

## ALTERNATE FORMAT QUESTIONS

I.
1. Which of the following are common signs and symptoms of heat exhaustion? Select all that apply. *(236)*
   1. Dizziness
   2. Muscle cramps
   3. Pale, dry skin
   4. Hot, dry skin
   5. Absent perspiration
   6. Seizures

2. Following a severe allergic reaction to an insect bite, which drugs are indicated to prevent anaphylaxis? Select all that apply. *(239)*
   1. Demerol
   2. Epinephrine
   3. Hydrocortisone
   4. Ibuprofen
   5. Benadryl

3. Which of the following are local effects of snake bites? Select all that apply. *(239)*
   1. Local itching
   2. Pain
   3. Mild to moderate edema
   4. Urticaria
   5. Discoloration

4. Which of the following are nursing diagnoses for a patient who is choking? Select all that apply. *(229)*
   1. Ineffective airway clearance
   2. Decreased cardiac output
   3. Ineffective tissue perfusion
   4. Risk for suffocation

5. Which of the following are goals and outcome criteria for a patient with cardiopulmonary arrest? Select all that apply. *(226)*
   1. Decreased coughing
   2. Improving skin color
   3. Spontaneous respirations
   4. Patent airway
   5. Palpable pulse

6. Which of the following are nursing diagnoses for a patient with hemorrhage? Select all that apply. *(229)*
   1. Ineffective tissue perfusion
   2. Decreased cardiac output
   3. Fear
   4. Ineffective breathing patterns

7. Which of the following are goals and outcome criteria for a patient with hemorrhage? Select all that apply. *(229)*
   1. Skin warm and dry
   2. Patent airway with normal respirations
   3. Adequate oxygenation
   4. Blood pressure within normal range

8. Which of the following are nursing diagnoses for a patient with a head injury? Select all that apply. *(231)*
   1. Risk for injury
   2. Risk for suffocation
   3. Ineffective breathing patterns
   4. Decreased cardiac output

9. Which of the following are manifestations that will aid in the prompt recognition of a patient with a head injury? Select all that apply. *(231)*
   1. Ineffective breathing pattern
   2. Unequal pupils
   3. Altered mental function
   4. Pain
   5. Abnormal response of pupils to light

10. Which of the following are nursing diagnoses for a patient with an abdominal injury? Select all that apply. *(234)*
    1. Impaired tissue integrity
    2. Ineffective breathing patterns
    3. Risk for injury
    4. Risk for infection

11. Which of the following are nursing diagnoses for a patient with a burn immediately after the burn injury? Select all that apply. *(235)*
    1. Impaired gas exchange
    2. Decreased cardiac output
    3. Risk for infection
    4. Pain
    5. Ineffective breathing pattern
    6. Impaired skin integrity

12. Which of the following are biologic agents most likely to be used as bioterrorism weapons? Select all that apply. *(238)*
    1. Tuberculosis
    2. Anthrax
    3. Smallpox
    4. Chlamydia
    5. *Staphylococcus aureus*
    6. Pneumonic plague
    7. Botulism

13. What are types of anthrax where symptoms may appear in 7–42 days? Select all that apply. *(242)*
    1. Heart
    2. Liver
    3. Skin
    4. Kidneys
    5. Digestive tract
    6. Lungs

# 17 Surgical Care

---

## OBJECTIVES

1. State the purpose of each type of surgery: diagnostic, exploratory, curative, palliative, and cosmetic.

2. List data to be included in the nursing assessment of the preoperative patient.

3. Assist in identifying the nursing diagnoses, goals and outcome criteria, and interventions during the preoperative phase of the surgical experience.

4. Outline a preoperative teaching plan.

5. List the responsibilities of each member of the surgical team.

6. Explain the nursing implications of each type of anesthesia.

7. Explain how the nurse can help prevent postoperative complications.

8. List data to be included in the nursing assessment of the postoperative patient.

9. Identify nursing diagnoses, goals and outcome criteria, and interventions for the postoperative patient.

10. Explain patient needs to be considered in discharge planning.

---

## LEARNING ACTIVITIES

A. **Age-Related Surgical Outcomes.** Which of the following are reasons that older adults are often at greater risk for surgical complications? Select all that apply. *(247)*

1. _____ Secretions are more copious.
2. _____ Impaired healing and recovery, if chronic illness is present.
3. _____ Takes longer to regain strength following periods of inactivity.
4. _____ Ciliary activity is less effective.
5. _____ Age-related changes in the heart and brain.

B.  **Pulmonary Complications.** Which of the following are reasons that smoking increases the risk of pulmonary complications? Select all that apply. *(248)*

1.  _____    Ineffective breathing patterns
2.  _____    Risk for suffocation
3.  _____    More tenacious secretions
4.  _____    Less effective ciliary activity

C.  **Lab Studies.** Which are diagnostic tests that are done preoperatively? Select all that apply. *(248)*

1.  _____    ECG
2.  _____    Urine tests
3.  _____    Culture and sensitivity tests
4.  _____    Chest radiograph
5.  _____    Thyroid function tests

D.  **Informed Consent.** Which of the following are components of a consent form for surgery? Select all that apply. *(251)*

1.  _____    Patient must be informed about the procedure to be done.
2.  _____    Results of preoperative work-up are explained.
3.  _____    Alternative treatments are discussed.
4.  _____    Discharge instructions are included.
5.  _____    Risks involved are mentioned.
6.  _____    Patient agrees to procedure.

E.  **Drug Therapy.** Refer to Table 17-1 in the textbook. Which drugs increase effects of general anesthetics? Select all that apply. *(249)*

1.  _____    Anticonvulsants
2.  _____    Antihistamines
3.  _____    Barbiturates
4.  _____    Antihypertensives
5.  _____    Potassium-wasting diuretics
6.  _____    Atropine
7.  _____    Aminoglycosides
8.  _____    Muscle relaxants

F.  **Pre-Op Medications.** Which are safety nursing interventions following administration of the preoperative medication? Select all that apply. *(256)*

1.  _____    Instruct patient to remain in bed.
2.  _____    Have the consent form signed.
3.  _____    Raise the side rails of the bed.
4.  _____    Have the patient void.

G. **Complications/Local Anesthesia.** Which are complications of local anesthesia? Select all that apply. *(259)*
   1. _____ Allergic responses
   2. _____ Seizures
   3. _____ Hypotension
   4. _____ Local tissue damage
   5. _____ Respiratory depression
   6. _____ Muscle relaxation

H. **General Anesthesia.** Which of the following are methods by which general anesthetic agents can be given? Select all that apply. *(259)*
   1. _____ Inhalation
   2. _____ Intravenous infusion
   3. _____ Oral administration
   4. _____ Rectal administration
   5. _____ Intramuscular injection

I. **Risk of Shock/Surgical Complications.** Which of the following are reasons why there is a risk of shock in the immediate postoperative period? Select all that apply. *(261)*
   1. _____ Loss of blood
   2. _____ Ineffective breathing patterns
   3. _____ Altered tissue perfusion
   4. _____ Effect of anesthesia

J. **Hypoxia/ Surgical Complications.** Which of the following are reasons why hypoxia may occur in the immediate postoperative period? Select all that apply. *(261)*
   1. _____ Tongue falls back and blocks the airway.
   2. _____ Secretions are more copious.
   3. _____ Cough and swallowing reflexes are depressed by anesthesia.
   4. _____ Ciliary activity is less effective.
   5. _____ Risk of laryngospasm or bronchospasm.

K. **Surgical Complications.** Match the condition in the numbered column with the effect in the lettered column.

   1. _____ Spasm of larynx or bronchi *(261)*
   2. _____ General anesthesia *(261)*
   3. _____ Patient is unconscious *(261)*

   A. Depresses respirations, cough, and swallowing reflex
   B. Narrows airway and obstructs air flow
   C. Tongue falls back and blocks airway

L. **Drug Therapy.** Which are classifications of pre-op and operative drugs that depress respiratory function and cause pulmonary secretions to be drier and thicker during the postoperative phase? Select all that apply. *(249)*
   1. _____ Preoperative anticholinergics
   2. _____ Opioid analgesics
   3. _____ Corticosteroids
   4. _____ General anesthetics
   5. _____ Antihypertensives

M. **Wound Complications.** Which of the following are complications of wound healing? Select all that apply. *(263)*

1. _____ Dehiscence
2. _____ Evisceration
3. _____ Infection
4. _____ Hypotension
5. _____ Bradycardia

N. **Shock/Surgical Complications.** Which measures are taken to prevent the postoperative complication of shock? Select all that apply. *(262)*

1. _____ Observe wound dressing
2. _____ Report excessive drainage or bleeding
3. _____ Adequate fluids and nutrition
4. _____ Assist to cough and deep breathe
5. _____ Monitor intake and output
6. _____ Note early changes in vital signs
7. _____ Withhold oral fluids until nausea subsides
8. _____ Splint incision during activity

O. **Impaired Peristalsis.** Which are factors that may cause peristalsis to be impaired after surgery? Select all that apply. *(274)*

1. _____ Hypertension
2. _____ Opioid analgesics
3. _____ Immobility
4. _____ Inability to cough
5. _____ Nausea

P. **Surgical Complications.** What are causes of urinary retention following surgery? Select all that apply. *(262)*

1. _____ Altered tissue perfusion
2. _____ Decreased cardiac output
3. _____ Anxiety about voiding
4. _____ Trauma to the urinary tract

Q. **Postoperative Recovery.** Which of the following are criteria that determine when the patient can be moved from the recovery room to the nursing unit? Select all that apply. *(266)*

1. _____ Patient is able to void.
2. _____ Gag reflex is present.
3. _____ Patient is able to ambulate.
4. _____ Vital signs are stable.
5. _____ Patient has minimal pain.
6. _____ Patient can be awakened easily.

R. **Safety Precautions.** What safety precautions should be taken when patients are transferred to their own bed on the nursing unit? Select all that apply. *(266)*

  1. _____ Lower the bed.

  2. _____ Place call button within reach.

  3. _____ Take vital signs every 4 hours.

  4. _____ Place head of bed in high Fowler's position.

S. **Post-Op Care/Coughing.** Which of the following are types of surgeries in which coughing is contraindicated? Select all that apply. *(273)*

  1. _____ Appendectomy

  2. _____ Cataracts

  3. _____ Brain surgery

  4. _____ Mastectomy

  5. _____ Hip replacement

  6. _____ Hernias

T. **Surgical Complications.** What measures are used to prevent thrombophlebitis and related pulmonary emboli? Select all that apply. *(273)*

  1. _____ Early ambulation

  2. _____ Leg exercises

  3. _____ Coughing and deep breathing

  4. _____ Monitor vital signs

  5. _____ Antiembolic stockings

U. **Pulmonary Emboli.** Which are signs and symptoms that would alert the nurse to possible pulmonary emboli? Select all that apply. *(273)*

  1. _____ Hypotension

  2. _____ Decreased respiratory rate

  3. _____ Chest pain

  4. _____ Dyspnea

  5. _____ Hemoptysis

V. **Paralytic Ileus.** Which are characteristics of paralytic ileus? Select all that apply. *(274)*

  1. _____ Abdominal pain

  2. _____ Presence of bowel sounds

  3. _____ Increased temperature

  4. _____ Increased blood pressure

  5. _____ Abdominal distention

**W. Risk for Infection.** Which criteria are used for evaluating the outcomes of nursing goals related to risk of infection? Select all that apply. *(265)*

1. _____ Absence of fever
2. _____ Intact wound margins
3. _____ Minimal swelling
4. _____ Patient statement of pain relief
5. _____ Presence of bowel sounds
6. _____ Normal serum electrolytes

**X. Wound Closure.** Using the figure below (Figure 17-10, p. 269), label each method of wound closure (A–F). *(269)*

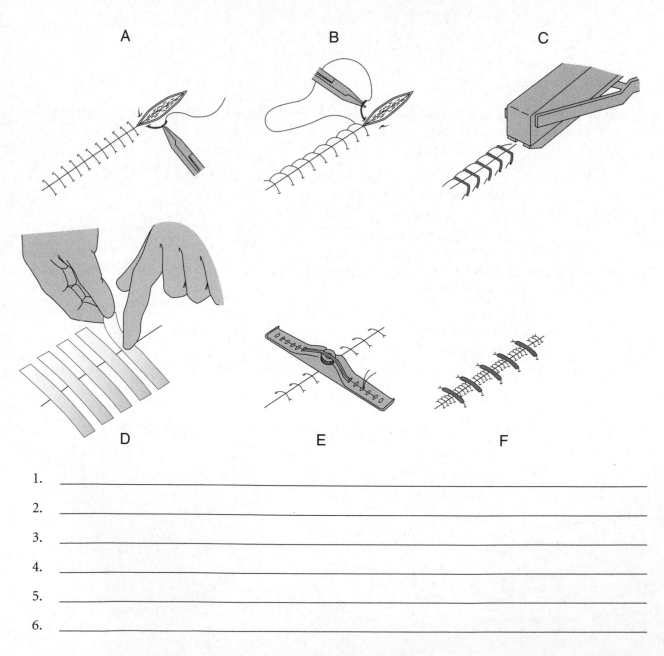

A    B    C

D    E    F

1. _____
2. _____
3. _____
4. _____
5. _____
6. _____

**Y.** **Complications of Wound Healing.** Using the figure below (Figure 17-9, p. 263), label each complication of wound healing (A and B). *(263)*

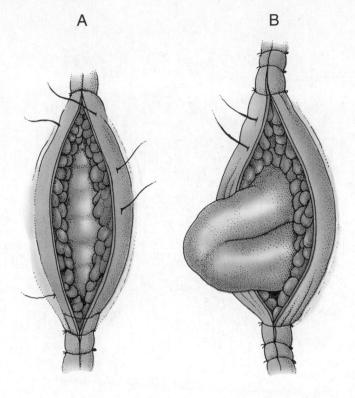

A                                          B

1. _____

2. _____

**Z.** **Complications of Wound Healing.** Match the description in the numbered column with the most appropriate term in the lettered column. Answers may be used more than once.

1. _____ Most likely to occur between the 5th and 12th postoperative days *(263)*

2. _____ Protrusion of body organs through the open wound *(263)*

3. _____ Reopening of the surgical wound *(263)*

4. _____ Likely to happen when there is excessive strain on the suture line *(263)*

A. Dehiscence
B. Evisceration

**AA. Endotracheal Tube.** Using the figure below (Figure 17-8, p. 260), label each part of the drawing representing inhalation anesthesia given through an endotracheal tube. *(260)*

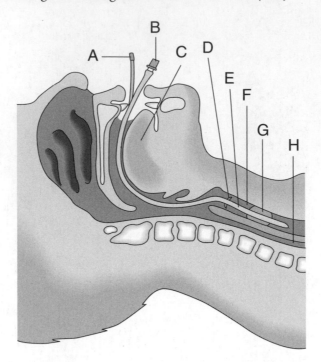

1. _____   5. _____

2. _____   6. _____

3. _____   7. _____

4. _____   8. _____

**BB. Drug Therapy/Preoperative Medications.** Match the preoperative drug in the numbered column with the most appropriate classification for use with preoperative surgical patients in the lettered column. Some answers may be used more than once. *(255-256)*

1. _____   Glycopyrrolate (Robinul)         A.   Tranquilizer
2. _____   Chloral hydrate (Noctec)         B.   Analgesic
3. _____   Promethazine hydrochlo-          C.   Anticholinergic
                ride (Phenergan)                 D.   Sedative or hypnotic
4. _____   Pentobarbital sodium             E.   Antiemetic
                (Nembutal Sodium)                F.   Skeletal muscle relaxant
5. _____   Diazepam (Valium)
6. _____   Atropine sulfate
7. _____   Meperidine hydrochloride
                (Demerol HCl)
8. _____   Secobarbital sodium (Se-
                conal Sodium)
9. _____   Morphine sulfate (MS
                Contin, Duramorph)

**CC. Surgical Complications.** Match the treatment in the numbered column with the complication it is used for in the lettered column. Some complications may be used more than once, and some treatments may match more than one complication. *(262)*

1. _____ Administer oxygen

2. _____ Pour warm water over perineum

3. _____ Give intravenous (IV) fluids as ordered; encourage oral intake when allowed

4. _____ Ambulate frequently when permitted; laxatives or enemas, or both, as ordered

5. _____ Vasopressors (drugs to raise blood pressure) as ordered

6. _____ Position to promote effective ventilation

7. _____ Cover the open wound with a sterile dressing; if organs protrude, saturate the dressing with normal saline, notify physician, and keep patient still and quiet

8. _____ Antiemetic drugs as ordered

9. _____ Encourage deep breathing and coughing

10. _____ Bed rest; anticoagulant therapy as ordered

11. _____ Rectal tube, heat to abdomen, bisacodyl suppositories as ordered; position on right side; nasogastric intubation with suction as ordered

12. _____ Fluid or blood replacement

13. _____ Rest; oxygen and antibiotics as ordered

14. _____ Additional surgery to control bleeding

15. _____ Suction as necessary

A. Fluid and electrolyte imbalances
B. Altered elimination
C. Impaired wound healing
D. Shock
E. Nausea and vomiting
F. Hypoxia
G. Thrombophlebitis
H. Inadequate oxygenation
I. Abdominal distention
J. "Gas" pains/constipation

## MULTIPLE-CHOICE QUESTIONS

**DD.** Choose the most appropriate answer.

1.  The surgical patient who is malnourished is at risk for: *(247)*
    1.  excessive bleeding and hemorrhage.
    2.  drug toxicity and ineffective metabolism.
    3.  cardiac complications and dyspnea.
    4.  poor wound healing and infection.

2.  Obese surgical patients are more likely to have postoperative: *(247)*
    1.  infection and increased temperature.
    2.  excessive bleeding and hemorrhage.
    3.  headache and bradycardia.
    4.  respiratory and wound healing complications.

3.  Excess body fluid in the surgical patient can overload the: *(247)*
    1.  brain.
    2.  heart.
    3.  muscles.
    4.  lungs.

4.  Electrolyte imbalances may predispose the surgical patient to: *(247)*
    1.  cardiac arrhythmias.
    2.  lung complications.
    3.  liver malfunction.
    4.  bone tissue loss.

5.  Before surgery, a patient must sign a legal document called a(n): *(251)*
    1.  bill of rights.
    2.  consent form.
    3.  advance directive.
    4.  living will.

6.  If the patient is a minor, who signs the surgical consent form? *(251)*
    1.  Physician
    2.  Registered nurse
    3.  Parent or guardian
    4.  Close relative

7.  Shaving the skin in preparation for surgery is often delayed until shortly before surgery in order to: *(253)*
    1.  improve wound healing.
    2.  control bleeding.
    3.  allow less time for organisms to multiply.
    4.  prevent postoperative edema.

8.  The use of local anesthetics that block the conduction of nerve impulses in a specific area is called: *(259)*
    1.  general anesthesia.
    2.  sedative anesthesia.
    3.  anticonvulsant anesthesia.
    4.  regional anesthesia.

9.  The injection of an anesthetic agent into and under the skin around the area of treatment is called: *(259)*
    1.  local infiltration.
    2.  topical administration.
    3.  nerve block technique.
    4.  intravenous infusion.

10. One complication of spinal anesthesia is: *(259)*
    1.  tachycardia.
    2.  hemorrhage.
    3.  headache.
    4.  shock.

11. Postspinal headache can be relieved by: *(259)*
    1.  elevating the head of the bed.
    2.  lying flat.
    3.  early ambulation.
    4.  coughing and deep breathing.

12. A "blood patch" may help treat: *(259)*
    1.  hemorrhage.
    2.  postspinal headache.
    3.  shock.
    4.  tachycardia.

13. Which of the following adverse effects of anesthetic agents may be reduced by giving preanesthetic medications? *(259)*
    1.  Tachycardia
    2.  Dry mouth
    3.  Urinary retention
    4.  Vomiting

14. Inhalation anesthetic agents and the endotracheal tube can cause irritation of the: *(260)*
    1. lungs.
    2. heart.
    3. kidney.
    4. larynx.

15. A life-threatening complication of inhalation anesthesia characterized by increasing body temperature and metabolic rate, tachycardia, hypotension, cyanosis, and muscle rigidity is called: *(260)*
    1. anaphylactic shock.
    2. malignant hyperthermia.
    3. hypotensive shock.
    4. hyperglycemia.

16. The patient develops rupture of the suture line and states: "My incision is breaking open." Which of the following actions should the nurse take to prevent complications in this patient? *(271)*
    1. Keep the patient in bed.
    2. Administer opioid analgesics as ordered.
    3. Have the patient cough and deep breathe every 2 hours.
    4. Auscultate breath sounds.

17. An infection of the lungs due to immobility is called: *(263)*
    1. hypovolemic pleurisy.
    2. atelectasis.
    3. hypostatic pneumonia.
    4. emphysema.

18. When peristalsis is slow, gas builds up, causing: *(263)*
    1. abdominal cramping and distention.
    2. diarrhea and tachycardia.
    3. fever and infection.
    4. nausea and vomiting.

19. "Gas pains" typically occur: *(263)*
    1. during surgery.
    2. immediately after surgery.
    3. 6 hours after surgery.
    4. on second or third day after surgery.

20. With urinary retention, the kidneys produce: *(263)*
    1. no urine and the patient is unable to empty the bladder.
    2. urine and the patient is able to empty the bladder.
    3. no urine and the patient is able to empty the bladder.
    4. urine but the patient is unable to empty the bladder.

21. The inflammation of veins with the formation of blood clots is: *(263)*
    1. hemorrhage.
    2. shock.
    3. thrombophlebitis.
    4. pericarditis.

22. Clots that cling to the walls of blood vessels are called: *(263)*
    1. emboli.
    2. platelets.
    3. thrombi.
    4. anticoagulants.

23. An outcome criterion related to absence of thrombophlebitis is: *(267)*
    1. adequate oxygenation.
    2. normal arterial blood gases.
    3. negative Homans' sign.
    4. normal wound healing.

24. If intravenous fluids are given too rapidly postoperatively, they can overload the circulatory system, causing: *(247)*
    1. lung failure.
    2. heart failure.
    3. brain failure.
    4. kidney failure.

25. What is used to monitor the oxygenation of the blood? *(264)*
    1. Sphygmomanometer
    2. Incentive spirometer
    3. Oximeter
    4. Stethoscope

26. When regional block anesthesia is used during surgery, the nurse must remember that after surgery: *(259)*
    1. sensation in the area is impaired.
    2. circulation in the area is impaired.
    3. infection is likely to occur.
    4. fever may make the patient drowsy.

27. Once the immediate postoperative phase has passed, which risks lessen? *(261)*
    1. Fever and infection
    2. Pneumonia and atelectasis
    3. Shock and hemorrhage
    4. Thrombophlebitis and decubitus ulcer

28. Two common narcotic analgesics that are given postoperatively are: *(268-269)*
    1. acetaminophen and aspirin.
    2. meperidine and morphine.
    3. codeine and tincture of opium.
    4. alprazolam and diazepam.

29. Clean sutured incisions heal by: *(269)*
    1. first intention.
    2. second intention.
    3. third intention.
    4. fourth intention.

30. After the first 24 hours following surgery, which finding should be reported to the physician if it is observed? *(269)*
    1. Respirations of 20/minute
    2. Temperature of 98.8° F
    3. Blood pressure of 110/70 mm Hg
    4. Continued or excessive bleeding

31. A soft tube that permits passive movement of fluids from the wound is called a(n): *(270)*
    1. active drain.
    2. Hemovac.
    3. Penrose drain.
    4. Jackson-Pratt drain.

32. In the immediate postoperative phase, wound drainage is often bright red; as the amount of blood in the drainage decreases, the fluid becomes: *(270)*
    1. straw-colored and then clear and pink.
    2. clear and then pink and straw-colored.
    3. pink and then clear and straw-colored.
    4. pink and then straw-colored and clear.

33. What may precede wound dehiscence? A sudden: *(271)*
    1. decrease in wound drainage.
    2. increase in wound drainage.
    3. increase in temperature.
    4. increase of purulent drainage.

34. If evisceration occurs, the usual practice is to cover the wound with: *(271)*
    1. dry sterile dressings.
    2. saline-soaked gauze with a dry dressing over it.
    3. antibiotic ointment and dry dressings.
    4. steroid ointment and dry dressings.

35. Signs and symptoms of wound infection usually do not develop until: *(271)*
    1. the first hour after surgery.
    2. 12 hours after surgery.
    3. the first and second days after surgery.
    4. the third to fifth day after surgery.

36. A postoperative patient complains of pain, fever, swelling, and purulent drainage. These signs and symptoms are indications of: *(272)*
    1. thrombophlebitis.
    2. evisceration.
    3. dehiscence.
    4. wound infection.

37. Which finding in a postoperative patient should be reported to the physician? *(272)*
    1. Redness that spreads to the surrounding area
    2. Redness at the wound suture site
    3. Low-grade fever
    4. Serosanguineous drainage

38. To prevent pneumonia, the patient must be assisted to turn initially every: *(272)*
    1. 5 minutes.
    2. 15 minutes.
    3. 2 hours.
    4. 6 hours.

39. A device used to promote lung expansion postoperatively is the: *(272)*
    1. Penrose drain.
    2. sphygmomanometer.
    3. inhaler.
    4. incentive spirometer.

40. Pulmonary emboli usually originate from thrombi that develop in veins of the: *(273)*
    1. chest.
    2. arms and shoulders.
    3. legs and pelvis.
    4. abdomen.

41. Emboli may be treated with: *(273)*
    1. phenytoin (Dilantin) and anticonvulsants.
    2. morphine and analgesics.
    3. heparin and thrombolytic agents.
    4. furosemide (Lasix) and diuretics.

42. Catheterization is usually done postoperatively if the patient does not void in: *(274)*
    1. 2 hours.
    2. 4 hours.
    3. 8 hours.
    4. 10 hours.

43. When a patient passes small amounts of urine frequently without feeling relief of fullness, this indicates: *(273)*
    1. retention with overflow.
    2. stress incontinence.
    3. urge incontinence.
    4. kidney failure.

44. Some agencies have policies that limit the amount of urine that can be drained from a full bladder at one time; these limits are usually: *(274)*
    1. 5–10 ml.
    2. 50–100 ml.
    3. 400–500 ml.
    4. 750–1000 ml.

45. Most patients pass flatus: *(274)*
    1. 15 minutes after surgery.
    2. 1 hour after surgery.
    3. 48 hours after surgery.
    4. 1 week after surgery.

46. The best way to prevent gastrointestinal discomfort postoperatively is: *(274)*
    1. administration of antacids.
    2. early, frequent ambulation.
    3. administration of laxatives.
    4. early, frequent meals.

47. Which surgical drain works by creating negative pressure when the receptacle is compressed? *(270)*
    1. Penrose
    2. Urinary
    3. Hemovac
    4. Passive

48. Which drug supplements the effects of local anesthetics? *(259)*
    1. Propranolol (Inderal)
    2. Atropine
    3. Morphine
    4. Epinephrine

49. A week after surgery, the patient develops pain, fever, swelling, and purulent drainage around the wound site. Which of the following actions should the nurse take to prevent complications? *(272)*
    1. Keep the patient in bed
    2. Early, frequent ambulation
    3. Monitor intake and output
    4. Good handwashing

50. A patient states that his wound feels as if it is "pulling apart." This is an indication of: *(271)*
    1. healing by first intention.
    2. dehiscence.
    3. evisceration.
    4. singultus.

51. One way to prevent shock as a surgical complication is to: *(262)*
    1. keep airway in place until patient is alert.
    2. splint incision during activity.
    3. keep IV fluid rate on schedule.
    4. change patient's position at least every 3 hours.

52. Which of the following postoperative drugs causes urinary retention? *(263)*
    1. Antibiotics
    2. Thrombolytics
    3. Opioid analgesics
    4. Anticoagulants

53. The use of IV drugs to reduce pain intensity or awareness without loss of reflexes is called: *(260)*
    1. regional anesthesia.
    2. conscious sedation.
    3. general anesthesia.
    4. balanced anesthesia.

54. Which is a commonly used IV drug for conscious sedation? *(260)*
    1. Succinylcholine
    2. Isoflurane
    3. Nitrous oxide
    4. Midazolam (Versed)

55. Which drug is often given along with a general anesthetic agent to prevent movement of muscles? *(260)*
    1. Midazolam (Versed)
    2. Succinylcholine
    3. Ketamine hydrochloride (Ketalar)
    4. Thiopental sodium (Pentothal)

56. Enflurane (Ethrane) and nitrous oxide are administered by: *(260)*
    1. inhalation.
    2. IV infusion.
    3. intramuscular (IM) injection.
    4. rectal insertion.

57. What is the priority nursing diagnosis during the immediate postoperative period? *(262)*
    1. Acute pain
    2. Impaired tissue integrity
    3. Shock
    4. Urinary retention

EE. Planning care for the postoperative patient. Refer to the Nursing Care Plan to answer these questions.

1. How often will you check her dressing during the first 24 hours? *(265)*
   1. Hourly
   2. Every 2 hours
   3. Every 4 hours
   4. Every 8 hours

2. What is the likely cause of her urinary retention postoperatively? *(273)*

---

## OBJECTIVES

1. List the indications for intravenous fluid therapy.

2. Describe the types of fluids used for intravenous fluid therapy.

3. Describe the types of venous access devices and other equipment used for intravenous therapy.

4. Given the prescribed hourly flow rate, calculate the correct drop rate for an intravenous fluid.

5. Explain the causes, signs and symptoms, and nursing implications of the complications of intravenous fluid or drug therapy.

6. Explain the nursing responsibilities when a patient is receiving intravenous therapy.

---

## LEARNING ACTIVITIES

**A.  Key Terms.** Match the definition in the numbered column with the most appropriate term in the lettered column. Not all answers may be used.

1. _____  A liquid containing one or more dissolved substances *(277)*

2. _____  A term used to describe a solution that has a higher concentration of electrolytes than normal body fluids *(277)*

3. _____  A term used to describe a solution that has the same concentration of electrolytes as normal body fluids *(277)*

4. _____  A term used to describe a solution that has a lower concentration of electrolytes than normal body fluids *(277)*

5. _____  A measure of the concentration of electrolytes in a fluid *(291)*

6. _____  Escape of fluid or blood from a blood vessel into body tissue *(285)*

A.  Hypotonic
B.  Cannula
C.  Solution
D.  Hypertonic
E.  Extravasation
F.  Isotonic
G.  Tonicity

**B.  Key Terms.** Match the definition or description in the numbered column with the most appropriate term in the lettered column.

1. _____  Used for single-dose therapy, therapy of short duration, for infants, and for adults with poor veins *(278)*

2. _____  Hickman-Broviac catheters inserted by physicians *(279)*

3. _____  Small plastic tubes that fit over or inside needles *(279)*

4. _____  Needles and catheters *(278)*

5. _____  Inserted in antecubital space and advanced into the axillary subclavian vein or superior vena cava *(278)*

A.  Catheters
B.  Winged infusion needle
C.  Central venous tunneled catheters
D.  Cannulas
E.  Peripherally inserted central catheters

C.  **Key Terms.** Match the definition or description in the numbered column with the most appropriate term in the lettered column.

1.  _____     Maintain infusion rate set by nurses; saves time and prevents accidental delivery of large amounts of fluid *(281)*

2.  _____     Implanted under skin; allows immediate access to vein without repeated venipunctures *(281)*

3.  _____     Short cannula with attached injection port; usually flushed with dilute heparin or saline solution *(281)*

4.  _____     Catheter and a chamber into which fluids are directly injected into vein or artery *(281)*

A.  Piggyback infusion
B.  Electronic infusion pump
C.  Heparin lock (saline lock)
D.  Infusion port

D.  **Complications.** Match the definition or description in the numbered column with the most appropriate term in the lettered column.

1.  _____     Leakage of fluid from a blood vessel *(285)*

2.  _____     Piece of catheter breaks off in vein *(288)*

3.  _____     Skin torn or irritated by tape or insertion of cannula *(285)*

4.  _____     Attached blood clot *(288)*

5.  _____     Obstruction caused by trapped embolus *(288)*

6.  _____     Collection of infused fluid in tissue surrounding the cannula *(285)*

7.  _____     Unattached blood clot *(287)*

8.  _____     Inflammation of the vein *(287)*

A.  Thrombus
B.  Embolism
C.  Infiltration
D.  Catheter embolus
E.  Embolus
F.  Trauma
G.  Phlebitis
H.  Extravasation

E. **Nursing Care.** Match the outcome criteria in the numbered column with the nursing diagnosis in the lettered column.

1. _____ Pulse and blood pressure within normal limits *(285)*

2. _____ Patient activities completed without disruption of intravenous therapy *(285)*

3. _____ Normal body temperature; no purulent drainage or redness at venipuncture site *(285)*

4. _____ Fluid output equal to intake; no dyspnea or edema *(285)*

A. Decreased cardiac output related to blood loss through disrupted intravenous line

B. Self-care deficit related to restricted movement of infusion site

C. Fluid volume excess related to rapid fluid infusion

D. Risk for infection related to disruption of skin integrity

F. **Nursing Diagnoses.** Which of the following are nursing diagnoses for patients receiving intravenous therapy? Select all that apply. *(285)*

1. _____ Decreased cardiac output

2. _____ Risk for injury

3. _____ Fluid volume excess

4. _____ Altered tissue perfusion

5. _____ Impaired gas exchange

6. _____ Risk for infection

7. _____ Risk for imbalanced fluid volume

## MULTIPLE-CHOICE QUESTIONS

G. Choose the most appropriate answer.

1. Tonicity of IV fluid is important because it affects: *(277)*
   1. acid-base balance.
   2. blood volume.
   3. buffer action.
   4. electrolytes.

2. Irrigation of an occluded IV cannula is not recommended because: *(288)*
   1. the IV cannula may become infiltrated.
   2. clots may be forced into the bloodstream.
   3. the IV cannula may become dislodged.
   4. thrombophlebitis may occur.

3. Normal saline is: *(278)*
   1. 0.25% sodium chloride.
   2. 0.45% sodium chloride.
   3. 0.9% sodium chloride.
   4. 1.5% sodium chloride.

4. An IV solution of 0.45% sodium chloride is: *(277)*
   1. hypertonic.
   2. isotonic.
   3. hypotonic.
   4. equivalent.

5. An IV solution of 0.45% sodium chloride is given if the patient has experienced: *(278)*
   1. excessive water loss.
   2. cerebral edema.
   3. excessive sodium loss.
   4. burns.

6. In which position should you place a patient if air accidentally enters a central line? *(288)*
   1. On the left side
   2. On the right side
   3. Semi-Fowler's
   4. Fowler's

7. Advantages of peripherally inserted central catheters (PICCs) over other central catheters include: *(279)*
   1. smaller needle, cost savings, and reduced risk of pneumothorax or air embolism.
   2. easier insertion, less expense, and reduced risk of infection.
   3. remaining in place longer, fewer dressing changes, and no risk of dislodgment.
   4. easier insertion, cost savings, and reduced risk of pneumothorax or air embolism.

8. Short peripheral cannulas and tubing are usually changed every: *(284)*
   1. 1–2 hours.
   2. 4–8 hours.
   3. 12–24 hours.
   4. 48–72 hours.

9. You notice that the IV on your patient is running in too fast. To slow the rate down, you: *(283)*
   1. vent the IV container.
   2. splint the arm with an armboard.
   3. turn the arm so that the IV site is free.
   4. lower the fluid container.

10. In order to calculate the IV infusion rate, you must know the: *(283)*
    1. ordered fluid volume per hour and number of drops equal to 1 ml in the tubing set.
    2. number of milliliters of fluid in a solution container.
    3. ordered fluid volume minus the urine output.
    4. ordered fluid volume and the prior 24 hours' IV intake.

11. Symptoms of an air embolus include: *(288)*
    1. pulmonary edema; frothy, pink sputum; and a feeling of doom.
    2. chest pain, diminished respirations, and lethargy.
    3. shortness of breath, hypotension, and possibly shock and cardiac arrest.
    4. nausea, vomiting and diarrhea, hepatomegaly, and pink sputum.

12. Edema, coolness, and pain at the IV insertion site are indications of: *(285)*
    1. thrombophlebitis.
    2. infection.
    3. air embolus.
    4. infiltration.

13. Which IV complication is characterized by redness, swelling, and warmth? *(287)*
    1. Phlebitis
    2. Infiltration
    3. Hemorrhage
    4. Catheter embolus

14. Signs of fluid volume excess include: *(287)*
    1. confusion.
    2. bounding pulse.
    3. inflammation.
    4. redness.

15. If signs of fluid volume excess occur, you should: *(287)*
    1. turn the patient to the right side.
    2. elevate the head of the bed.
    3. check the vital signs.
    4. lower the head of the bed.

16. The patient with an air embolus is placed on the left side to trap air in the: *(288)*
    1. left atrium so that it can be gradually absorbed.
    2. right ventricle so that it is not transferred to the lungs.
    3. left ventricle so that it is not transferred to the lungs.
    4. right atrium so that it can be gradually absorbed.

17. When a central catheter is inserted or re-moved, the patient is instructed to: *(288)*
    1. take a deep breath and hold it for 30 seconds.
    2. take a deep breath and bear down.
    3. breathe normally.
    4. take a normal breath and hold it for 30 seconds.

18. When a central catheter is inserted or removed, the patient is asked to take a deep breath and bear down in order to help: *(288)*
    1. prevent air from entering the lungs.
    2. prevent air from entering the blood-stream.
    3. air enter the bloodstream.
    4. air enter the lungs.

19. Outcome criteria for evaluating the nursing care of a patient with an IV include the absence of: *(285)*
    1. palpitations, pain, and redness at the infusion site.
    2. blood return, swelling, and pain at the infusion site.
    3. edema, pallor, redness, and drainage at the infusion site.
    4. movement, erythema, and firmness at the infusion site.

20. As you are making your morning rounds at 7:00 AM, you note that your patient's IV has 900 ml and is running at 75 ml/hour as ordered. When you check the IV on your 10:00 AM rounds, you note that there is only 100 ml remaining. Which signs and symptoms do you need to be alert for with this patient? *(268)*
    1. Flushing of the face
    2. Nausea and vomiting
    3. Bounding pulse
    4. Diarrhea

21. Which nursing intervention may prevent fluid volume excess during IV therapy? *(286)*
    1. Encourage the patient to ambulate.
    2. Encourage the patient to cough.
    3. Time-tape the IV bag and monitor closely.
    4. Keep an accurate intake and output record.

22. Your patient complains of crushing chest pain and difficulty breathing and has a rapid, thready pulse. You suspect that he is experiencing an air embolism. Which interventions are appropriate? *(288)*
    1. Turn the patient onto his left side, raise the head of the bed, and notify the charge nurse or physician.
    2. Turn the patient onto his left side, lower the head of the bed, and notify the charge nurse or physician.
    3. Place the patient on his back, lower the head of the bed, and notify the charge nurse.
    4. Ambulate the patient for 15 minutes and notify the charge nurse.

23. The hand in which an IV is infusing is puffy and cool. This is a sign of: *(285)*
    1. phlebitis.
    2. infection.
    3. infiltration.
    4. air embolus.

24. When the IV line has infiltrated, which nursing interventions are appropriate? *(287)*
    1. Discontinue IV, apply ice, and place area lower than the heart.
    2. Slow down the IV rate, apply ice, and elevate affected arm.
    3. Discontinue IV and restart in a different vein; elevate affected arm.
    4. Slow down the IV rate, apply warm compresses, and place the area lower than the heart.

25. You check your patient's IV site and find that her vein is cord-like. The IV is running well, but the site is red; the patient tells you that the site is "sore when touched." These are signs of: *(287)*
    1. infiltration.
    2. catheter embolus.
    3. air embolus.
    4. phlebitis.

26. What does a "drop factor of 15" mean? *(283)*
    1. The infusion set will deliver 15 ml of fluid for every drop.
    2. The infusion set will deliver 1 ml of fluid for every 15 drops.
    3. The infusion set will deliver 1 ml of fluid in 15 minutes.
    4. The infusion set will deliver 15 ml of fluid in 1 minute.

27. You checked the patient's IV 1 hour ago, and it was running at the correct rate of 50 ml/hour. Now you find that the IV is running at 100 ml/hour. What may be the cause of this increased rate? *(282)*
    1. The tubing has a kink in it.
    2. The clamp has slipped.
    3. The fluid container is too low.
    4. The filter is blocked.

28. How much air does it take to cause an air embolism in an adult? *(288)*
    1. 5 cc
    2. 10 cc
    3. 15 cc
    4. 25 cc

29. An IV fluid container should not be used for more than: *(284)*
    1. 12 hours.
    2. 24 hours.
    3. 48 hours.
    4. 72 hours.

30. Because older people often have less efficient cardiac function, you should monitor an older person with an IV for: *(285)*
    1. fluid volume excess.
    2. bleeding.
    3. infection.
    4. infiltration.

31. A cannula with a clot in it should not be irrigated because it could cause: *(288)*
    1. extravasation.
    2. infiltration.
    3. air embolism.
    4. pulmonary embolism.

32. Administering a hypertonic IV solution causes fluid to be pulled from: *(277)*
    1. blood into the cells.
    2. cells into the blood.
    3. cells into interstitial tissue.
    4. blood into interstitial tissue.

33. An older patient is receiving IV fluids to treat dehydration. When he complains of pain and a burning sensation at the IV site, your assessment reveals that the IV site is pale, puffy, and cool. Which complication do you suspect? *(285)*
    1. Phlebitis
    2. Infiltration
    3. Fluid volume excess
    4. Embolism

34. Which vein is usually used for administering solutions through a central vein? *(280)*
    1. Subclavian vein
    2. Brachial vein
    3. Femoral vein
    4. Pulmonary vein

35. Your patient is an 80-year-old male with a history of high blood pressure. When you come in to give him a bath, you notice that his IV of $D_5W$, which was hung 1 hour before you came into his room, contains 500 ml. 1000 ml was ordered to run in over 8 hours. You should observe him for signs of: *(287)*
    1. infection.
    2. shock.
    3. hemorrhage.
    4. heart failure.

36. What concern is the most important factor that led to the development of devices to reduce needlestick risks? *(279)*
    1. Concern about thrombophlebitis
    2. Concern about infiltration
    3. Concern about imbalanced fluid volume
    4. Concern about blood-borne pathogens

**H.  Nursing Care Plan Questions.** Refer to Nursing Care Plan.

1.  While Mr. E. is receiving his IV, his BP is 145/90, his pulse is 110 and bounding, and he reports difficulty breathing. After you slow the infusion, what nursing intervention is appropriate? *(286)*
    1.  Monitor his vital signs hourly.
    2.  Inspect the infusion site for swelling and bleeding.
    3.  Elevate the head of his bed.
    4.  Check connections to be sure they are secure.

2.  Mr. E.'s IV started at 1:00 PM. How much fluid should have been administered by 3:30 PM that same day? _____ *(286)*

## OBJECTIVES

1. List the types of shock.

2. Describe the pathophysiology of each type of shock.

3. List the signs and symptoms of each stage of shock.

4. Explain the first aid emergency treatment of shock outside the medical facility.

5. Identify general medical and nursing interventions for shock.

6. Explain the rationale for medical/surgical treatment of shock.

7. Assist in developing care plans for patients in each type of shock.

## LEARNING ACTIVITIES

**A. Key Terms.** Match the definition in the numbered column with the correct term in the lettered column.

1. _____  Presence of systemic inflammatory response syndrome (SIRS) with a confirmed infection *(300)*

2. _____  Generalized inflammatory condition that follows serious physiologic threat; characterized by damage to vascular endothelium and hypermetabolic state *(298)*

3. _____  Deficiency of blood flow *(293)*

4. _____  Failure of more than one organ as a result of SIRS *(300)*

5. _____  A state of acute circulatory failure and impaired tissue perfusion *(290)*

6. _____  A pathologic condition associated with an increase in acid relative to bicarbonate content; increased hydrogen ion concentration *(293)*

A.  Ischemia
B.  Metabolic acidosis
C.  Multiple organ dysfunction syndrome (MODS)
D.  Sepsis
E.  Shock
F.  Systemic inflammatory response syndrome (SIRS)

B. **Types of Shock.** Match the description in the numbered column with the type of shock in the lettered column. Answers may be used more than once.

1. _____ Caused by hemorrhage, severe diarrhea or vomiting, and excessive perspiration *(290)*

2. _____ Complicated by increased capillary permeability *(291)*

3. _____ Occurs with physical impairment to blood flow *(290)*

4. _____ Associated with pulmonary embolism and tension pneumothorax *(290)*

5. _____ Occurs when the circulating blood volume is inadequate to maintain the supply of oxygen and nutrients to tissue *(290)*

6. _____ Fluid pools in dependent areas of the body *(291)*

7. _____ Related to excessive blood or fluid loss, inadequate fluid intake, or a shift of plasma from blood into body tissues *(290)*

8. _____ Occurs when heart fails as a pump *(290)*

9. _____ Problem is with excessive dilation of blood vessels *(291)*

10. _____ Related to burns, peritonitis, and intestinal obstruction *(290)*

11. _____ Associated with congestive heart failure (CHF), acute myocardial infarction (MI), and heart rhythm disturbances *(290)*

A. Hypovolemic
B. Cardiogenic
C. Distributive
D. Obstructive

C. **Drug Therapy.** Refer to Drug Therapy Table on pp. 294-295 in the textbook. Which medications are commonly used in the treatment of cardiogenic shock? Select all that apply. *(294-295)*

1. _____ Inotropics

2. _____ Vasopressors

3. _____ Corticosteroids

4. _____ Histamine 1 blockers

5. _____ Venodilators

6. _____ Antimicrobials

**D. Mechaical Devices.** Refer to Table 19-2 (Mechanical Devices) in the textbook. Which mechanical devices are used in the treatment of shock? Select all that apply. *(297)*

1. _____ Ventricular assist devices
2. _____ Extracorporeal membrane oxygenation (ECMO)
3. _____ Medical antishock trousers
4. _____ Intra-aortic balloon pump

**E. Response to Shock.** Refer to Table 19-1 in the textbook. Which are compensatory mechanisms in shock related to the sympathetic nervous system response? Select all that apply. *(292)*

1. _____ Decreased heart rate
2. _____ Peripheral vasodilation
3. _____ Constriction of renal arteries
4. _____ Renin-angiotensin-aldosterone system activated
5. _____ Increased ADH secretion
6. _____ Increased water excretion

**F. First Aid for Shock.** List in order of priority the steps to be taken in the first aid treatment for a patient in shock. *(293)*

1. _____ Control external bleeding with direct pressure or pressure dressing.
2. _____ Keep the patient in a flat position, with legs elevated (unless further injury could be caused by raising legs).
3. _____ Summon medical assistance.
4. _____ Protect the patient from cold but do not overheat.
5. _____ Establish/maintain patent airway.

## MULTIPLE-CHOICE QUESTIONS

**G.** Choose the most appropriate answer.

1. Anaphylactic, septic, and neurogenic are examples of which types of shock? *(291)*
   1. Hypovolemic
   2. Cardiogenic
   3. Obstructive
   4. Distributive

2. Following an automobile accident, a 35-year-old man experienced severe hemorrhage. This type of shock is classified as: *(290)*
   1. hypovolemic.
   2. cardiogenic.
   3. obstructive.
   4. distributive.

3. A woman experiences burns over 80% of her body. You suspect she has: *(290)*
   1. hypovolemic shock.
   2. cardiogenic shock.
   3. obstructive shock.
   4. distributive shock.

4. Inadequate tissue perfusion deprives cells of essential oxygen, forcing cells to rely on: *(290)*
   1. anabolic metabolism.
   2. catabolic metabolism.
   3. aerobic metabolism.
   4. anaerobic metabolism.

5. A person has a severe allergic reaction that results in bronchoconstriction and increased capillary permeability. This type of shock is: *(291)*
   1. anaphylactic.
   2. cardiogenic.
   3. hypovolemic.
   4. septic.

6. Which type of shock occurs suddenly, following exposure to a substance for which the patient had already developed antibodies? *(291)*
   1. Neurogenic
   2. Septic
   3. Anaphylactic
   4. Cardiogenic

7. Following a spinal cord injury, a 24-year-old man develops hypotension and bradycardia. This type of shock is: *(291)*
   1. hypovolemic.
   2. septic.
   3. anaphylactic.
   4. neurogenic.

8. The body of a patient with neurogenic shock is unable to compensate with vasoconstriction because: *(291)*
   1. the vasomotor center is incapacitated.
   2. chemicals released as a result of tissue ischemia depress the myocardium.
   3. bronchoconstriction and airway obstruction occur.
   4. systemic inflammatory response syndrome occurs.

9. One of the effects of shock on the neuroendocrine system is: *(291)*
   1. release of catecholamines.
   2. decreased ADH.
   3. increased cerebral blood flow.
   4. decreased aldosterone.

10. One of the effects of shock on the respiratory system is: *(291)*
    1. metabolic alkalosis.
    2. tissue hypoxia.
    3. depressed immune system.
    4. bronchodilation.

11. Assessment findings in the compensatory stage are likely to include: *(292)*
    1. drowsiness.
    2. slightly increased blood pressure.
    3. increased blood glucose.
    4. increased bowel sounds.

12. The stage of shock during which cells resort to anaerobic metabolism producing lactic acid is called: *(292-293)*
    1. compensatory.
    2. progressive.
    3. irreversible.
    4. refractory.

13. Which assessment data would you expect to find in a patient in the progressive stage of shock? *(292-293)*
    1. Increased pulse pressure
    2. Weak, thready pulse
    3. Warm, flushed skin
    4. Increased blood pressure

14. The stage of shock in which death is imminent is known as: *(293)*
    1. compensatory.
    2. refractory.
    3. progressive.
    4. hypovolemic.

15. Assessment data in the irreversible stage of shock include: *(293)*
    1. loss of consciousness.
    2. a drop in diastolic blood pressure to 50.
    3. rapid, shallow respirations.
    4. warm, flushed skin.

16. A priority in shock treatment is to: *(293)*
    1. correct acid-base balances.
    2. manage cardiac dysrhythmias.
    3. administer antishock drugs.
    4. improve blood flow and oxygen supply to vital organs.

17. Which position is best to maintain blood flow to vital organs for a patient with shock? *(293)*
    1. Supine with head lowered
    2. Fowler's
    3. Supine with legs elevated 45 degrees
    4. Left side-lying

18. The purpose of giving blood and fluids to improve cardiac output in a patient with cardiogenic shock is to: *(297)*
    1. promote delivery of oxygen to cells.
    2. correct acid-base imbalances.
    3. improve fluid and electrolyte imbalances.
    4. decrease the incidence of infection.

19. Which type of shock does *not* have replacement of fluid as a priority? *(294)*
    1. Distributive
    2. Neurogenic
    3. Hypovolemic
    4. Cardiogenic

20. Vasopressin is given to patients with septic shock because it is a: *(295)*
    1. vasoconstrictor.
    2. vasodilator.
    3. bronchodilator.
    4. positive inotropic.

21. Which patient condition is likely to have a history of severe vomiting and diarrhea? *(290)*
    1. Hypovolemic shock
    2. Cardiogenic shock
    3. Distributive shock
    4. Progressive shock

22. For which type of shock are antimicrobials prescribed? *(299)*
    1. Hypovolemic
    2. Cardiogenic
    3. Distributive
    4. Septic

23. Why is atropine prescribed for neurogenic shock? *(299)*
    1. Raise heart rate
    2. Raise blood pressure
    3. Treat pain
    4. Dilate blood vessels

24. Why is improving blood flow and oxygen supply to the vital organs a priority in shock treatment? *(294)*
    1. Brain cells begin to die after 4 minutes without oxygen.
    2. Cells resort to anaerobic metabolism, producing lactic acid immediately.
    3. Acidosis has a depressant effect on myocardial cells.
    4. If compensatory mechanisms are effective, the blood pressure will remain normal.

25. Why is Trendelenburg's (head down) position *not* recommended for shock treatment? *(299)*
    1. It can stimulate respirations and filling of coronary arteries.
    2. It can impair cerebral blood flow and increase intracranial pressure.
    3. It can cause fluid overload.
    4. It can lead to metabolic acidosis.

26. For which type of shock are inotropic and antidysrhythmic agents ordered? *(294-295)*
    1. Neurogenic
    2. Distributive
    3. Cardiogenic
    4. Anaphylactic

27. A patient in shock has a pulse of 120, BP of 80/40, and respirations of 28. These signs represent: *(294)*
    1. deficient fluid volume.
    2. ineffective tissue perfusion.
    3. decreased cardiac output.
    4. electrolyte imbalance.

28. Hypermetabolism in shock causes which type of malnutrition? *(300)*
    1. Decreased carbohydrate
    2. Decreased protein
    3. Decreased glucose
    4. Increased nitrogen

29. Which assessment finding would you expect to see in a patient with septic shock that would not be present in a patient with hypovolemic shock? *(290-291)*
    1. Cool skin
    2. Fever
    3. Low blood pressure
    4. Dizziness

30. A patient with a wound infection is likely to develop which type of shock? *(291)*
    1. Hypovolemic
    2. Cardiogenic
    3. Septic
    4. Neurogenic

# CHAPTER 20 Falls

---

## OBJECTIVES

1. Define falls.

2. Give the incidence of falls.

3. Describe factors that increase the risk of falls.

4. Discuss the relationship between restraint use and falls, types of restraints, and regulations for restraint use.

5. Describe fall prevention techniques.

6. Describe nursing interventions to use when a fall occurs.

---

## LEARNING ACTIVITIES

**A. Key Terms.** Match the definition in the numbered column with the most appropriate term in the lettered column.

1. _____E_____ Anything that restricts movement *(304)*

2. _____C_____ Circumstance in which one unintentionally falls to the ground or hits an object such as a chair or stair *(302)*

3. _____F_____ Factors related to the internal functioning of an individual, such as the aging process or physical illness that can cause falls *(302)*

4. _____A_____ Psychotropic medication given to subdue agitated or confused patients *(305)*

5. _____D_____ Law enacted in 1987 to protect patients from unnecessary restraints in nursing homes *(304)*

6. _____B_____ Factors in the environment that can cause falls *(302)*

A. Chemical restraints
B. Extrinsic factors
C. Fall
D. Omnibus Reconciliation Act (OBRA)
E. Physical restraint
F. Intrinsic factors

**B. Risk Factors.** Which of the following are factors associated with people at greatest risk for injury from falls? Select all that apply. *(302-303)*

1. __×__ Peripheral neuropathy
2. _____ Pneumonia
3. __×__ Parkinson's disease
4. __×__ Loss of consciousness
5. _____ Hypertension
6. __×__ Osteoporosis

7. _____ Anticoagulation therapy
8. _____ Antibiotic therapy
9. __×__ Sensory impairment
10. __×__ Decreased muscle strength
11. _____ Increased reaction time
12. __×__ Decreased balance

**C. Restraints.** Which of the following are damaging psychological effects of restraints on older patients? Select all that apply. *(304)*

1. __×__ Decreased dependency
2. __×__ Anger
3. __×__ Increased confusion
4. __×__ Decreased disorientation
5. __×__ Withdrawal

6. __×__ Aggressive behavior
7. __×__ Loss of self-image
8. __×__ Fear
9. _____ Security

**D. Nursing Interventions.** Match each risk factor in the numbered column with the most appropriate intervention in the lettered column. *(306)*

1. __H__ Musculoskeletal disorders
2. __A__ Impaired adaptation to the dark
3. __J__ Balance disorders
4. __K__ Stroke
5. __F__ Reduced visual acuity
6. __I__ Postural hypotension
7. __D__ Impacted cerumen (earwax)
8. __G__ Peripheral neuropathy
9. __E__ Impaired color perception
10. __B__ Foot disorders
11. __C__ Presbycusis

A. Maintain adequate lighting; reduce glare from shiny floors and allow time for eyes to adjust to light levels (e.g., from a dark room to outside); use night-light in bedroom and bathroom
B. Trim toenails; use appropriate footwear
C. Speak slowly; use low voice; decrease background noise; encourage use of hearing aid
D. Remove earwax
E. Use bright colors as markers, especially orange, yellow, and red
F. Be sure that individual wears glasses, if appropriate; keep glasses clean; encourage regular eye examinations
G. Use correctly sized footwear with firm soles
H. Encourage balance, gait training, and muscle-strengthening exercises
I. Encourage dorsiflexion exercises; use pressure-graded stockings; elevate head of bed; teach individual to get up from chair or bed slowly to avoid tipping head backward
J. Encourage balance exercises
K. Place call bell in visual field and within reach of arm that has use; anticipate needs for toileting, dressing, eating, and bathing; assist with transfer; provide passive range of motion exercises to improve functional ability

E. **Prevention.** Which of the following are basic strategies for reducing all types of falls? Select all that apply. *(307)*

1. _____ Decrease physical activities
2. ___X____ Increase exercise
3. ___X____ Modify the environment
4. ___X____ Reduce visual impairment

F. **Documentation.** What factors are important to document at the time when a fall occurs? Select all that apply. *(306)*

1. ___X____ What the patient was doing
2. _____ Vital signs of the patient at the time of the fall
3. ___X____ Mental status of the patient
4. _____ Nutritional status of the patient
5. ___X____ Environmental factors

G. **Nursing Interventions.** What are interventions to prevent falls for a patient with impaired dark adaptation? Select all that apply. *(306)*

1. ___X____ Be sure the patient wears glasses, if appropriate.
2. ___X____ Maintain adequate lighting.
3. ___X____ Reduce glare from shiny floors.
4. ___X____ Allow time to adjust to light levels (as patient moves from a dark room to outside).
5. ___X____ Keep glasses clean.
6. ___X____ Encourage regular eye examinations.
7. ___X____ Use a night-light in the bathroom.

H. **Intrinsic Risk Factors.** Which are intrinsic risk factors for falling? Select all that apply. *(306)*

1. ___X____ Impaired hearing
2. ___X____ Balance and gait problems
3. _____ Environmental factors
4. _____ Loose rugs
5. ___X____ Foot disorders
6. ___X____ Postural hypotension
7. _____ Glare from shiny floors

I. **Prevention.** Which are environment-oriented fall prevention techniques used in long-term care facilities? Select all that apply. *(307)*

1. ___X____ Assist patient to void every 4 hours.
2. ___X____ Check for proper fit of slippers and footwear.
3. ___X____ Keep rooms and hallways free from clutter.
4. ___X____ Place TV controls within reach.
5. ___X____ Clean up spills, including urine.
6. ___X____ Encourage exercise to strengthen muscles and prevent weakness.

**J.   Prevention in Home Setting.** Which are fall prevention guidelines for the home? Select all that apply. *(307)*

1. _____✗_____    Watch for pets underfoot and scattered pet food.
2. _____✗_____    Check for even, nonglare lighting in every room.
3. _____    Use 60 watt light bulbs to provide proper lighting in rooms.
4. _____    Make sure there is a telephone in the room next to the bedroom.

## MULTIPLE-CHOICE QUESTIONS

**K.**   Choose the most appropriate answer.

1.  What is the estimated ratio of people aged 65 or older who fall in a given year? *(302)*
    1.  1 in 3
    2.  1 in 10
    3.  1 in 20
    4.  1 in 100

2.  After what age does there appear to be a steady increase in the number of falls? *(302)*
    1.  40
    2.  65
    3.  75
    4.  85

3.  Of the total number of deaths due to falls, which percentage of the victims is elderly? *(302)*
    1.  10%
    2.  20%
    3.  50%
    4.  72%

4.  Which percentage of deaths due to falls does the U.S. Public Health Service state are preventable? *(302)*
    1.  one-fifth
    2.  one-third
    3.  one-half
    4.  two-thirds

5.  Factors such as the aging process and physical illness that increase the possibility of falling are called: *(302)*
    1.  extrinsic factors.
    2.  environmental factors.
    3.  intrinsic factors.
    4.  physical factors.

6.  Factors that increase the opportunity to fall are called: *(302)*
    1.  extrinsic factors.
    2.  aging process factors.
    3.  intrinsic factors.
    4.  physical illness factors.

7.  Of all reported falls, what percentage does not result in injury? *(303)*
    1.  10–20%
    2.  25–35%
    3.  40–50%
    4.  65–75%

8.  What is the most frequent type of injury from falls, occurring in 25–30% of all falls? *(303)*
    1.  Deep tissue damage
    2.  Contusions, cuts, or lacerations
    3.  Concussion
    4.  Fractures

9.  Geriatric chairs and side rails are examples of: *(304)*
    1.  environmental restraints.
    2.  social restraints.
    3.  physical restraints.
    4.  chemical restraints.

10. Older patients are more likely than younger patients to be physically restrained because of their greater likelihood of: *(304)*
    1.  mental decline and weight loss.
    2.  chronic illness and physical decline.
    3.  heart disease and insomnia.
    4.  falling and confusion.

11. The major complications from using physical restraints include: *(304)*
    1. sedation from medications administered and accidental aspiration.
    2. falls from wheelchairs and beds (when patients are able to untie restraints or wriggle out of them) and accidental strangulation.
    3. fatigue from fighting the restraints and confusion resulting from fatigue.
    4. skin breakdown from friction and wound development.

12. The Omnibus Reconciliation Act of 1987 (OBRA) states that nursing home residents have the right to be free from any physical restraints imposed or psychoactive drug administered for the purposes of: *(304)*
    1. discipline or convenience.
    2. safety or public health.
    3. exercise or physical therapy.
    4. strict confinement.

13. Physical restraints should be removed and released every: *(304)*
    1. hour for 10 minutes.
    2. 2 hours for 10 minutes.
    3. 4 hours for 10 minutes.
    4. 8 hours for 10 minutes.

14. Psychoactive drugs should never be used for the purpose of: *(305)*
    1. relief of headaches.
    2. insomnia.
    3. discipline.
    4. hallucinations.

15. In the "roll" method of getting up from a fall, after rolling onto the right side and bending the right knee, the patient should: *(308)*
    1. crawl to a chair.
    2. pull to a sitting position on the floor.
    3. get up on all fours.
    4. leverage upward to the kneeling position by pressing down on the right forearm.

16. In the "crawl" method of getting up from a fall, after rolling to a prone position, getting up on all fours, and crawling to a sturdy couch, the patient should: *(308)*
    1. pull to a sitting position on the floor.
    2. bring one foot forward, putting the foot flat on the floor.
    3. stand up.
    4. gradually move up and backward to a stair height.

17. In the "stair shuffle" method of getting up from a fall, after pulling to a sitting position on the floor and shuffling on the buttocks to the stairs, the patient should: *(308)*
    1. turn around and kneel on the lowest stair.
    2. get up on all fours.
    3. turn around and place arms on waist-height stair to support body.
    4. gradually move up and backward to a stair height suitable for standing.

18. Keeping the bed at the lowest level and using the least restrictive restraints are interventions related to: *(304)*
    1. Impaired skin integrity.
    2. Risk for injury.
    3. Altered urinary function.
    4. Risk for infection.

19. The first step in preventing falls and injury is to determine: *(303-304)*
    1. which medications the patient is taking.
    2. the hazards in the environmental setting.
    3. who is at greatest risk.
    4. whether the patient has alcohol or drug problems.

20. Why are older adults at particular risk for injury from their accidents? *(302)*
    1. They are more confused.
    2. They are more disoriented.
    3. They are likely to have poorer clinical outcomes.
    4. They are not as coordinated.

21. What percentage of falls occurs in older persons staying in long-term residential care facilities? *(303)*
    1.  20%
    2.  30%
    3.  50%
    4.  60%

22. In all reported falls, which is the percentage of falls resulting in no injury? *(303)*
    1.  30%
    2.  50%
    3.  60%
    4.  75%

23. What percentage of falls result in fractures in older adults? *(303)*
    1.  1%
    2.  5%
    3.  20%
    4.  30%

L.  **Nursing Care Plan.** Refer to Nursing Care Plan, The Patient with a History of Falls, p. 303 in the textbook.

1.  Which factor in her health history put this patient most at risk for a fracture from a fall? *(303)*
    1.  Emphysema
    2.  Dementia
    3.  High blood pressure
    4.  History of several falls at home

2.  What is the priority intervention for this patient to prevent her from falling? *(303)*
    1.  Assess patient and the environment for possible hazards and remove.
    2.  Keep bed at lowest level.
    3.  Orient patient frequently to person, place, and time.
    4.  Remove restraints at least every 2 hours for 10 minutes for range of motion exercises.

# 21 Immobility

---

## OBJECTIVES

1. Describe common problems associated with immobility.

2. Discuss the impact of exercise and positioning on preventing complications related to immobility.

3. Identify the risk factors for pressure ulcers.

4. Describe the stages of pressure ulcers.

5. Describe methods of preventing and treating pressure ulcers.

6. Discuss the effects of immobility on respiratory status, nutrition, and elimination.

---

## LEARNING ACTIVITIES

**A. Key Terms.** Match the definition in the numbered column with the most appropriate term in the lettered column.

1. ____D____  The inability to move; imposed restriction on entire body *(310)*

2. ____E____  Exercise in which each joint is moved in various directions to the farthest possible extreme *(312-313)*

3. ____I____  Exercise of the patient that is carried out by the therapist or nurse without the assistance of the patient *(312)*

4. ____C____  Muscle contraction without movement used to maintain muscle tone *(314)*

5. ____F____  Exercise carried out by the patient *(312)*

6. ____A____  Redness of the skin; usually a sign that capillaries have become congested because of impaired blood flow *(315)*

7. ____G____  Shortening of the muscles and tendons *(313)*

8. ____H____  Two contacting parts sliding on each other *(315)*

9. ____B____  An open wound caused by pressure on a bony prominence; also called a "bed sore" or "decubitus ulcer" *(314)*

A. Erythema
B. Pressure ulcer
C. Isometric exercise
D. Immobility
E. Range of motion
F. Active exercise
G. Contracture
H. Shearing forces
I. Passive exercise

**B. Preventing Pressure Ulcers.** Which of the following are elements of a pressure sore prevention protocol? Select all that apply. *(315-316)*

1. ____—____  Reposition bed patient at least every 4 hours.

2. ____X____  Apply sheepskin to prevent shearing forces.

3. ____X____  Utilize trapeze bars to enhance patient mobility.

4. ____X____  Teach wheelchair patients to shift their weight every 15 minutes if able.

5. ____—____  Position patients so that they are resting on pressure points of the skin.

6. ____—____  When the patient is in bed, keep the head raised as much as possible to reduce shearing force.

7. ____|____  Do not use rubber rings to elevate heels or sacral areas.

C.  **Pressure Ulcers.** Match the characteristic in the numbered column with the most appropriate stage of pressure ulcer in the lettered column. Answers may be used more than once. *(316-317)*

1.  ___C___  Wound may be infected and is usually open and draining

2.  ___B___  Some skin loss in the epidermis and/or dermis

3.  ___A___  Irregular, ill-defined area of pressure reflecting the shape of the object creating the pressure

4.  ___C___  Crater-like sore with a distinct outer margin

5.  ___A___  Ulcer is surrounded by a broad, indistinct, painful, reddened area that is hot or warmer than normal

6.  ___A___  Nonblanchable erythema

7.  ___B___  A shallow ulcer develops and appears blistered, cracked, or abraded

8.  ___D___  Ulcer is usually infected and may appear black with exudation, foul odor, and purulent drainage

9.  ___C___  Full-thickness skin loss involving damage or necrosis of the dermis and subcutaneous tissues

10. ___A___  Little destruction of tissue; condition is reversible

11. ___D___  Full-thickness skin loss with extensive destruction of the deeper underlying muscle and possible bone tissue

12. ___A___  Pain and tenderness may be present, with swelling and hardening of the tissue and associated heat

A.  Stage I
B.  Stage II
C.  Stage III
D.  Stage IV

**D. Consequences of Immobility.** Match the consequences of immobility in the numbered column with the body system in the lettered column. Answers may be used more than once. *(311)*

1. ___D___   Increased risk of atelectasis and infection

2. ___E___   Decreased glomerular filtration rate

3. ___G___   Decreased tactile stimulation

4. ___C___   Thickening of joint capsule

5. ___A___   Pressure ulcers

6. ___B___   Constipation

7. ___F___   Increased storage of fat

8. ___H___   Increased peripheral resistance

9. ___F___   Decreased glucose tolerance

10. ___C___   Loss of smoothness of cartilage surface

A.   Integumentary
B.   Gastrointestinal
C.   Musculoskeletal
D.   Pulmonary
E.   Urinary
F.   Metabolic
G.   Sensory
H.   Cardiovascular

E. **Pressure Ulcer Locations.** Refer to the figure below, Possible Locations of Pressure Ulcers (Figure 21-1, p. 314). Label the bony prominences (A–Z). *(314)*

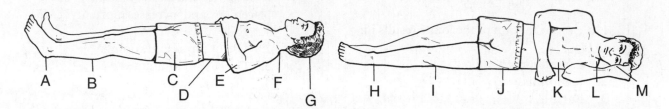

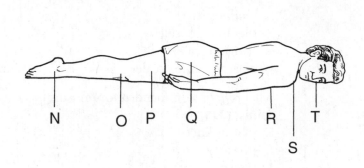

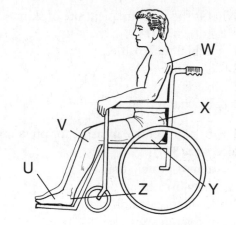

A. Heels

B. Posterior calf

C. Sacrum

D. spinous processes

E. Elbows

F. scapulae

G. Back of head

H. Malleolus

I. Lateral and Medial condyles

J. Greater trochanter

K. Ribs

L. Acromion process

M. Ear

N. Dorsum foot & Ankle

O. Knees

P. thigh

Q. Iliac crest

R. Anterior chest

S. Acromion process

T. cheek and ear

U. Plantar foot

V. Heels

W. popliteal

X. Ischial Tuberosities

Y. Sacrum & coccyx

Z. scapula

## MULTIPLE-CHOICE QUESTIONS

**F.**   Choose the most appropriate answer.

1. Little or no motion of the joints results in: *(313)*
   1. contractures.
   2. tendonitis.
   3. bursitis.
   4. skin breakdown.

2. What is the most frequent site of skin breakdown? *(314)*
   1. Ischial tuberosities
   2. Sacrum
   3. Heels
   4. Trochanter

3. The best preventive measure for pressure ulcers is: *(314)*
   1. a high-protein diet.
   2. deep breathing.
   3. frequent position changes.
   4. moderate exercise.

4. The medical term used for bed sores is: *(315)*
   1. wound infection.
   2. cellulitis.
   3. pressure ulcer.
   4. bony pressure.

5. An area of redness that is the beginning of a pressure ulcer is called: *(315)*
   1. erythema.
   2. inflammation.
   3. a wound.
   4. hemorrhage.

6. Erythema progresses rapidly to an ulcerated stage in patients who are malnourished, obese, or aged, who have: *(315)*
   1. skin infection.
   2. poor skin turgor.
   3. lacerations.
   4. circulatory disease.

7. The action on tissues that occurs when a patient slumps down while sitting in bed is called: *(315)*
   1. lacerating.
   2. shearing.
   3. projectile.
   4. slanting.

8. Which of the following conditions is expensive to treat, results in longer hospital stays, increases the likelihood of nursing home placement, and increases mortality? *(315)*
   1. Falls
   2. Use of physical restraints
   3. Overuse of antibiotics
   4. Pressure ulcers

9. A useful instrument for identifying those at risk for developing pressure ulcers is the: *(315)*
   1. pain scale.
   2. neurologic scale.
   3. Norton scale.
   4. Glasgow coma scale.

10. What is *not* recommended for pressure points? *(316)*
    1. Sheepskin
    2. Massage
    3. Egg crate mattress
    4. Trapeze bars

11. Which of the following causes concentrated areas of pressure that puts patients at higher risk for developing pressure ulcers? *(316)*
    1. Sheepskin
    2. Egg crate mattress
    3. Trapeze bar
    4. Rubber ring

12. When a person remains immobile or does not take deep breaths, which of the following is most likely to occur to the respiratory status? *(318)*
    1. An accumulation of carbon dioxide that collects in the alveoli
    2. An accumulation of thick secretions that pool in the lower respiratory structures
    3. Decreased circulation to the lungs
    4. Decreased oxygen entering the lungs

13. When thick secretions pool in the lower respiratory structures, they interfere with the: *(318)*
    1. exchange of white blood cells and red blood cells in the capillaries.
    2. circulation of blood to the extremities.
    3. detoxification process in the liver.
    4. exchange of oxygen and carbon dioxide in the lungs.

14. Which of the following is contraindicated in the care of patients with pressure ulcers? *(316)*
    1. Use of moisturizers
    2. Heat lamp
    3. Egg crate mattress
    4. Sheepskin boots

15. What is the most common problem associated with immobility in relation to food and fluid intake? *(318)*
    1. Hypoproteinemia
    2. Hypokalemia
    3. Anorexia
    4. Nausea

16. For patients with pressure ulcers, the diet should be high in: *(318)*
    1. potassium.
    2. fiber.
    3. protein.
    4. vitamins.

17. Inactivity, decreased fluid intake, and lack of fiber in the diet cause: *(319)*
    1. anorexia.
    2. nausea.
    3. constipation.
    4. diarrhea.

18. Which of the following is recommended for the treatment of stage I ulcers? *(316)*
    1. Disinfectants
    2. Mild soap
    3. Alcohol
    4. Powder

19. The urinary system functions best when the person is: *(319)*
    1. sitting.
    2. upright.
    3. side-lying.
    4. lying prone.

20. The most effective way to prevent urinary incontinence associated with immobility is to establish a: *(319)*
    1. high-protein diet.
    2. coughing and deep-breathing program.
    3. restriction of fluid intake.
    4. schedule for toiletings.

21. Which of the following is contraindicated in the treatment of patients with stage II ulcers? *(316)*
    1. Mild soap
    2. Normal saline
    3. Water
    4. Heat lamp

22. The use of slip-on shoes, loose pullover shirts, and Velcro closures assists the immobile patient to: *(311)*
    1. prevent atelectasis.
    2. gain independence.
    3. improve respirations.
    4. decrease pressure ulcers.

## ALTERNATE FORMAT QUESTIONS

G. 1. Which of the following are therapeutic reasons for immobility? Select all that apply. *(310)*
    1. Reduce the workload of the heart
    2. Prevent atelectasis and hypostatic pneumonia
    3. Treat urinary incontinence
    4. Obtain relief from pain
    5. Treat abdominal hernias
    6. Prevent further injury of a body part
    7. Obtain relief from joint contractures

2. Which side effects of drugs may contribute to factors causing immobility? Select all that apply. *(310)*
    1. Vertigo
    2. Hypertension
    3. Loss of sensory function
    4. Hyperglycemia
    5. Tachycardia

**H. Nursing Care Plan.** Refer to the Nursing Care Plan, Preventing Hazards of Immobility, p. 312 of the textbook.

1.  Which additional nursing diagnoses is this woman likely to have? *(312)*
    1.  Risk for latex allergy response
    2.  Risk for compromised human dignity
    3.  Impaired gas exchange
    4.  Sedentary lifestyle
    5.  Risk for loneliness
    6.  Complicated grieving

2.  List seven factors in the assessment of this woman that put her at risk for injury. *(312)*

---

## OBJECTIVES

1. Define delirium and dementia.

2. Identify the causes of acute confusion.

3. Explain the differences between delirium and dementia.

4. Discuss nursing assessment and interventions related to delirium and dementia.

---

**LEARNING ACTIVITIES**

A. **Key Terms.** Match the definition in the numbered column with the most appropriate term in the lettered column. Answers may be used more than once. *(322)*

| 1. | A | Short-term confusional state | A. | Delirium |
|---|---|---|---|---|
| 2. | B | Often irreversible confusion | B. | Dementia |
| 3. | A | Acute confusional state | | |
| 4. | B | Chronic confusion | | |
| 5. | A | Often reversible confusion | | |
| 6. | A | Characterized by disturbances in attention, thinking, and perception | | |
| 7. | B | Characterized by impairment of intellectual function | | |
| 8. | B | Caused by some underlying illness | | |
| 9. | A | Develops over a short period of time | | |
| 10. | A | Clearly defined hallucinations may be present | | |
| 11. | B | Flat or indifferent affect | | |
| 12. | A | Intermittent fear, perplexity, or bewilderment | | |

B. **Delirium.** Which of the following are systemic causes of delirium? Select all that apply. *(323)*

1. _____ Alzheimer's disease
2. ___X___ Postoperative status
3. ___X___ Trauma
4. _____ Huntington's disease
5. _____ AIDS
6. _____ Cardiovascular disease

C. **Dementia.** Which concepts should be used as a basis for providing care for patients with dementia? Select all that apply. *(324)*

1. ___X___ Patients usually forget things relatively quickly.
2. _____ Orient the patients to time and person with clocks and calendars.
3. ___X___ Patients are usually unable to learn new things.
4. _____ Break down tasks into individual steps to be done one at a time.

D. **Dementia.** Match the criteria for dementia definitions in the numbered column with the correct term in the lettered column. *(324)*

1. ___C___ Impaired ability to carry out motor activities despite intact motor function
2. ___B___ Language disturbance
3. ___D___ Trouble with planning and sequencing
4. ___A___ Failure to recognize objects despite intact sensory function

A. Agnosia
B. Aphasia
C. Apraxia
D. Disturbed executive functioning

E. **Disturbed Sleep Patterns.** Match the nursing diagnoses about disturbed sleep pattern in the numbered column with the most appropriate term in the lettered column. Answers may be used more than once. *(323, 326)*

1. ___A___ Disturbed sleep pattern related to agitation
2. ___A___ Disturbed sleep pattern related to drugs
3. ___B___ Disturbed sleep pattern related to neurologic changes
4. ___B___ Disturbed sleep pattern related to altered perceptions
5. ___A___ Disturbed sleep pattern related to mood alterations

A. Delirium
B. Dementia

**F. Risk for Injury.** Match the nursing diagnoses about risk for injury in the numbered column with the most appropriate term in the lettered column. Answers may be used more than once. *(323, 326)*

1. _A_ Risk for injury related to disorientation
2. _A_ Risk for injury related to unfamiliar setting
3. _B_ Risk for injury related to poor judgment
4. _B_ Risk for injury related to physical decline
5. _A_ Risk for injury related to agitation
6. _B_ Risk for injury related to sensorimotor changes

A. Delirium
B. Dementia

**G. Disturbed Thought Processes.** Match the nursing diagnoses about disturbed thought processes in the numbered column with the most appropriate term in the lettered column. Answers may be used more than once. *(323, 326)*

1. _A_ Disturbed thought processes related to drugs
2. _A_ Disturbed thought processes related to infection
3. _B_ Disturbed thought processes related to memory loss
4. _B_ Disturbed thought processes related to altered perception

A. Delirium
B. Dementia

## MULTIPLE-CHOICE QUESTIONS

**H.** Choose the most appropriate answer.

1. The first priority of nursing interventions for the patient with delirium is to: *(324)*
   1. provide safety and comfort.
   2. take vital signs.
   3. force fluids.
   4. provide therapeutic touch.

2. Because adequate sleep is important for the patient with delirium, which would be most appropriate to help the patient fall asleep? *(325)*
   1. A glass of wine, a shower, and a long walk
   2. Pain medication, milk and cookies, and watching a movie
   3. A back rub, a glass of warm milk, and soothing conversation
   4. A sedative, a large dinner, and physical activity

3. When one is dealing with a delirious patient who is experiencing hallucinations, the best response of the nurse would be: *(325)*
   1. "What is it that you are seeing on the wall?"
   2. "You are sick in the hospital, and what you are seeing is part of the illness."
   3. "The time is 2:00 PM and the date is _____."
   4. "Tell me what you are seeing."

4. The use of physical restraints should be avoided with patients with delirium because restraints tend to: *(326)*
   1. increase anxiety.
   2. disturb thought processes.
   3. increase impaired thinking.
   4. disturb sleep patterns.

5.  When a patient with dementia resists activities such as bathing or dressing, the nurse should: *(327)*
    1.  orient the patient to reality.
    2.  avoid confrontations.
    3.  state clearly what needs to be done.
    4.  offer a variety of choices to encourage decision-making.

6.  Patients with dementia should be offered: *(328)*
    1.  three full meals a day.
    2.  low-fiber foods.
    3.  a diet high in salt.
    4.  finger foods high in protein and carbohydrates.

7.  When you are taking care of patients with dementia, it is helpful to remember that they usually: *(327)*
    1.  benefit from reality orientation.
    2.  forget things quickly.
    3.  do not forget things quickly.
    4.  are able to learn new things.

8.  If patients with dementia start to become very restless or agitated, an effective nursing intervention is to: *(328)*
    1.  discuss the cause of their discomfort with them.
    2.  speak calmly and reassure them constantly.
    3.  orient them to time and place.
    4.  divert their attention and gently guide them to a new activity.

9.  Which approach may agitate people with dementia? *(327)*
    1.  A nonconfrontational manner
    2.  Use of calm, gentle mannerisms
    3.  Reality orientation
    4.  Use of simple, direct communication

10. If a patient with dementia is afraid of bathtubs, you should: *(329)*
    1.  reassure the patient that there is nothing to be afraid of.
    2.  explain the reason for taking a bath in the bathtub.
    3.  offer a variety of choices to the patient about taking a bath.
    4.  arrange another way to give personal care.

11. In caring for a patient with delirium, you should: *(326)*
    1.  provide frequent, routine toileting.
    2.  provide frequent orientation to surroundings.
    3.  cut the food into small portions.
    4.  break tasks down into individual steps to be done one at a time.

I.  **Nursing Care Plan.** Refer to Nursing Care Plan for the Patient with Delirium, p. 325 in the textbook.

1.  What is the first priority of nursing interventions for this patient? *(325)*
    1.  State clearly what needs to be done.
    2.  Speak calmly and reassure the patient constantly.
    3.  Provide reality orientation frequently.
    4.  Provide safety and comfort.

2.  What is the probable cause of this patient's delirium? *(325)*

3.  What is the most appropriate nursing diagnosis for this type of delirium? *(325)*
    1.  Acute confusion
    2.  Chronic confusion
    3.  Risk for acute confusion
    4.  Altered thought process

J.  **Nursing Care Plan.** Refer to the Nursing Care Plan for the Patient with Dementia, p. 328 in the textbook.

1.  Which concept is used as a basis for breaking down self-care tasks for this patient? *(328)*
    1.  Patients can learn new things with repetition.
    2.  Patients usually forget things quickly.
    3.  Patients should be reoriented frequently and consistently.
    4.  Patients should have family members stay with them.

2.  Why is this patient at risk for injury? *(328)*
    1.  Poor judgment
    2.  Impaired verbal communication
    3.  Anxiety
    4.  Agitation and mood alterations

# Incontinence

---

## OBJECTIVES

1. Identify the types of urinary and fecal incontinence.

2. Explain the pathophysiology and treatment of specific types of incontinence.

3. Identify common therapeutic measures used for the incontinent patient.

4. List nursing assessment data needed to assist in the evaluation and treatment of incontinence.

5. Assist in developing a nursing care plan for the patient with incontinence.

---

## LEARNING ACTIVITIES

**A. Key Terms.** Match the definition in the numbered column with the most appropriate type of urinary incontinence in the lettered column. *(338)*

1. _F_    Involuntary loss of urine during physical exertion

2. _C_    Loss of urine due to reflexive contraction

3. _A_    Inappropriate voiding in the presence of normal bladder and urethral function

4. _B_    Involuntary loss of urine associated with a full bladder

5. _D_    The inability to control the passage of urine

6. _E_    Involuntary loss of urine, usually shortly after a strong urge to void

 

A. Functional urinary incontinence
B. Overflow urinary incontinence
C. Reflex urinary incontinence
D. Total urinary incontinence
E. Urge urinary incontinence
F. Stress urinary incontinence

B. **Voiding.** Which factors are required for normal controlled voiding? Select all that apply. *(331)*

1. __☓__ Patent urethra
2. _____ Underactive detrusor muscle
3. __☓__ Mental alertness
4. _____ Constricted bladder sphincter
5. __☓__ Nerve impulse transmission

C. **Urinary Urge Incontinence.** Which methods of treatment are used for urinary urge incontinence? Select all that apply. *(338)*

1. __☓__ Anticholinergics
2. _____ Adrenergic drugs
3. _____ Tricyclic antidepressants
4. _____ Catheterization
5. __☓__ Behavior modification

D. **Overflow Incontinence.** Which factors contribute to overflow incontinence? Select all that apply. *(338)*

1. _____ Urethral obstruction
2. __☓__ Spinal cord injury
3. _____ Overactive detrusor muscle
4. __☓__ Impaired nerve impulse transmission
5. __☓__ Postanesthesia
6. _____ Dementia

E. **Drug Therapy.** Which drugs may cause urinary retention? Select all that apply. *(339)*

1. _____ Sedatives or hypnotics
2. _____ Antipsychotics
3. __☓__ Anticholinergics
4. __☓__ Antihistamines
5. __☓__ Theophylline (xanthines)
6. __☓__ Epinephrine

F. **Intermittent Catheterization.** Which type of patient usually requires intermittent catheterization only once or twice before normal bladder function returns? Select all that apply. *(338)*

1. __☓__ Postoperative patient
2. _____ Spinal cord injury patient
3. _____ Alzheimer's patient
4. __☓__ Postpartum patient

G. **Stress Incontinence.** Which activities may lead to stress incontinence? Select all that apply. *(339)*

1. __☓__ Coughing
2. __☓__ Laughing
3. __☓__ Lifting
4. _____ Nervous system disorder
5. _____ Urethral obstruction
6. __☓__ Sneezing

H. **Stress Incontinence.** Which are contributing factors to stress incontinence? Select all that apply. *(339)*

1. __☓__ Postpartum pelvic floor muscle relaxation
2. _____ Spinal cord injury
3. _____ Postanesthesia
4. __☓__ Obesity
5. __☓__ Aging

I. **Stress Incontinence.** Which of the following are methods of treatment for a person with stress incontinence? Select all that apply. *(338)*

1. __☓__ Scheduled voiding
2. __☓__ Pelvic muscle exercises
3. _____ Decreased fluid intake
4. __☓__ Avoid fluids with caffeine
5. __☓__ Use of Contigen (collagens)

J. **Diagnostic Procedures.** Match the definition or description in the numbered column with the most appropriate diagnostic test or procedure in the lettered column. *(332-333)*

1. ___C___ Used to evaluate the neuromuscular function of the bladder
2. ___B___ May be ordered to create images of the urinary structures
3. ___F___ Clean-catch urinalysis and blood urea nitrogen measurement
4. ___A___ Used to determine whether the patient is emptying the bladder completely
5. ___H___ Measures voiding duration and the amount and rate of urine voided
6. ___E___ Uses a scope inserted through the urethra to visualize the urethra and bladder
7. ___G___ Detects involuntary passage of urine when abdominal pressure increases
8. ___D___ Used to assess neuromuscular function of the urinary tract

A. Postvoiding residual
B. Imaging procedures
C. Cystometry
D. Urodynamic testing
E. Cystoscopy
F. Laboratory tests
G. Provocative stress testing
H. Uroflowmetry

K. **Therapeutic Measures.** Match the definition or description in the numbered column with the most appropriate therapeutic measure in the lettered column. *(333-334)*

1. ___G___ Intended to help the patient recognize incontinence and to ask caregivers for help with toileting
2. ___D___ Voiding schedule based on the patient's usual pattern
3. ___E___ Includes anticholinergics and smooth muscle relaxants
4. ___C___ Uses patient education, scheduled voiding, and positive reinforcement
5. ___H___ Sometimes employed by people with spinal cord injury
6. ___F___ Uses electronic or mechanical sensors to give feedback about physiologic activity
7. ___A___ Commonly called Kegel exercises
8. ___B___ Retained in the vagina to strengthen muscles of pelvic floor

A. Pelvic muscle exercises
B. Vaginal cones
C. Bladder training
D. Habit training
E. Drug therapy
F. Biofeedback
G. Prompted voiding
H. Reflex training

**L. Nursing Diagnoses.** Match the nursing diagnosis in the numbered column with the most appropriate cause in the lettered column. *(341)*

1. ___C___   Functional incontinence
2. ___A___   Reflex incontinence
3. ___B___   Risk for infection

A. Neurologic impairment
B. Chronic bladder distention or catheterization
C. Physical, cognitive, or environmental barriers

**M. Drug Therapy.** Match the name or classification of the drugs in the numbered column with the corresponding type of incontinence they treat in the lettered column. Answers may be used more than once. *(335-336)*

1. ___C___   Alpha-adrenergic blockers
2. ___B___   Cholinergics
3. ___C___   Beta-adrenergic blockers
4. ___B___   Anticholinergics
5. ___C___   Alpha-adrenergics
6. ___A___   5-alpha reductase inhibitors
7. ___C___   Propranolol (Inderal)
8. ___A___   Bethanechol chloride (Urecholine)
9. ___A___   Prazosin (Minipress)
10. ___C___   Ephedrine
11. ___B___   Oxybutynin (Ditropan)
12. ___B___   Propantheline bromide (Pro-Banthine)
13. ___A___   Finasteride (Proscar)
14. ___C___   Collagen (Contigen)

A. Overflow incontinence
B. Urge incontinence
C. Stress incontinence

**N. Types of Urinary Incontinence.** Match the cause of incontinence in the numbered column with the type of incontinence in the lettered column. Answers may be used more than once.

1. ___A___   UTI *(337)*
2. ___C___   Spinal cord injury above T10 *(338)*
3. ___D___   Relaxation of pelvic floor muscles *(339)*
4. ___E___   Dementia *(339)*
5. ___E___   CVA *(339)*
6. ___D___   Urethral trauma *(339)*
7. ___B___   Postanesthesia *(337)*

A. Urge
B. Overflow
C. Reflex
D. Stress
E. Functional

## MULTIPLE-CHOICE QUESTIONS

**O.** Choose the most appropriate answer.

1. Drugs that may cause urinary retention include: *(337)*
   1. chlorothiazides and loop diuretics.
   2. antihypertensives and insulin.
   3. anticholinergics and epinephrine.
   4. antibiotics and antiviral drugs.

2. The amount of urine remaining in the bladder after voiding is called the: *(332)*
   1. urodynamic series.
   2. clean catch.
   3. voiding duration.
   4. postvoid residual.

3. Which treatment is contraindicated for patients with reflex incontinence? *(338)*
   1. Cutaneous triggering
   2. Tapping the suprapubic area
   3. Stroking the inner thigh
   4. Credé's method

4. How much urine normally remains in the bladder after voiding? *(332)*
   1. 50 ml or less
   2. 100 ml or less
   3. 200 ml or less
   4. 250 ml or less

5. If the bladder becomes overdistended, the patient with reflex incontinence may have a very serious reaction called: *(339)*
   1. stress incontinence.
   2. orthostatic hypotension.
   3. autonomic dysreflexia.
   4. tachycardia.

6. Which is considered to be the last resort in the management of overflow incontinence? *(334)*
   1. Credé's method
   2. Valsalva maneuver
   3. Indwelling catheter
   4. Anal stretch maneuver

7. When a person voids inappropriately because of an inability to get to the toilet, this is called: *(339)*
   1. urge incontinence.
   2. functional incontinence.
   3. reflex incontinence.
   4. stress incontinence.

8. Stimuli that may encourage voiding include: *(342)*
   1. decreasing the fluid intake to less than 2000 ml/day.
   2. drinking caffeine and cola drinks.
   3. pressing down on the abdomen.
   4. pouring warm water over the perineum, and drinking water while on the toilet.

9. The patient who is incontinent of urine is at risk for: *(344)*
   1. urinary tract infection and urinary calculi (stones).
   2. upper respiratory infection and pelvic infection.
   3. bradycardia and thrombophlebitis.
   4. diarrhea and skin breakdown.

10. Which constipating drug would be effective in treating neurogenic incontinence if given once a day in the morning? *(346)*
    1. Senna
    2. Milk of magnesia
    3. Codeine
    4. Metamucil

11. The first step in the medical management of fecal overflow incontinence is to: *(346)*
    1. treat the underlying medical condition.
    2. teach pelvic muscle exercises and biofeedback.
    3. cleanse the colon, often with enemas and suppositories.
    4. schedule toileting based on the patient's usual time of defecation.

12. What type of incontinence is present in patients with dementia who do not voluntarily delay defecation? *(346)*
    1. Overflow
    2. Anorectal
    3. Neurogenic
    4. Symptomatic

13. The treatment for fecal neurogenic incontinence is to: *(346)*
    1. cleanse the colon, usually with enemas and suppositories.
    2. treat the underlying medical condition.
    3. schedule toileting based on the patient's usual time of defecation.
    4. teach pelvic muscle exercises and biofeedback.

14. A patient has blood and mucus in his stool. This type of fecal incontinence is: *(346)*
    1. neurogenic.
    2. symptomatic.
    3. anorectal.
    4. overflow.

15. Fecal incontinence associated with nerve damage that causes the muscles of the pelvic floor to weaken is: *(346)*
    1. symptomatic.
    2. neurogenic.
    3. anorectal.
    4. overflow.

16. Causes of overflow fecal incontinence include: *(345)*
    1. nerve damage that causes weak pelvic muscles.
    2. colon or rectal disease.
    3. loss of anal reflexes in patients with dementia.
    4. constipation in which the rectum is constantly distended.

17. A patient with fecal incontinence may need laxatives to: *(345)*
    1. relieve constipation.
    2. establish bowel control.
    3. improve the loss of anal sphincter tone.
    4. reverse the loss of the anal reflex.

18. In order to prevent constipation, the patient with fecal incontinence is advised to consume increased fluids and: *(345)*
    1. protein.
    2. fiber.
    3. carbohydrates.
    4. potassium.

19. What is a common reason for urethral obstruction in males? *(338)*
    1. Vasoconstriction
    2. Hypertension
    3. Kidney obstruction
    4. Prostate enlargement

**P.  Nursing Care Plan.** Refer to Nursing Care Plan, The Patient with Stress Incontinence, p. 340 in your textbook.

1. Which symptoms are indicative of stress incontinence in this patient? *(340)*

2. What are factors that have contributed to her stress incontinence? *(340)*

# Loss, Death, and End-of-Life Care

---

## OBJECTIVES

1. Describe beliefs and practices related to death and dying.

2. Describe responses of patients and their families to terminal illness and death.

3. Identify nursing diagnoses that are appropriate for the terminally ill.

4. Identify nursing goals that are appropriate for the terminally ill.

5. Identify nursing interventions to meet the needs of terminally ill and dying patients.

6. Discuss the needs of the terminally ill patient's significant others.

7. Discuss the ways nurses can intervene to meet the needs of the terminally ill patient's significant others.

8. Explore the responses of the nurse who works with the terminally ill.

9. Explore the needs of the nurse who works with terminally ill patients.

10. Identify issues related to caring for the dying patient, including advance directives, do-not-resuscitate decisions, brain death, organ donations, and pronouncement of death.

---

## LEARNING ACTIVITIES

A. **Beliefs About Death.** Which of the following are common beliefs about death for a 68-year-old person? Select all that apply. *(354)*

1. _____ Seldom thinks about death
2. _____ Death is temporary and reversible
3. _____ Afraid of prolonged death
4. _____ Faces death of family members and peers
5. _____ Sees death as inevitable
6. _____ Examines death as it relates to various meanings, such as freedom from discomfort
7. _____ Own death can be avoided
8. _____ Afraid of prolonged health problems

**B. Key Terms.** Match the physical manifestations of approaching death in the numbered column with the most appropriate term in the lettered column. *(357)*

1. _____ Breathing is rapid and deep with periods of apnea

2. _____ Breathing becomes irregular, gradually slowing down to terminal gasps

3. _____ Grunting and noisy tachypnea

A. Death rattle
B. Cheyne-Stokes breathing
C. "Guppy breathing"

**C. Grieving Process.** Match the definition or description in the numbered column with the most appropriate stage of grieving in the lettered column. Answers may be used more than once. *(354)*

1. _____ Patient or family members may become outraged with situations

2. _____ Peaceful acknowledgment of the loss

3. _____ Patient realizes the loss is final and the situation cannot be altered

4. _____ Patient refuses to acknowledge the loss

5. _____ Patient wishes for more time or wishes to avoid the loss

6. _____ Patient expresses feelings that the loss is occurring as a punishment for past actions and may try to negotiate with a higher power for more time

7. _____ Protects the patient and family from the reality of the loss

A. Depression
B. Anger
C. Denial
D. Acceptance
E. Bargaining

**D. Stages of Grief and Dying.** Match Martocchios's stages of grief in the numbered column with Kübler-Ross's stages of grief in the lettered column. *(354)*

1. _____ Yearning and protest

2. _____ Anguish, disorganization, and despair

3. _____ Shock and disbelief

4. _____ Reorganization and restoration

5. _____ Identification of bereavement

A. Depression
B. Denial
C. Acceptance
D. Anger
E. Bargaining

E. **Beliefs About Death.** Match the belief about death in the numbered column with the most appropriate age group in the lettered column. Answers may be used more than once. *(354)*

1. _____ Sees death as inevitable

2. _____ Faces death of parents and family members

3. _____ Examines death as it relates to various meanings, such as freedom from discomfort

4. _____ Sees death as future event

5. _____ Faces death of peers

6. _____ May experience death anxiety

A. Young adulthood
B. Middle adulthood
C. Older adulthood

F. **Terminal Illness.** Match the definition or description in the numbered column with the most appropriate state of awareness of terminal illness in the lettered column. *(355)*

1. _____ Patients and others involved freely discuss the impending death.

2. _____ Patient and family know of a terminal prognosis but do not discuss the issue openly.

3. _____ Patient and family recognize that patient is ill but do not understand severity of illness.

A. Mutual pretense
B. Closed awareness
C. Open awareness

G. **Fears of Dying.** Match the action in the numbered column with the relevant fear in the lettered column. Answers may be used more than once. *(356)*

1. _____ Assure patient that medication will be given promptly, as needed

2. _____ Express worth of dying person's life

3. _____ Simple presence of person to provide support and comfort

4. _____ Holding hands, touching, and listening

5. _____ Provide consistent pain control

6. _____ Dying person reviews his or her life

7. _____ Prayers, thoughts, and feelings provide comfort

A. Fear of loneliness
B. Fear of meaninglessness
C. Fear of pain

**H. Key Terms.** Match the definition in the numbered column with the most appropriate term in the lettered column. *(358)*

1. _____    The body's cooling after death
2. _____    Discoloration in the skin after death
3. _____    Stiffening of the body after death

A.    Rigor mortis
B.    Livor mortis
C.    Algor mortis

## MULTIPLE-CHOICE QUESTIONS

I.    Choose the most appropriate answer.

1.    Which change occurs preceding death? *(357)*
    1.    Blood pressure rises.
    2.    Breathing sounds are quiet.
    3.    Pulse slows.
    4.    Extremities turn red.

2.    Mouth breathing and the accumulation of mucus preceding death result in noisy, wet-sounding respirations called: *(357)*
    1.    suffocation.
    2.    death rattle.
    3.    tightness in the chest.
    4.    pneumonia.

3.    Livor mortis is generally most obvious in the: *(358)*
    1.    skin in extremities.
    2.    fingers and toes.
    3.    face and chest.
    4.    back and buttocks.

4.    Most states have replaced the idea of living wills with: *(362)*
    1.    euthanasia acts.
    2.    natural death acts.
    3.    self-disclosure acts.
    4.    DNR acts.

5.    Which cultural group values stoicism at death? *(356)*
    1.    Greeks
    2.    Mexicans
    3.    Vietnamese
    4.    Swedes

6.    What is the last sense to remain intact during the death process? *(357)*
    1.    Vision
    2.    Smell
    3.    Hearing
    4.    Touch

7.    Where does the sense of touch decrease first in a dying person? *(357)*
    1.    Face
    2.    Abdomen
    3.    Arms
    4.    Legs

8.    Why does the patient who is dying appear to stare? *(357)*
    1.    The blink reflex is lost gradually.
    2.    Vision is blurred.
    3.    There is decreased lubrication of the eye.
    4.    Decreased circulation to the eye occurs progressively.

9.    Which body function ceases first in the dying person? *(357)*
    1.    Heartbeat
    2.    Respiration
    3.    Brain function
    4.    Kidney function

10.    Which is *not* a criterion to determine death? *(358)*
    1.    Unresponsiveness to external stimuli that would usually be painful
    2.    Complete absence of spontaneous breathing
    3.    Total lack of reflexes
    4.    A flat EEG for 8 hours

11. Which criterion must be present for brain death to be pronounced and life support disconnected by the physician? *(358)*
    1. All brain function must cease.
    2. Coma or unresponsiveness must be present.
    3. Absence of all brain stem reflexes must be noted.
    4. Apnea must be present.

12. After death, what happens to the body as it cools? *(358)*
    1. Respirations are noisy and labored.
    2. Reflex jerking movements of the extremities occur.
    3. Pupils are not reactive to light.
    4. Skin loses elasticity and is easily broken.

13. What causes livor mortis after death? *(358)*
    1. Skin loses elasticity and breaks down easily.
    2. There is a breakdown of red blood cells.
    3. Chemical changes prevent muscle relaxation.
    4. Circulation decreases and the body cools.

14. Which religious group believes that the body should not be shrouded until sacraments have been performed? *(361)*
    1. Muslims
    2. Orthodox Jews
    3. Protestants
    4. Roman Catholics

15. The durable power of attorney for health care can be used only if the physician certifies in writing that the person is: *(364)*
    1. incapable of making decisions.
    2. brain dead.
    3. unresponsive or in a coma.
    4. lacking reflexes.

16. What decision involves the use of medications for resuscitation without the use of CPR? *(364)*
    1. Chemical code
    2. No code
    3. DNR
    4. Advance directive

17. The Patient Self-Determination Act requires that institutions must inform patients about: *(362)*
    1. rules and regulations about CPR.
    2. the right to have an autopsy.
    3. the right to initiate advance directives.
    4. rules and regulations about the delivery of hospice care.

## ALTERNATE FORMAT QUESTIONS

**J. Ordered Response.**

1. Place sequential order (from 1-5) the Kübler-Ross stages of grieving. *(354)*
   A. _____        Acceptance
   B. _____        Depression
   C. _____        Bargaining
   D. _____        Denial
   E. _____        Anger

2. Place in sequential order (from 1-3) the Rando stages of grieving. *(355)*
   A. _____        Confrontation
   B. _____        Avoidance
   C. _____        Accommodation

**K.** Which are physical manifestations of approaching death? Select all that apply. *(357)*
   1. Decreased pain and touch perception
   2. Involuntary blinking of the eyes
   3. Eyelids remain open
   4. Cold, clammy skin
   5. Jaw is clenched
   6. Swallowing is difficult
   7. Gag reflex is stimulated
   8. Drop in blood pressure

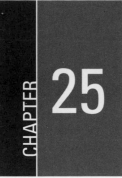

CHAPTER

# 25 The Patient with Cancer

---

## OBJECTIVES

1. Explain the differences between benign and malignant tumors.

2. List the most common sites of cancer in men and women.

3. Describe measures to reduce the risk of cancer.

4. Define terms used to name and classify cancer.

5. List nursing responsibilities in the care of patients having diagnostic tests to detect possible cancer.

6. Explain the nursing care of patients undergoing each type of cancer therapy: surgery, radiation, chemotherapy, and biotherapy.

7. Assist in developing a nursing care plan for the terminally ill patient with cancer and the patient's family.

---

## LEARNING ACTIVITIES

A. **Key Terms.** Match the definition in the numbered column with the most appropriate term in the lettered column.

1. _____ Tending to progress in virulence; has the characteristics of becoming increasingly undifferentiated, invading surrounding tissues, and colonizing distant sites *(369)*

2. _____ Cancer-causing agent *(370)*

3. _____ The use of radiation in the treatment of cancer and other diseases *(376)*

4. _____ Process by which cancer spreads to distant sites *(370)*

5. _____ Drugs used to treat cancer, including hematopoietic growth factors, biologic response modifiers, and monoclonal antibodies *(387)*

6. _____ An agent that inhibits the maturation or reproduction of malignant cells *(378)*

7. _____ Tumor; may be benign or malignant *(369)*

8. _____ Use of chemicals to treat illness *(378)*

9. _____ Not malignant *(369)*

A. Radiotherapy
B. Benign
C. Chemotherapy
D. Metastasis
E. Neoplasm
F. Malignant
G. Antineoplastic
H. Carcinogen
I. Biotherapy

B. **Radiation Therapy.** Which of the following normal cells are most sensitive to radiation? Select all that apply. *(378)*

1. _____ Nail beds

2. _____ Digestive and urinary tract linings

3. _____ Respiratory tract lining

4. _____ Skin

5. _____ Lymph tissue

6. _____ Ovaries

7. _____ Kidneys

8. _____ Lungs

9. _____ Testes

10. _____ Hair follicle

11. _____ Bone marrow

C. **Drug Therapy.** Of the following drugs, which types of antineoplastic drugs are frequently used in chemotherapy? Select all that apply. *(378)*

1. _____   Diuretics

2. _____   Bronchodilators

3. _____   Hormones

4. _____   Mitotic inhibitors

5. _____   Narcotics

6. _____   Alkylating agents

7. _____   Antithyroid drugs

8. _____   Antiemetics

9. _____   Sedatives

10. _____   Antihypertensives

11. _____   Antitumor antibiotics

12. _____   Hypnotics

13. _____   Biologic response modifiers

D. **Drug Therapy.** Which of the following are major systemic side effects of antineoplastic drugs? Select all that apply. *(381)*

1. _____   Dry mouth

2. _____   Bone marrow suppression

3. _____   Urinary retention

4. _____   Sedation

5. _____   Nausea and vomiting

6. _____   Constipation

7. _____   Dizziness

8. _____   Alopecia

9. _____   Electrolyte imbalance

10. _____   Tachycardia

E. **Warning Signs of Cancer.** Which of the following are warning signs of cancer? Select all that apply. *(372)*

1. _____   Nausea and vomiting

2. _____   Nagging cough and hoarseness

3. _____   Change in bowel or bladder habits

4. _____   Heart palpitations and tachycardia

5. _____   Sores that do not heal

6. _____   Dyspnea and trouble breathing

7. _____   Change in warts or moles

F. **Types of Tumors.** Match the tissue affected in the numbered column with the type of tumor in the lettered column. *(371)*

| | | |
|---|---|---|
| 1. _____ | Bone | A. Chondrosarcoma |
| 2. _____ | Pigment cells in the skin | B. Fibroma |
| 3. _____ | Fat tissue | C. Melanoma |
| 4. _____ | Cartilage | D. Osteosarcoma |
| 5. _____ | Smooth muscle tissue | E. Leiomyoma |
| 6. _____ | Fibrous connective tissue | F. Lipoma |
| 7. _____ | Tissues in the skin, glands, and linings of the digestive, urinary, and respiratory tracts | G. Leukemias and lymphoma |
| | | H. Sarcoma |
| | | I. Carcinoma |
| 8. _____ | Blood-forming tissues | |
| 9. _____ | Bone, muscle, and other connective tissue | |

G. **Stages of Tumors.** Match the definition in the numbered column with the most appropriate stage in the lettered column. *(371)*

| | | |
|---|---|---|
| 1. _____ | There is limited spread of the cancer in the local area, usually to nearby lymph nodes | A. Stage I |
| | | B. Stage II |
| | | C. Stage III |
| | | D. Stage IV |
| 2. _____ | The malignant cells are confined to the tissue of origin; there is no invasion of other tissues | |
| 3. _____ | The cancer has metastasized to distant parts of the body | |
| 4. _____ | The tumor is larger or has spread from the site of origin into nearby tissues, or both; regional lymph nodes are likely to be involved | |

H. **Diagnostic Procedures.** Match the definition or description in the numbered column with the most appropriate term in the lettered column. *(374)*

1. _____ Used to detect cancers of digestive and urinary tracts

2. _____ Useful for diagnosing tumors in the head or trunk

3. _____ Insertion of lighted tubes into hollow organs or body cavities

4. _____ Used to detect cancers of the central nervous system, spinal column, neck bones, and joints

5. _____ Used to detect tissue abnormalities of cancers of the thyroid, liver, and lung

6. _____ Used to detect solid tumors in the brain and breast

A. Magnetic resonance imaging
B. Computed tomography (CT Scan)
C. Endoscopy
D. Positron emission tomography (PET)
E. Contrast radiographs
F. Radionuclide scans

I. **Drug Therapy.** Match the side effect in the numbered column with the most appropriate drug in the lettered column. *(380-382)*

1. _____ Pulmonary inflammation and fibrosis

2. _____ Neurotoxicity resulting in numbness and tingling of extremities

3. _____ Toxic effects on the heart that may lead to heart failure

4. _____ Hypersensitivity

A. Vincristine (Oncovin)
B. Doxorubicin (Adriamycin)
C. Bleomycin (Blenoxane)
D. Paclitaxel (Taxol)

## MULTIPLE-CHOICE QUESTIONS

J. Choose the most appropriate answer.

1. What is the second most common cause of death in the United States? *(368)*
   1. Heart disease
   2. Cancer
   3. Accident
   4. Stroke

2. The type of invasion that involves the movement of cancer cells into adjoining tissue is: *(370)*
   1. regional.
   2. systemic.
   3. localized.
   4. centralized.

3. What is the effect on cells and tissue when DNA of a normal cell is exposed to a carcinogen and irreversible changes occur in the DNA? *(370)*
   1. The cell appears abnormal but continues to function normally.
   2. The cell is in a latent period before increased growth forms tumors.
   3. A tumor develops.
   4. Transformed cells relocate to remote sites.

4. A patient whose primary tumor has grown and spread to regional lymph nodes but not to distant sites is staged: *(371)*
   1. T1, N2, M1.
   2. T2, N1, M0.
   3. T0, N3, M1.
   4. T4, N0, M0.

5. The recommended diet that may reduce the risk of some cancers is one that is: *(369)*
   1. high-protein.
   2. high-fat.
   3. high-fiber.
   4. low-carbohydrate.

6. Your patient has cancer that has been staged T1, N0, M0. You would interpret this information as: *(371)*
   1. minimal size and extension of tumor.
   2. no sign of tumor.
   3. malignancy in epithelial tissue but not in basement membrane.
   4. progressively increasing size and extension.

7. A treatment likely to be curative when tumors are confined in one area is: *(375)*
   1. radiotherapy.
   2. chemotherapy.
   3. immunotherapy.
   4. surgery.

8. The use of ionizing radiation in the treatment of disease is called: *(376)*
   1. biotherapy.
   2. chemotherapy.
   3. radiotherapy.
   4. immunotherapy.

9. Radiation has immediate and delayed effects on cells; the immediate effect is: *(376)*
   1. cell death.
   2. alteration of DNA, which impairs cell's ability to reproduce.
   3. interruption of the clotting cascade.
   4. cell starvation.

10. Androgenic steroids and certain estrogens are known to be: *(371-372)*
    1. anti-inflammatory.
    2. carcinogenic.
    3. biologic response modifiers.
    4. appetite stimulants.

11. A patient experiences erythema and peeling of skin while receiving radiation therapy. The appropriate nursing intervention is to: *(379)*
    1. increase fluid intake.
    2. not use lotions.
    3. watch for excessive bruising and bleeding.
    4. report fever.

12. Which side effect occurs in patients undergoing radiotherapy and also in patients taking antineoplastic drugs? *(379, 381)*
    1. Phlebitis at infusion site
    2. Erythema and peeling of skin
    3. Alopecia
    4. Cardiomyopathy

13. The highest rate of death from prostate, colon, and breast cancer occurs among: *(373)*
    1. Caucasians.
    2. Latinos.
    3. Native Americans.
    4. African-Americans.

14. What is the most dangerous side effect of antineoplastic drugs? *(381)*
    1. Alopecia
    2. Nausea and vomiting
    3. Electrolyte imbalance
    4. Bone marrow suppression

15. A drug that boosts the body's natural defenses to combat malignant cells is: *(380)*
    1. vincristine.
    2. interferon.
    3. doxorubicin (Adriamycin).
    4. paclitaxel (Taxol).

16. The outcome criterion, a patient's completion of essential activities without dyspnea or tachycardia, is related to patients with: *(386)*
    1. alopecia.
    2. loss of a body part.
    3. anemia.
    4. denial.

17. The priority care for patients experiencing neurotoxicity from antineoplastic drugs is to: *(381)*
    1. monitor for edema.
    2. protect the patient from infection.
    3. protect extremities from injury.
    4. assess skin turgor.

18. Invasive procedures are minimized in patients with: *(381)*
    1. leukopenia.
    2. thrombocytopenia.
    3. anemia.
    4. agranulocytosis.

19. Compromised host precautions may be needed for patients with: *(385)*
    1. leukopenia.
    2. thrombocytopenia.
    3. anemia.
    4. weight loss.

20. What is appropriate teaching for the patient who is having external radiation therapy? *(378-379)*
    1. The treatment may be painful for the first 5 minutes, but the pain will subside.
    2. You will be radioactive as long as the machine is turned on.
    3. Skin markings made by the radiologist are used to mark areas that will not be irradiated.
    4. Skin over the area being treated may become discolored and irritated.

21. Which is the early detection period of cancer, when normal cells are transforming into malignant cells? *(370)*
    1. Cell appears somewhat abnormal.
    2. Latent period before increased growth forms tumors.
    3. Progression of tumor development.
    4. Cells mutate so that they are not at all identical.

22. When tumor cells metastasize, where do the tumor cells become trapped, forming a fibrin meshwork that prevents detection by the immune system? *(370)*
    1. Mucous membranes
    2. Lung tissue
    3. Capillary beds
    4. Lymph nodes

23. Which of the following tumors are malignant? *(371)*
    1. Fibroma
    2. Lipoma
    3. Melanoma
    4. Myoma

## ALTERNATE FORMAT QUESTIONS

**K.** 1. Which of the following are characteristics of malignant tumors? Select all that apply. *(369-370)*
    1. Usually slow growth rate
    2. Invades surrounding tissue
    3. Cells closely resemble those of tissue of origin
    4. Recurrence is common after removal
    5. Metastasis frequently occurs
    6. Little tissue destruction

2. Which of the following are common oncologic emergencies? Select all that apply. *(393)*
    1. Superior vena cava syndrome
    2. Pulmonary edema
    3. Hypertension
    4. Hypercalcemia
    5. Syndrome of inappropriate antidiuretic hormone (SIADH)
    6. Spinal cord compression
    7. Disseminated intravascular coagulation

**L. Nursing Care Plan.** Refer to Nursing Care Plan, The Patient with Cancer, pp. 385-386 in your textbook.

1. Which patient teaching points will you emphasize with this patient, regarding his radiotherapy? Select all that apply. *(379)*
   1. Do not wash off skin markings.
   2. Do not apply lotion to irritated skin.
   3. Advise him to avoid crowds and people with infection.
   4. Eat small, frequent meals.
   5. Do frequent, gentle mouth care.

2. Anzemet is ordered for the nausea and vomiting he experiences while undergoing chemotherapy. What are the main side effects of this drug? Select all that apply. *(390)*
   1. Abdominal pain
   2. Dizziness
   3. Headache
   4. Bradycardia

3. This patient has a Stage II tumor. What is the meaning of the Stage II classification? *(371)*
   1. Malignant cells are confined to the tissue of origin.
   2. The cancer has metastasized to distant parts of the body.
   3. The tumor is larger and has spread from the site of origin into nearby tissues.
   4. There is limited spread of the cancer in the local area, usually to nearby lymph nodes.

4. This patient develops signs of bone marrow suppression as a result of his chemotherapy. What is the priority nursing intervention? *(381)*
   1. Avoid exposure to sun and harsh chemicals.
   2. Use a soft toothbrush.
   3. Schedule activities to prevent overtiring.
   4. Protect from injury.

# CHAPTER 26

# The Patient with an Ostomy

---

## OBJECTIVES

1. List the indications for ostomy surgery to divert urine or feces.

2. Describe nursing interventions to prepare the patient for ostomy surgery.

3. Explain the types of procedures used for fecal diversion.

4. Assist in developing a nursing process to plan care for the patient with each of the following types of fecal diversion: ileostomy, continent ileostomy, ileoanal reservoir, and colostomy.

5. Explain the types of procedures done for urinary diversion.

6. Assist in developing a nursing care plan for the patient with each of the following types of urinary diversion: ureterostomy, ileal conduit, continent internal reservoir.

7. Discuss content to be included in teaching patients to learn to live with ostomies.

---

## LEARNING ACTIVITIES

A.  **Key Terms.** Match the definition in the numbered column with the most appropriate term in the lettered column.

1.  _____   Opening created to drain contents of an organ *(396)*

2.  _____   Surgically created opening in the kidney to drain urine *(413)*

3.  _____   Surgically created opening into the urinary bladder *(413)*

4.  _____   Surgical procedure that creates an opening into a body structure *(396)*

5.  _____   Capable of controlling natural impulses; in relation to an ostomy, able to retain feces or urine *(401)*

6.  _____   Surgically created opening in the ureter *(409)*

7.  _____   Downward displacement *(405)*

8.  _____   Communication or connection between two organs or parts of organs *(398)*

9.  _____   Surgically created opening in the ileum *(397)*

10. _____   Surgically created opening in the colon *(404)*

A.   Anastomosis
B.   Colostomy
C.   Continent
D.   Ileostomy
E.   Nephrostomy
F.   Ostomy
G.   Prolapse
H.   Stoma
I.   Ureterostomy
J.   Vesicostomy

**B. Supplies Needed for Ostomy.**

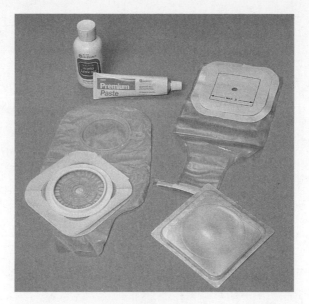

1. What are the supplies needed to pouch an intestinal ostomy that are included in this picture (Figure 26-1A, p. 400)? *(400)*

2. Following ileostomy surgery, the stoma is inspected for bleeding and: *(398)*
   1. edema.
   2. rough edges.
   3. temperature.
   4. color.

3. Refer to Figure 26-1B, p. 400 in your textbook. What color is the stoma in this figure? *(400)*

4. What color would the stoma be if the circulation is poor? *(398)*

5. Following ileostomy surgery, what should you examine when checking the base of the stoma? Select all that apply. *(398)*
   1. _____  Purulent drainage
   2. _____  Redness
   3. _____  Amount of drainage present
   4. _____  Skin breakdown

6. If the color of the stoma is pale or blue following ileostomy surgery, what should the nurse do? *(398)*
   1. Cleanse skin around stoma with soap and water.
   2. Apply a protective skin barrier before replacing the pouch.
   3. Notify the physician.
   4. Check the pouch hourly to detect leakage.

**C.   Application of Ostomy Pouch.**

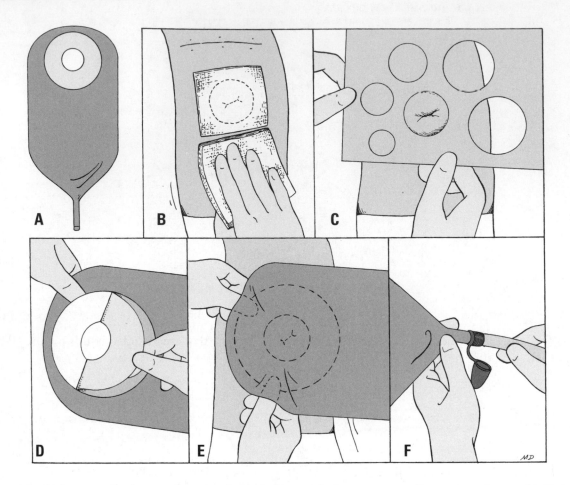

1.  Match the steps in the numbered column below with the corresponding correct letters (A-F) in the figure above (Figure 26-6, p. 411). *(411)*

    1. _____    Gently press into place with the pouch drain pointed toward the floor.
    2. _____    Remove the backing from the adhesive of the new pouch.
    3. _____    Connect the drain to the tubing or close the drain, if appropriate.
    4. _____    Gather supplies.
    5. _____    Use a stoma template to measure the size of the stoma.
    6. _____    Wash hands and put on gloves.
    7. _____    Remove the old pouch and clean the area around the stoma.
    8. _____    Cut an opening the same size as the stoma into the skin barrier and adhesive.
    9. _____    Place a gauze square over the stoma to absorb the drainage.
    10. _____   Place the opening in the new pouch over the stoma.
    11. _____   Secure the tubing to the sheets or according to agency policy.

2.  Why is sizing the ostomy pouch so important during the first 6–8 weeks postoperatively? *(398)*


3.  What does a small amount of bleeding around the base of a new stoma indicate? *(398)*
    1.  Infection
    2.  Tissue injury
    3.  Adequate blood supply
    4.  Poor circulation

4. If edema occurs after the first week postoperatively, this most likely indicates: *(398)*
   1. improperly fitting collection device.
   2. infection.
   3. capillary hemorrhage.
   4. poor circulation.

5. When does ileostomy drainage occur after surgery? *(398)*
   1. First 6 hours
   2. 10–12 hours
   3. 24–48 hours
   4. After 72 hours

6. Which manifestation indicates mental status changes in the postoperative ileostomy patient indicating electrolyte imbalances? *(399)*
   1. Twitching
   2. Weakness
   3. Poor tissue turgor
   4. Confusion

7. Postoperative ileostomy patients may experience electrolyte imbalances due to: *(399)*
   1. passage of liquid stool.
   2. bleeding around the stoma.
   3. poor circulation.
   4. infection.

8. Which foods should patients with continent ileostomies avoid initially? Select all that apply. *(403)*
   1. _____ Pasta
   2. _____ Coffee
   3. _____ Berries
   4. _____ Nuts
   5. _____ Boiled rice
   6. _____ Fresh fruit

**D. Colostomy Types.**

1.  Using the figure below (Figure 26-4, p. 405), label each type of colostomy (A–D) and indicate which type of drainage is passed by each (E–G). Match the characteristics (H–I) to the appropriate type of colostomy. *(405)*

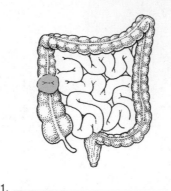

1. _____
   _____

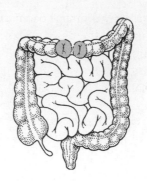

2. _____
   _____

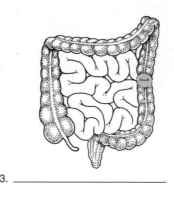

3. _____
   _____

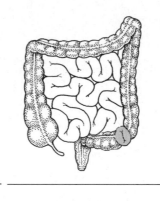

4. _____
   _____

    A.  Descending colostomy

    B.  Ascending colostomy

    C.  Transverse colostomy

    D.  Sigmoid colostomy

    E.  Passes liquid to semisolid stool

    F.  Passes softly formed stool

    G.  Passes liquid material

    H.  Done for right-sided tumors

    I.  Often used in emergencies such as intestinal obstruction, because it can be done quickly

2.  What are the two main long-term complications of colostomies? *(405)*

3. What type of medication can be inserted into a colostomy stoma to stimulate evacuation? *(408)*
    1. Laxative liquid
    2. Hyperosmolar laxative
    3. Rectal suppository
    4. Nystatin

4. What are factors that contribute to a prolapsed stoma in a colostomy? Select all that apply. *(405)*
    1. _____    Increased abdominal pressure
    2. _____    Coughing
    3. _____    Poor blood supply
    4. _____    Peristomal hernia
    5. _____    Poorly attached stoma
    6. _____    Abdominal opening that is too small

## E.  Types of Urinary Diversions.

1. Using the figure below (Figure 26-5, p. 408), label the types of urinary diversion procedures (A–E) using the following terms. *(408)*

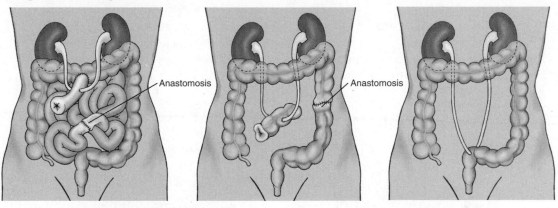

Anastomosis    Anastomosis

1. _____    2. _____    3. _____

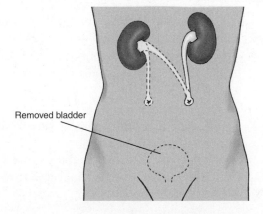

Removed bladder

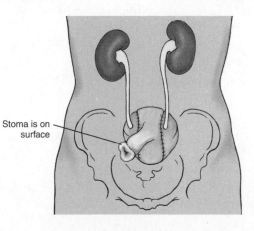

Stoma is on surface

4. _____    5. _____

A. Continent internal ileal reservoir
B. Colon conduit
C. Ureterosigmoidostomy
D. Ileal conduit
E. Cutaneous ureterostomy

2. What are two serious consequences of urinary tract infections following ureterostomy? *(409)*

3. What is the treatment for yeast infections around the ureterostomy stoma? *(410)*
   1. Nystatin powder
   2. Antibiotic ointment
   3. Steroid ointment
   4. Soap and water

4. If odor is a problem with ureterostomy, the pouch can be soaked for 20–30 minutes in: *(410)*
   1. 50% alcohol.
   2. normal saline.
   3. vinegar water.
   4. baking soda and water.

## MULTIPLE-CHOICE QUESTIONS

F. Choose the most appropriate answer.

1. A colostomy is performed by bringing a loop of the intestine through the wall of the: *(405)*
   1. bladder.
   2. rectum.
   3. abdomen.
   4. stomach.

2. Which complication of colostomy involves the narrowing of the abdominal opening around the base of the stoma? *(405)*
   1. Prolapse
   2. Stenosis
   3. Obstruction
   4. Evisceration

3. A nursing diagnosis for the colostomy patient is Risk for injury related to: *(406)*
   1. hemorrhage or infection.
   2. dyspnea or tachycardia.
   3. hypotension or bradycardia.
   4. prolapse or stenosis.

4. What should you do if you notice that the colostomy is not draining properly? *(408)*
   1. Place a gloved finger in the stoma to dilate it.
   2. Use a larger catheter to irrigate.
   3. Inform the physician.
   4. Push the catheter in 3 inches.

5. The loss of bicarbonate in ileostomy drainage can result in: *(399)*
   1. hypokalemia.
   2. hypercalcemia.
   3. metabolic acidosis.
   4. fluid volume excess.

6. If the ileal conduit stoma turns gray or black, the physician should be notified immediately, as it may mean that: *(412)*
   1. ureteral obstruction has occurred.
   2. circulation is impaired.
   3. wound infection is present.
   4. prolapse has occurred.

7. After bowel resection for the ileal conduit procedure, you should expect: *(412)*
   1. necrosis of the wound.
   2. temporary ileus (absence of bowel activity).
   3. gray-black stoma.
   4. ureteral calculi.

8. In which procedure would the nurse expect to find mucus in the drainage? *(412)*
   1. Ureterostomy
   2. Vesicostomy
   3. Cystostomy
   4. Ileal conduit

9. A patient with an ileoanal reservoir is at risk for injury related to: *(404)*
   1. peritonitis.
   2. inflammation of the reservoir.
   3. leaking of suture lines.
   4. obstruction of pouch drainage.

10. With a temporary ileostomy, abdominal distention, nausea and vomiting, and decreased bowel sounds are signs and symptoms of: *(403)*
    1. inflammation of the ileoanal reservoir.
    2. peritonitis.
    3. small bowel obstruction.
    4. hemorrhage.

11. The Kock pouch is made with a section of: *(402)*
    1. sigmoid colon.
    2. jejunum.
    3. ileum.
    4. ascending colon.

12. A patient with an ileostomy one week postoperatively has a pulse of 120, respirations 28, temperature of 101° F, and a rigid abdomen. You suspect that this patient has which complication? *(403)*
    1. Obstruction
    2. Peritonitis
    3. Inflammation
    4. Evisceration of the site

13. Which foods tend to produce thicker stools? *(404)*
    1. Milk and cottage cheese
    2. Fresh fruits
    3. Green, leafy vegetables
    4. Pasta and boiled rice

14. Why is a nasogastric tube placed in a patient with bowel obstruction? *(404)*
    1. Dilate the digestive tract
    2. Decompress the bowel
    3. Provide method of feeding
    4. Improve peristalsis

15. What is a complication of colostomy irrigation? *(406)*
    1. Obstruction
    2. Diarrhea
    3. Infection
    4. Perforated bowel

16. The reason metronidazole (Flagyl) is given to patients with an ileoanal reservoir is that it treats: *(404)*
    1. pain.
    2. bleeding.
    3. inflammation.
    4. fluid volume deficit.

17. Which condition in a patient with a colostomy requires the nurse to contact the physician immediately? *(405)*
    1. Prolapse
    2. Perforated bowel
    3. Diarrhea
    4. Red stoma

18. Which of the following is a sign of bowel obstruction? *(403)*
    1. Bloody stools
    2. Fever
    3. Abdominal distention
    4. Hypotension

19. Which of the following is a major long-term complication caused by coughing in a patient with a colostomy? *(405)*
    1. Prolapse
    2. Stenosis
    3. Obstruction
    4. Inflammation

20. Which is a complication of ureterostomy? *(409)*
    1. Obstruction
    2. Perforation
    3. Hydronephrosis
    4. Prolapse

21. Which drug is used to treat a rash around the stoma of a patient with an ureterostomy? *(410)*
    1. Tetracycline
    2. Neosporin
    3. Benadryl
    4. Nystatin

22. Which group has the highest rate of colon and rectal cancers, which are commonly treated with ostomies? *(397)*
    1. Asians
    2. African-Americans
    3. Caucasians
    4. Native Americans

23. Which type of patient with a colostomy should be given a two-piece appliance that allows frequent pouch changes without skin trauma? *(404)*
    1. Jewish
    2. Native American
    3. Asian
    4. Muslim

**G. Nursing Care Plan.** Refer to the Nursing Care Plan, The Patient with a Colostomy, p. 407 in y our textbook.

1. How often do you check his pouch to detect leakage? *(407)*

2. A physician orders 1000 ml of $D_5W$ to infuse over 8 hours. The drop factor is 15 drops per 1 ml. The nurse sets the flow rate at how many drops per minute? (Round to the nearest tenth). *(407)*

# CHAPTER 27

# Neurologic Disorders

---

## OBJECTIVES

1. Identify common neurologic changes in the older person and the implications of these for nursing care.

2. Describe the diagnostic tests and procedures used to evaluate neurologic dysfunction and the nursing responsibilities associated with each.

3. Identify the uses, side effects, and nursing interventions associated with common drug therapies employed in patients with neurologic disorders.

4. Describe the signs and symptoms associated with increased intracranial pressure and the medical therapies used in treatment.

5. List the components of the nursing assessment of the patient with a neurologic disorder.

6. Describe the pathophysiology, signs and symptoms, complications, and medical or surgical treatment for patients with selected neurologic disorders.

7. Assist in developing a nursing care plan for the patient with a neurologic disorder.

---

## LEARNING ACTIVITIES

A. **Key Terms.** Match the definition in the numbered column with the most appropriate term in the lettered column.

1. _____ Abnormal extension of the upper extremities with extension of the lower extremities; accompanies increased pressure on the entire cerebrum and the motor tract structures of the brain stem *(433)*

2. _____ Weakness on one side of the body *(433)*

3. _____ Abnormal flexion of the upper extremities with extension of the lower extremities; accompanies increased pressure on the frontal lobes *(433)*

4. _____ Pain in a nerve or along the course of a nerve *(456)*

5. _____ Inflammation of brain tissue *(444)*

6. _____ Effects on the autonomic nervous system *(416)*

7. _____ Affecting the same side *(426)*

8. _____ Paralysis on one side of the body *(433)*

9. _____ Affecting the opposite side *(426)*

10. _____ Within the skull *(433)*

A. Dysautonomia
B. Contralateral
C. Extension (decerebrate) posturing
D. Abnormal flexion (decorticate) posturing
E. Encephalitis
F. Hemiparesis
G. Hemiplegia
H. Intracranial
I. Ipsilateral
J. Neuralgia

B. **Neurotransmitters.** Which of the following are neurotransmitters? Select all that apply. *(416)*

1. _____ Acetylcholine
2. _____ Thyroxine
3. _____ Epinephrine
4. _____ Norepinephrine
5. _____ Insulin
6. _____ Myosin

C. **Age-Related Changes.** List how the four parts of the nervous system listed below change with normal aging. *(418)*

1. Nerve cells (number):_____

2. Brain (weight): _____

3. Ventricles (size): _____

4. Nerve tissues: _____

D. **Pupillary Evaluation.** Which of the following are normal characteristics of pupils that are noted in pupillary evaluation? Select all that apply. *(422)*
1. _____ Size: 6 mm
2. _____ Shape: Round
3. _____ Reactivity: React quickly to light

E. **Intracranial Pressure.**

1. Which measures are indicated for patients with increased ICP? Select all that apply. *(433)*
    1. _____ Raise the head of the bed 90 degrees.
    2. _____ Employ mechanical ventilation to eliminate $CO_2$.
    3. _____ Increase fluids and monitor carefully.
    4. _____ Monitor for changes in LOC.
    5. _____ Check pupillary reactivity.

2. Which drugs are commonly used in the treatment of patients with increased ICP? Select all that apply. *(434)*
    1. _____ Hyperosmolar agents (Mannitol)
    2. _____ Corticosteroids
    3. _____ Diuretics (furosemide)
    4. _____ Antihypertensives
    5. _____ Barbiturates

F. **Amyolateral Sclerosis.** Complete the table below by filling in the appropriate "related to" statements and nursing goals for the patient with amyotrophic lateral sclerosis (ALS). *(453)*

| Nursing Diagnosis | Related To: | Nursing Goals/Outcome Criteria |
| --- | --- | --- |
| Ineffective airway clearance | | |
| Impaired physical mobility | | participation in activities to maintain mobility |
| Imbalanced nutrition: less than body requirements | dysphagia | |
| Impaired verbal communication | | effective communication |
| Anticipatory grieving | progressive, fatal disease | |
| Situational low self-esteem | | |
| Altered family processes | | |

**G. Age-Related Changes.** In each of the physical examination areas in the numbered column, indicate the possible age-related change by matching it to a term in the lettered column. Some terms may be used more than once, and some terms may not be used. *(418)*

1. _____   Pupil of the eye
2. _____   Pupillary response to light
3. _____   Tracking movement of eye
4. _____   Reflexes
5. _____   Achilles tendon jerk
6. _____   Reaction time

A. Slower
B. Decrease(s)
C. Remain(s) intact
D. Larger
E. Faster
F. May be absent
G. Smooth
H. Increase(s)
I. Jerky
J. Smaller

**H. Levels of Consciousness.** Complete the statements in the numbered column with the most appropriate term in the lettered column. Some terms may be used more than once, and some terms may not be used. *(422)*

1. Decreased responsiveness accompanied by lack of spontaneous motor activity is _____.

2. A patient who cannot be aroused even by powerful stimuli is _____.

3. The most accurate and reliable indicator of neurologic status is the _____.

4. Excessive drowsiness is _____.

5. If a patient is stuporous but can be aroused, the patient is _____.

6. Unnatural drowsiness or sleepiness is _____.

A. Agitation
B. Level of consciousness
C. Combativeness
D. Somnolence
E. Neuromuscular response
F. Lethargy
G. Comatose
H. Pupillary evaluation
I. Semicomatose
J. Stupor

**I. Neurologic Disorders.** Complete the statements in the numbered column with the most appropriate term in the lettered column. Some terms may be used more than once, and some terms may not be used.

1. The most common type of pain is _____. *(435)*

2. Inflammation of the coverings of the brain and spinal cord caused by either viral or bacterial organisms is called _____. *(442)*

3. Inflammation of brain tissue usually caused by a virus is _____. *(444)*

4. A rapidly progressing disease that affects the motor component of the peripheral nervous system is _____. *(444)*

5. A progressive degenerative disorder that results in an eventual loss of coordination and control over involuntary motor movement is _____. *(446)*

A. Meningitis
B. Parkinson's disease
C. Seizure disorder
D. Cerebral palsy
E. Guillain-Barré syndrome
F. Headache
G. Encephalitis

**J. Neurologic Disorders.** Complete the statements in the numbered column with the most appropriate term in the lettered column. Some terms may be used more than once, and some terms may not be used.

1. The amount of acetylcholine available at the neuromuscular junction is reduced in _____. *(454)*

2. A chronic, progressive, degenerative disease that attacks the protective myelin sheath around axons and disrupts motor pathways of the CNS is _____. *(449)*

3. A degenerative neurologic disease, which is also known as Lou Gehrig's disease, is _____. *(452)*

4. Young adults have the highest rate of incidence, with women affected more frequently than men, in _____. *(449)*

5. A disease that affects males more than females, striking most often between 40 and 70 years of age, is _____. *(452)*

6. An inherited degenerative neurologic disorder that begins with abnormal movements in middle adulthood is _____. *(454)*

7. A chronic, progressive disease in which there is a defect at the neuromuscular junction, where electrical impulses are transmitted to muscle tissue, is _____. *(454)*

A. Amyolateral sclerosis (ALS)
B. Huntington's disease
C. Parkinson's disease
D. Myasthenia gravis
E. Multiple sclerosis (MS)
F. Cerebral palsy
G. Guillain-Barré syndrome

**K. Autonomic Nervous System.** Indicate whether the following responses are controlled by the (A) sympathetic or (B) parasympathetic nervous system. *(420)*

1. _____ Bronchial dilation

2. _____ Pupil constriction

3. _____ Increased gut peristalsis and tone in lumen

4. _____ Decreased rate and force of cardiac contractions

5. _____ Pupil dilation

6. _____ Bronchial constriction

7. _____ Decreased gut peristalsis and tone in lumen

8. _____ Increased rate and force of cardiac contractions

9. _____ Flight-or-fight response

10. _____ Mediates rest response

**L.  Brain Dysfunctions.** Match the dysfunctions in the numbered column with the corresponding part of the brain in the lettered column. Some terms may be used more than once, and some terms may not be used. *(426)*

1. _____    Loss of steady gait

2. _____    Dysfunction occurring on the same side as the offending lesion

3. _____    Motor dysfunction on the opposite side from the lesion

4. _____    Loss of steady, balanced posture

A.  Cerebellum
B.  Hypothalamus
C.  Cerebral cortex
D.  Spinal cord

**M.  Diagnostic Procedures.** Match the intervention or description in the numbered column with the appropriate diagnostic test in the lettered column. Some diagnostic tests may be used more than once, and some tests may not be used.

1. _____    People who are confused or claustrophobic may require mild sedation before this test. *(424, 430)*

2. _____    A shampoo is done before the test, and medications, such as anticonvulsants and stimulants, are withheld 24–48 hours before the test. *(433)*

3. _____    Tell the patient to expect to lie still on a stretcher while the dye is injected and radiographs are taken of the head. *(424, 429)*

4. _____    Keep the patient flat, and "log-roll" the patient for up to 48 hours. *(424)*

5. _____    A cannula is usually inserted into the femoral artery, and a catheter is advanced to the carotid or vertebral arteries. *(424, 429)*

6. _____    Needle electrodes are placed on several points over a nerve and muscles supplied by the nerve. *(429, 433)*

7. _____    Special infusion pumps, oxygen equipment, and ventilators are used. *(424, 430)*

8. _____    Encourage fluid intake following the procedure to minimize headache. *(423)*

A.  Brain scan
B.  Lumbar puncture
C.  Magnetic resonance imaging
D.  Pneumoencephalography
E.  CT scan
F.  Cerebral angiography
G.  Electromyography (EMG)
H.  Pupillary evaluation
I.  Electroencephalogram (EEG)

9. _____ Inform the radiologist about any allergies to iodine, shellfish, or contrast media. *(424, 429)*

10. _____ Patient must remain on one side in a knee-to-chest position. *(423)*

11. _____ Potassium chloride is given 2 hours before the isotope is given for this test to prevent excessive isotope uptake. *(429, 433)*

12. _____ Because air, blood, bone, tissue, and CSF have varying densities, they appear in various shades of gray in this test. *(424, 429)*

13. _____ A contrast dye is injected, followed by a series of radiographs. *(424, 429)*

14. _____ Tell the patient to expect to hear a noise like a muffled drumbeat while in the machine. *(424, 430)*

N. **Brain Surgery.** Match the definition or description in the numbered column with the most appropriate term in the lettered column. *(430)*

1. _____ Surgery that requires opening the skull

2. _____ Excision of a segment of the skull

3. _____ Procedure done to repair a skull defect

   A. Cranioplasty
   B. Craniotomy
   C. Craniectomy

O. **Head Trauma.** Match the definition in the numbered column with the most appropriate term in the lettered column. Some terms may be used more than once, and some terms may not be used. *(438)*

1. _____ Head trauma in which there is no visible injury to the skull or brain

2. _____ Head trauma in which there is actual bruising and bleeding in the brain tissue

3. _____ A collection of blood, usually clotted, which may be classified as subdural or epidural

   A. Contusion(s)
   B. Seizure(s)
   C. Amnesia
   D. Hematoma
   E. Concussion

**P. Scalp Injuries.** Which of the following are common scalp injuries? Select all that apply. *(438)*

1. _____   Lacerations
2. _____   Fissures
3. _____   Contusions
4. _____   Abrasions
5. _____   Hematomas
6. _____   Tumors

**Q. Meningitis.** Match the nursing diagnosis for patients with meningitis in the numbered column with the "related to" statement in the lettered column. *(443)*

1. _____   Ineffective cerebral tissue perfusion
2. _____   Ineffective breathing pattern
3. _____   Acute pain
4. _____   Risk for injury
5. _____   Deficient fluid volume
6. _____   Risk for disuse syndrome

A. Confusion, seizures, restlessness
B. Irritation of the meninges
C. Bed rest
D. Increased intracranial pressure
E. Vomiting and fever
F. Depression of the respiratory center

**R. Clinical Manifestations of Parkinson's Syndrome.**

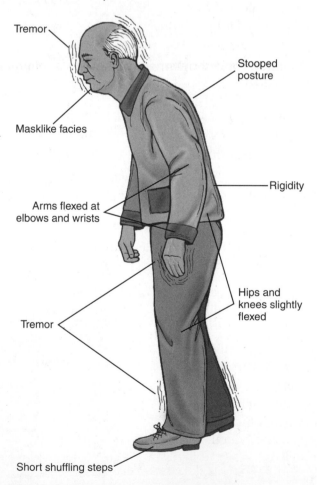

Tremor

Masklike facies

Stooped posture

Rigidity

Arms flexed at elbows and wrists

Hips and knees slightly flexed

Tremor

Short shuffling steps

Refer to Figure 27-17 (p. 447 in the textbook) on previous page. Match the description of symptoms of Parkinson's disease in the numbered column with the most appropriate term in the lettered column. Some terms may be used more than once, and some may not be used. *(447)*

1. _____   Trembling, shaking type of movement usually seen in upper extremities

2. _____   Stiffness

3. _____   Extremely slow movements

4. _____   Movement of thumb against fingertips

A.   Bradykinesia
B.   Tremor
C.   Bradycardia
D.   Rigidity
E.   Pill-rolling
F.   Dementia

S.   **Signs and Symptoms of Parkinson's Syndrome.**

1.   Refer to Figure 27-17 (p. 447 in the textbook) on previous page. What are the three major symptoms (major triad) of Parkinson's syndrome? Select all that apply. *(447)*
   1. _____   Aching
   2. _____   Monotone voice
   3. _____   Tremors at rest
   4. _____   Rigidity
   5. _____   Slumped posture
   6. _____   Bradykinesia

2.   What is characteristic of the tremors of a patient with Parkinson's syndrome? *(447)*


3.   What are the two main goals for the patient with Parkinson's disease? *(448)*


4.   What physical therapy programs are most helpful for patients with Parkinson's disease? Select all that apply. *(448)*
   1. _____   Crutch walking
   2. _____   Massage
   3. _____   Cold compresses
   4. _____   Exercise
   5. _____   Gait retraining

5.   What are ways to improve mobility for a patient with Parkinson's disease? Select all that apply. *(448)*
   1. _____   Scoot to the edge of a chair before trying to stand.
   2. _____   March in place before starting to walk.
   3. _____   Use cotton sheets to make it easier to move in and out of bed.
   4. _____   Practice lifting the foot as if to step over an object on the floor to initiate walking.

**T. Drug Therapy.** Match the uses of drugs in the numbered column with names of drugs used for multiple sclerosis in the lettered column. *(450)*

1. _____ Anti-inflammatory drug used during period of exacerbation

2. _____ Anti-inflammatory drug used to encourage remission

3. _____ Drug used to decrease the frequency of recurrent neurologic episodes in relapsing-remitting MS

4. _____ Drug used to treat the spasticity experienced by MS patients

A. Betaseron (interferon beta-1b)
B. Prednisone
C. Baclofen
D. ACTH

**U. Neurologic Diseases.** Match the definition in the numbered column with the most appropriate neurologic disease in the lettered column. Some diseases may be used more than once, and some diseases may not be used.

1. _____ A disease characterized by intense pain along nerve lines in the face *(457)*

2. _____ A disease characterized by multiple tumors of peripheral, spinal, and cranial nerves *(457)*

3. _____ Acute paralysis of the seventh cranial nerve *(457)*

4. _____ Paralysis associated with a loss in motor coordination caused by cerebral damage *(457)*

5. _____ Progressive muscle weakness, fatigue, pain, and respiratory problems years after the initial infection, illness, and recovery *(458)*

A. Myasthenia gravis
B. Neurofibromatosis
C. Cerebral palsy
D. Bell's palsy
E. Parkinson's disease
F. Postpolio syndrome
G. Trigeminal neuralgia
H. Multiple sclerosis

**V. Divisions of Trigeminal Nerve (Figure 27-20, p. 457).**

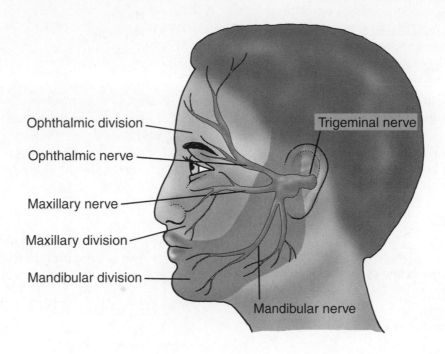

1. What disease is characterized by intense pain along one of the three branches of the trigeminal nerve? *(456)*


2. What is the main focus of nursing care for the patient with trigeminal neuralgia? *(457)*


3. What other problems does this patient have due to nerve involvement? Select all that apply. *(457)*
   1. _____     Imbalanced nutrition
   2. _____     Social isolation
   3. _____     Increased ICP
   4. _____     Hypertension
   5. _____     Ineffective tissue perfusion

4. What condition occurs when a patient has paralysis of Cranial Nerve VII? *(457)*

## MULTIPLE-CHOICE QUESTIONS

**W.** Choose the most appropriate answer.

1. To minimize headache following a lumbar puncture, what should be increased? *(423)*
   1. Calcium
   2. Fluid intake
   3. Potassium
   4. Ambulation

2. The family should be advised that a craniotomy can take as long as: *(430)*
   1. 2 hours.
   2. 6 hours.
   3. 12 hours.
   4. 24 hours.

3. As ICP increases and perfusion is reduced, oxygen delivery to cerebral tissue is: *(433)*
   1. increased.
   2. bypassed.
   3. reduced.
   4. stopped.

4. Classic pupillary changes are seen in increasing ICP. Sometimes a "blown pupil" is observed, which means that the pupil: *(433)*
   1. is dilated.
   2. is pinpoint.
   3. reacts to light.
   4. is unequal to the other pupil.

5. The pupils may become dilated and fixed as ICP rises due to pressure on the: *(433)*
   1. oculomotor nerve.
   2. cerebellum.
   3. hypothalamus.
   4. optic nerve.

6. Which neurons transmit information toward the CNS? *(415)*
   1. Sensory
   2. Motor
   3. Efferent
   4. Axon

7. A type of headache in which the pain is usually unilateral and has a warning is called: *(435)*
   1. cluster.
   2. migraine.
   3. tension.
   4. sinus.

8. Seizure activity involves a large number of hyperactive neurons that use excessive: *(435)*
   1. calcium and vitamin D.
   2. potassium and chloride.
   3. sodium and iron.
   4. oxygen and glucose.

9. Management of bacterial meningitis revolves around prompt recognition and treatment with: *(443)*
   1. corticosteroids.
   2. antihistamines.
   3. anticholinergics.
   4. antimicrobials.

10. One common source of anxiety for many patients with Guillain-Barré syndrome is impaired: *(445)*
    1. communication.
    2. self-esteem.
    3. circulation.
    4. elimination.

11. In order to reduce the symptoms of Parkinson's disease, L-dopa crosses the blood-brain barrier and is converted to: *(447)*
    1. epinephrine.
    2. dopamine.
    3. norepinephrine.
    4. acetylcholine.

12. Which cranial nerve is tested by asking the patient to swallow on command? *(426)*
    1. Vagus (CN X)
    2. Trigeminal (CN V)
    3. Facial (CN VII)
    4. Glossopharyngeal (CN IX)

13. In myasthenia gravis, rapid improvement of muscle strength after administration of edrophonium chloride (Tensilon) indicates an underlying: *(455)*
    1. hypertensive crisis.
    2. adrenergic crisis.
    3. myasthenic crisis.
    4. cholinergic crisis.

X. **Nursing Care Plan.** Refer to the Nursing Care Plan, The Patient with a Head Injury, p. 440 in the textbook.

1. What is the most reliable indicator of mental status in this patient? *(440)*
   1. Blood pressure
   2. Pulse
   3. Level of consciousness
   4. Pupil quality

2. What is a late sign of increased intracranial pressure, due to pressure on the third cranial nerve? *(440)*
   1. Jerky tracking of eyes
   2. Altered motor function
   3. Dilated pupils
   4. Hemiparesis

3. How high should this patient's bed be raised to prevent increased ICP? *(440)*
   1. 15 degrees
   2. 30 degrees
   3. 45 degrees
   4. 90 degrees

4. What nursing measures are likely to be the most helpful in the management of seizures for this patient? Select all that apply. *(440)*
   1. Keep the patient flat on his back.
   2. Remove any objects that could cause harm.
   3. Call a medical emergency if a generalized tonic-clonic seizure lasts more than 4 minutes
   4. Hold the patient down so that he is not thrashing.
   5. Place a padded tongue blade between his teeth.

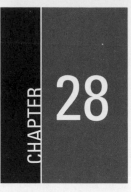

# Cerebrovascular Accident

## OBJECTIVES

1. Discuss the risk factors for cerebrovascular accident (CVA).

2. Identify two major types of CVA.

3. Describe the pathophysiology, signs and symptoms, and medical treatment for each type of CVA.

4. Describe the neurologic deficits that may result from CVA.

5. Explain the tests and procedures used to diagnose a CVA, and nursing responsibilities for patients undergoing those tests and procedures.

6. List data to be included in the nursing assessment of the CVA patient.

7. Assist in developing a nursing process for a CVA patient during the acute and rehabilitation phases.

8. Specify criteria used to evaluate the outcomes of nursing care for the CVA patient.

9. Identify resources for the CVA patient and family.

# LEARNING ACTIVITIES

A. **Key Terms.** Match the definition in the numbered column with the most appropriate term in the lettered column. Not all answers may be used.

1. _____ Inability to speak clearly because of neurologic damage that impairs normal muscle control *(468)*

2. _____ Drooping of the upper eyelid *(477)*

3. _____ Difficulty speaking, reading, and writing *(468)*

4. _____ Double vision *(477)*

5. _____ The inability to understand words or the inability to respond with words, or both *(468)*

6. _____ Loss of half the field of vision; loss is on the side opposite the brain lesion *(469)*

7. _____ Partial inability to initiate coordinated voluntary motor acts *(468)*

8. _____ Ability to speak clearly but without meaning *(468)*

9. _____ Difficulty swallowing *(468)*

10. _____ Paralysis of one side of the body *(468)*

A. Hemiplegia
B. Nonfluent aphasia
C. Dyspraxia
D. Dysarthria
E. Ptosis
F. Homonymous hemianopsia
G. Expressive aphasia
H. Receptive aphasia
I. Aphasia
J. Dysphagia
K. Diplopia

B. **Central Nervous System.** Match the definition or description in the numbered column with the most appropriate term in the lettered column. Some terms may be used more than once, and some terms may not be used.

1. _____ The part of the brain that controls the left side of the body *(460)*

2. _____ The part of the brain that controls the right side of the body *(460)*

3. _____ The part of the brain that controls vital basic functions, including respiration, heart rate, and consciousness *(460)*

4. _____ The part of the brain that coordinates movement, balance, and posture *(461)*

5. _____ The circulatory system in the cerebrum *(460)*

6. _____ The part of the brain that controls analytic mental processes such as language ability, mathematics, and reasoning powers *(460)*

7. _____ The part of the brain that includes the midbrain, pons, and medulla *(460)*

8. _____ The part of the brain that controls emotional and artistic tendencies *(460)*

A. Cerebellum
B. Brainstem
C. Spinal cord
D. Cerebrovascular system
E. Right hemisphere
F. Cerebrum
G. Left hemisphere

C.  **Control Zones of the Brain (figure 28-1, p. 461).**

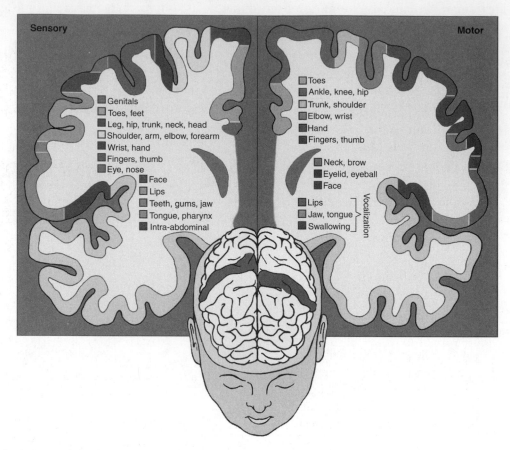

1.  Which part of the brain receives and interprets sensory information? *(460)*
    1.  Frontal lobe
    2.  Parietal lobe
    3.  Occipital lobe
    4.  Temporal lobe

2.  Which part of the cerebrum initiates motor activity for various parts of the body? *(460)*
    1.  Frontal lobe
    2.  Parietal lobe
    3.  Occipital lobe
    4.  Temporal lobe

3.  Which part of the brain controls balance, coordination, and posture? *(461)*
    1.  Frontal lobe
    2.  Cerebellum
    3.  Thalamus
    4.  Cerebrum

4.  Which of the following are signs of a stroke? Select all that apply. *(462)*
    1.  _____    Sudden, severe headache with no known cause
    2.  _____    Sudden trouble seeing
    3.  _____    Tremors of extremities at rest
    4.  _____    Rigidity of movement
    5.  _____    Sudden trouble speaking
    6.  _____    Numbness or weakness of the face, arm, or leg

D. **Types of Stroke (Figure 28-4, p. 467).**

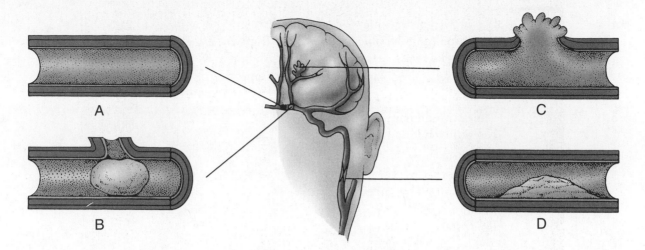

1. _____ Which figure represents blood flowing freely through a normal artery?
2. _____ Which figure represents a thrombotic stroke?
3. _____ Which figure represents a hemorrhagic stroke?
4. _____ Which figure represents an embolic stroke?

E. **Types of Stroke.** Match the definition in the numbered column with the most appropriate term In the lettered column.

1. _____ Caused by cerebral arterial wall rupture *(466)*

    A. Thrombotic stroke
    B. Ischemic stroke
    C. Hemorrhagic stroke

2. _____ Caused by obstruction of blood vessel by plaque, blood clot, or both *(467)*

3. _____ Caused by obstruction forming in blood vessel of the brain *(467)*

F. **Key Terms.** Match the definition or description in the numbered column with the most appropriate term in the lettered column. Some terms may be used more than once, and some terms may not be used.

1. _____ An important warning condition for a possible later stroke *(462)*

2. _____ A buildup of fatty deposits in the blood vessels *(462)*

3. _____ The common name for cerebrovascular accident *(461)*

4. _____ A temporary neurologic deficit caused by impairment of cerebral blood flow *(462)*

5. _____ A "swooshing" noise in a clogged carotid artery that can be auscultated in diagnosing a TIA *(464)*

6. _____ Opening an obstructed blood vessel and removing the plaque *(466)*

A. Bruit
B. Transient ischemic attack (TIA)
C. Angioplasty
D. Stroke
E. Endarterectomy
F. Atherosclerosis

G. **Cincinnati Prehospital Stroke Scale.** Refer to Figure 28-2, p. 471 in the textbook, Cincinnati Prehospital Stroke Scale.

1. What is an abnormal finding when the patient is asked to show teeth or smile? *(471)*

2. What is an abnormal finding when the patient is asked to close both eyes and hold both arms straight out for 10 seconds? *(471)*

3. What are abnormal findings when the patient is asked to repeat a simple phrase, such as "You can't teach an old dog new tricks"? Select all that apply. *(471)*
   1. _____ Uses correct words, but speaks slowly
   2. _____ Slurs words together
   3. _____ Uses the wrong words
   4. _____ Speaks with a lisp
   5. _____ Unable to speak

H. **Nurse's Role in Stroke Prevention.** According to *Healthy People 2010*, what is the role of the nurse in stroke prevention and treatment? Select all that apply. *(463)*

1. _____ Spread the word about risk factors for and warning signs of stroke.

2. _____ Participate in stroke and blood pressure screenings.

3. _____ Engage in and promote physical activity.

4. _____ Assist patients to locate anti-smoking campaigns.

5. _____ Encourage yearly eye exams.

6. _____ Help patients obtain treatment for depression following a stroke.

I. **NIH Stroke Scale.** Refer to Table 28-3, p. 475 in the textbook, NIH Stroke Scale. What variables are assessed in the NIH Stroke Scale? Select all that apply. *(475)*

1. _____ Level of consciousness
2. _____ Visual field testing
3. _____ Motor function of arms
4. _____ Best language
5. _____ Blood pressure
6. _____ Sensory comparison side to side
7. _____ Temperature
8. _____ Pupillary reaction

## MULTIPLE-CHOICE QUESTIONS

J. Choose the most appropriate answer.

1. A folded layer of nerve cells that covers each hemisphere of the brain is called the: *(460)*
   1. cerebellum.
   2. cerebrum.
   3. gyrus.
   4. cortex.

2. One of the most important needs of the acute stroke patient is to be turned and repositioned at least every: *(478)*
   1. 2 hours.
   2. 4 hours.
   3. 8 hours.
   4. 12 hours.

3. Turning and repositioning the stroke patient will reduce the incidence of: *(478)*
   1. hypertension.
   2. skin breakdown.
   3. headache.
   4. cerebral edema.

4. A warning condition for a possible later stroke is: *(462)*
   1. TIA.
   2. paralysis.
   3. hemorrhage.
   4. cyanosis.

5. Which diagnostic test shows narrowing of cerebral blood vessels? *(463)*
   1. CT scan
   2. MRI
   3. EEG
   4. Angiography

6. Diminished or lost sensation in body parts occurs in many stroke patients. The patient who does not feel pressure or pain is susceptible to: *(468)*
   1. injury.
   2. infection.
   3. pneumonia.
   4. dyspnea.

7. Constipation may develop in the stroke patient due to dehydration, drug therapy, and: *(479)*
   1. infection.
   2. cerebral edema.
   3. loss of sensation on one side.
   4. immobility.

8. In the acute phase following a stroke, if the patient has homonymous hemianopsia, the environment is arranged so that the important items are available on the: *(481)*
   1. unaffected side.
   2. affected side.
   3. left side.
   4. right side.

9. The main focus of the rehabilitation phase following a stroke is to: *(480)*
   1. cure the disease process.
   2. assist the patient into remission.
   3. prevent another stroke from occurring.
   4. return the patient to the highest functional level possible.

10. The most frequent cause of death following a stroke is: *(476)*
    1. kidney failure.
    2. pneumonia.
    3. seizure.
    4. heart attack.

11. What (approximate) percentage of individuals who experience a TIA will have a stroke within 5 years? *(463)*
    2. 10%
    3. 20%
    4. 30%
    5. 40%

12. What is a priority problem immediately following a stroke? *(470)*
    1. Oxygenation
    2. Hydration
    3. Nutrition
    4. Thermoregulation

13. What is a common sensory-perceptual problem in a patient with a stroke? *(477)*
    1. Weakness
    2. Paralysis
    3. Diplopia
    4. Dysphagia

14. A patient who does not feel pressure or pain due to lost sensation following a stroke is at risk for: *(478)*
    1. aphasia.
    2. paralysis.
    3. injury.
    4. infection.

15. A patient experiencing a TIA should received full medical attention within: *(463)*
    1. 12 hours.
    2. 24 hours.
    3. 36 hours.
    4. 48 hours.

16. Which term is used to describe speech impaired to the point that the person has almost no ability to communicate? *(468)*
    1. Global aphasia
    2. Expressive aphasia
    3. Receptive aphasia
    4. Nonfluent aphasia

## ALTERNATE FORMAT QUESTIONS

K. Which factors create problems related to physical mobility for a patient with a stroke? Select all that apply. *(468, 469)*
   1. Edema
   2. Dyspraxia
   3. Hypertension
   4. Visual field disturbances
   5. Hemiplegia

L. **Drug Therapy.** Match the uses of drugs in the numbered column with the drugs used for treatment of stroke in the lettered column.

1. _____ Used to treat cerebral edema *(464)*

2. _____ Used to treat hemorrhagic stoke by dilating and preventing spasms in cerebral blood vessels *(463)*

3. _____ Used to reduce intracranial pressure by reducing cerebral inflammation *(464)*

4. _____ Used to prevent strokes caused by thrombi *(465)*

5. _____ Used to dissolve clots that cause acute ischemic stroke *(465)*

6. _____ Used to treat seizures, if seizures are present with stroke *(470)*

7. _____ Used to destroy thrombi *(465)*

A. Anticonvulsants, such as phenytoin and phenobarbital
B. Platelet aggregation inhibitors, such as aspirin
C. Hyperosmotic agents, such as mannitol
D. Streptokinase
E. Calcium channel blockers, such as nimodipine
F. Tissue plasminogen activator (tPA), and rt-PA
G. Corticosteroids

M. **Nursing Care Plan.** Refer to the Nursing Care Plan, The Patient with a Stroke, p. 472 in the textbook. Match the uses of drugs in the numbered column with the drugs used for treatment of stroke in the lettered column. Match the nursing diagnosis for the patient with a stroke in the numbered column with the most appropriate "related to" statement in the lettered column. *(472)*

1. _____ Risk for injury

2. _____ Deficient fluid volume

3. _____ Anxiety

4. _____ Imbalanced nutrition: less than body requirements

5. _____ Altered family processes

6. _____ Impaired verbal communication

7. _____ Impaired physical activity

A. Dysphagia, inability to feed self
B. Loss of function, fear of disability
C. Inadequate intake, dysphagia
D. Weakness, paralysis, impaired balance
E. Paralysis
F. Anticipated need for assistance after discharge
G. Aphasia

N. **Nursing Care Plan.** Refer to the Nursing Care Plan, The Patient with a Stroke, p. 472 in the textbook. In which stage of treatment of a stroke is this patient? *(472)*
1. Acute period
2. Subacute period
3. Rehabilitation phase
4. Primary prevention phase

# CHAPTER 29

# Spinal Cord Injury

---

## OBJECTIVES

1. Explain the impact of spinal cord injury.

2. Describe the diagnostic tests used to evaluate spinal cord injuries and related nursing responsibilities.

3. Explain the physical effects of spinal cord injury.

4. Describe the medical and surgical treatment during the acute phase of spinal cord injury.

5. List the data to be included in the nursing assessment of the patient with a spinal cord injury.

6. Identify nursing diagnoses, goals, interventions, and outcome criteria for the patient with a spinal cord injury.

7. Describe the nursing care for the patient undergoing a laminectomy.

8. State the goals of rehabilitation for the patient with spinal cord injury.

---

## LEARNING ACTIVITIES

A. **Key Terms.** Match the definition in the numbered column with the most appropriate term in the lettered column.

1. _____ Loss of motor and sensory function in all four extremities due to damage to the spinal cord *(491)*

2. _____ Soft, in relation to muscle, lacking tone *(493)*

3. _____ Abnormally exaggerated response of the autonomic nervous system to a stimulus *(493)*

4. _____ Loss of motor and sensory function due to damage to the spinal cord that spares the upper extremities but, depending on the level of the damage, affects the trunk, pelvic, and lower extremities *(491)*

5. _____ Increased muscle tone characterized by sudden, involuntary muscle spasms *(494)*

6. _____ Area of skin supplied by sensory nerve fibers from a single posterior spinal root *(499)*

7. _____ Surrounded with a sheath *(487)*

A. Paraplegia
B. Myelinated
C. Quadriplegia; tetraplegia
D. Dermatome
E. Flaccid
F. Spasticity
G. Autonomic dysreflexia

**B.** Complete the statements in the numbered column with the most appropriate term in the lettered column. Some terms may be used more than once, and some terms may not be used.

1. As spinal shock begins to subside and reflex activity returns, the patient is at risk for _____. *(493)*

2. Cervical injuries below the level of C4 spare the diaphragm, but they can involve the impairment of the _____. *(493)*

3. An immediate, transient response to injury in which reflex activity below the level of the injury temporarily ceases is called _____. *(493)*

4. A very serious and potentially dangerous problem for the patient with a spinal cord injury, which is described as an exaggerated response of the autonomic nervous system in the patient whose injury is at or above the T6 level, is called _____. *(493)*

5. When the abdomen becomes distended and bowel sounds are absent, peristalsis has ceased, this is a condition called _____. *(502)*

A. Spinal shock
B. Respiratory arrest
C. Autonomic dysreflexia
D. Intercostal muscles
E. Ileus
F. Coma

**C.** Match the description in the numbered column with the most appropriate stage in the lettered column. Some stages may be used more than once, and some may not be used. *(496)*

1. _____ When the patient is ready to tackle the work of rehabilitation

2. _____ When the patient is in emotional shock and may express a desire to die

3. _____ When the patient is ready to begin to plan for the future

4. _____ When the patient begins to face the injury and deal with it realistically

5. _____ When the patient becomes aware of the devastating changes that have taken place

6. _____ The stage marked by depression and withdrawal as the patient considers the implications of the injury

A. Impact
B. Denial
C. Acknowledgment
D. Retreat
E. Reconstruction
F. Remediation

**D.** Complete the statements in the numbered column with the most appropriate term in the lettered column. Some terms may be used more than once, and some terms may not be used.

1. Removal of all or part of the posterior arch of the vertebra is called _____. *(505)*

2. The placement of a piece of donor bone, commonly taken from the hip, into the area between the involved vertebrae is called _____. *(505)*

3. Sensory loss is best determined by the use of a _____. *(500)*

4. The surgical procedure that is done to alleviate compression of the spinal cord or nerves is called _____. *(505)*

A. Dermatome chart
B. Immobilization
C. Spinal fusion
D. Proprioception
E. Laminectomy
F. Traction

**E.  Spinal Cord Injury (p. 492).**

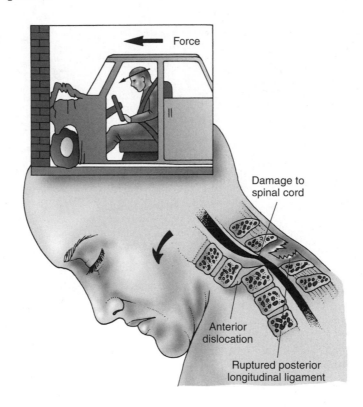

1. Where do most spinal injuries occur? Select all that apply. *(491)*
   1. _____   Cervical
   2. _____   Thoracic
   3. _____   Lumbar
   4. _____   Sacral

2. What is the greatest priority in the acute phase of a spinal cord injury? *(496)*
   1. Keep a patent airway.
   2. Prevent further cord injury.
   3. Preserve cord function.
   4. Immobilize the patient.

3. During the acute phase, what procedure may be done to decrease pressure on the spinal cord? *(497)*
   1. Placement of halo device
   2. Decompressive laminectomy
   3. Placement of Crutchfield tongs
   4. Lumbar puncture

F. Explain why most spinal cord–injured patients can maintain bowel function. *(604)*



G. List three factors that contribute to problems with the integumentary system of the spinal cord–injured patient. *(604)*

   1. _____

   2. _____

   3. _____

H. Explain why the traditional head-tilt–chin-lift method of opening the airway is inappropriate in spinal cord–injured patients. *(604)*



I. Match the nursing diagnosis for the spinal cord–injured patient in the numbered column with the "related to" statements in the lettered column. Some statements may be used more than once. *(498)*

| | | |
|---|---|---|
| 1. _____ Risk for infection | A. | Sensory motor impairment |
| 2. _____ Disturbed sensory perception (kinesthetic, tactile) | B. | Altered body function |
| | C. | Involuntary muscle spasms, lack of motor and sensory function, orthostatic hypotension |
| 3. _____ Ineffective thermoregulation | D. | Skeletal traction pins |
| 4. _____ Self-care deficit (feeding, dressing, grooming) | E. | Overwhelming losses and limited potential for recovered function |
| 5. _____ Sexual dysfunction | F. | Neurologic impairment |
| 6. _____ Dysreflexia | G. | Altered sensory transmission |
| 7. _____ Risk for disuse syndrome | H. | Impaired conduction of impulses |
| 8. _____ Bowel incontinence | I. | Bladder or bowel distention, renal calculi, pressure ulcers |
| 9. _____ Impaired urinary elimination | J. | Pathologic or prescribed immobility, or both |
| 10. _____ Ineffective individual coping | K. | Spinal cord trauma |
| 11. _____ Ineffective breathing patterns | | |
| 12. _____ Risk for injury | | |

## MULTIPLE-CHOICE QUESTIONS

**J.** Choose the most appropriate answer.

1. The halo device is used to provide immobilization and alignment of the: *(497)*
   1. cervical vertebrae.
   2. thoracic vertebrae.
   3. lumbar vertebrae.
   4. sacral vertebrae.

2. For the patient maintained in cervical traction while on a conventional bed, position changes must be accomplished by: *(501)*
   1. assisted ambulation.
   2. range-of-motion exercises.
   3. "log-rolling."
   4. grasping the muscles.

3. Prompt intervention following autonomic dysreflexia (AD) must be directed toward severe: *(502)*
   1. hypertension.
   2. hypotension.
   3. infection.
   4. lung compromise.

4. Patients with skull tongs are maintained on: *(502)*
   1. bed rest with ambulation three times a day.
   2. isolation precautions.
   3. high-roughage diets.
   4. strict bed rest.

5. When the patient has spasticity, nursing management is directed toward the prevention of contractures and: *(502)*
   1. infection.
   2. muscle atrophy.
   3. dyspnea.
   4. heart failure.

6. During the time of flaccid paralysis, the nurse must be diligent in performing: *(502)*
   1. active range-of-motion exercises.
   2. passive range-of-motion exercises.
   3. coughing and deep-breathing exercises.
   4. early ambulation.

7. Following an ileus, the patient will be given oral fluids and food when: *(502)*
   1. the swallow reflex returns.
   2. the patient is no longer anorexic.
   3. bladder continence returns.
   4. peristalsis returns.

8. Using the "Grading Scale for Muscle Strength," the nurse would score a finding of full active range of motion against gravity and resistance as: *(499)*
   1. 1.
   2. 2.
   3. 3.
   4. 5.

9. Which finding is reported to the physician in the postlaminectomy patient? *(505)*
   1. WBC of 7,000
   2. Blood pressure 125/80
   3. Clear drainage from incision site
   4. Respirations of 18

10. Applying pneumatic stockings, assisting patients with ROM exercises, and auscultating breath sounds are done in the postoperative laminectomy patient to promote: *(505)*
    1. tissue perfusion.
    2. resistance to infection.
    3. pain relief.
    4. physical immobility.

11. Which type of spinal cord injury will result in a loss of motor control below the waist? *(494)*
    1. C4
    2. C7
    3. T4
    4. T10

12. Which action is indicated in the management of spasticity in the spinal cord–injured patient? *(502)*
    1. Increase tactile stimuli.
    2. Administer antihypertensive medications.
    3. Perform passive ROM exercises at least four times a day.
    4. Turn and reposition the patient at least every 4 hours.

13. Which procedure is a visualization of the spinal cord and vertebrae through the injection of a radiopaque dye directly into the subarachnoid space of the spinal cord? *(490)*
    1. Myelography
    2. Electromyography
    3. Lumbar puncture
    4. Electroencephalography

14. Injuries at or above C5 may result in instant death because the: *(494)*
    1. innervation to the phrenic nerve is interrupted.
    2. sympathetic innervation to the heart is blocked.
    3. sensory nerves to the brain are interrupted.
    4. saphenous nerve can no longer transmit impulses.

15. The spinal cord–injured patient may have difficulty maintaining body temperature within a normal range because: *(498)*
    1. the hypothalamus can no longer regulate temperature.
    2. regulatory mechanisms of vasoconstriction and sweating are lost.
    3. the peripheral nerves to the skin are interrupted.
    4. the skin is not able to lose heat through evaporation.

16. At the scene of an accident involving a patient with spinal cord injury, emergency personnel will apply a hard cervical collar around the patient's neck to immobilize the: *(496)*
    1. skull.
    2. spinal column.
    3. brain.
    4. upper part of the body.

17. Which type of traction is applied to a fiberglass jacket and is used to immobilize and align the cervical vertebrae and relieve compression of nerve roots? *(496)*
    1. Philadelphia collar
    2. Gardner-Wells tongs
    3. Crutchfield tongs
    4. Halo ring

18. Which condition is an exaggerated sympathetic response to stimuli, such as bladder distention, that produces severe hypertension with the potential for seizures and stroke? *(493)*
    1. Spinal cord injury
    2. Autonomic dysreflexia
    3. Meningitis
    4. Amyotrophic lateral sclerosis

# 30 Acute Respiratory Disorders

---

## OBJECTIVES

1. Identify data to be collected in the nursing assessment of the patient with a respiratory disorder.

2. Identify the nursing implications of age-related changes in the respiratory system.

3. Describe diagnostic tests or procedures for respiratory disorders and nursing interventions.

4. Explain nursing care of patients receiving therapeutic treatments for respiratory disorders.

5. For selected respiratory disorders, describe the pathophysiology, signs and symptoms, complications, diagnostic measures, and medical treatment.

6. Assist in developing a nursing care plan for the patient who has an acute respiratory disorder.

---

## LEARNING ACTIVITIES

A. **Key Terms.** Match the definition in the numbered column with the most appropriate term in the lettered column.

1. _____ Dry, rattling sound caused by partial bronchial obstruction *(514)*

2. _____ Rapid respiratory rate *(528)*

3. _____ Presence of air in the pleural cavity that causes the lung on the affected side to collapse *(514)*

4. _____ Temporary cessation of breathing *(511)*

5. _____ Low oxygen level in body tissues *(513)*

6. _____ Movement of air in and out of the lungs *(528)*

7. _____ Rales; abnormal lung sounds heard on auscultation *(514)*

8. _____ Difficulty breathing when lying down *(511)*

9. _____ Accumulation of blood in the pleural space *(544)*

10. _____ Low level of oxygen in the blood *(524)*

11. _____ Blood flow through blood vessels of tissue *(547)*

12. _____ Collapsed lung or part of a lung *(514)*

13. _____ Difficulty breathing *(511)*

14. _____ Excess carbon dioxide in the blood *(538)*

A.  Atelectasis
B.  Crackles
C.  Dyspnea
D.  Hemothorax
E.  Hypercapnia
F.  Hypoxemia
G.  Hypoxia
H.  Orthopnea
I.  Pneumothorax
J.  Rhonchus
K.  Tachypnea
L.  Tissue perfusion
M.  Ventilation
N.  Apnea

B. **Lower Respiratory Tract.**

1. Using the figure below (Figure 30-1, p. 510), label the structures (A–I). *(510)*

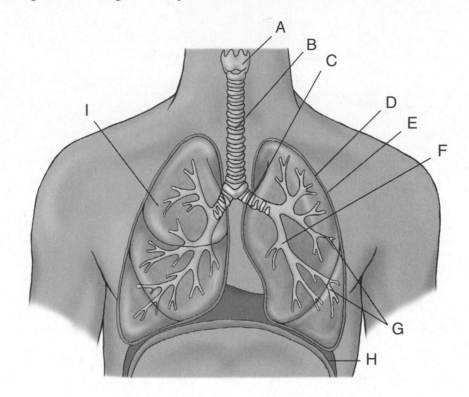

A. _____

B. _____

C. _____

D. _____

E. _____

F. _____

G. _____

H. _____

I. _____

2. How many lobes are in the right and left lungs? *(511)*


3. Which characteristics of the right bronchus explain why foreign bodies from the trachea are more likely to enter the right bronchus than the left bronchus? Select all that apply. *(511)*

   1. _____    The right bronchus is longer.

   2. _____    The right bronchus is wider.

   3. _____    The right bronchus is straighter vertically.

   4. _____    The right bronchus has a greater horizontal slant.

## C.  Age-Related Changes.

1.   Which of the following are age-related changes that occur in the pharynx and the larynx? Select all that apply. *(512)*

    1.   _____     Loss of elasticity of laryngeal muscles
    2.   _____     Louder voice
    3.   _____     Thickening of the voice cords
    4.   _____     Muscle atrophy
    5.   _____     Gravelly voice

2.   Which of the following are age-related changes in the respiratory system? Select all that apply. *(512)*

    1.   _____     Increased lung elasticity
    2.   _____     Enlargement of bronchioles
    3.   _____     Decreased number of functioning alveoli
    4.   _____     Rib cage becomes more rigid
    5.   _____     Diaphragm widens
    6.   _____     Atrophy of respiratory muscles

3.   Which of the following age-related respiratory system changes cause the older adult to be more susceptible to lung infections? Select all that apply. *(512)*

    1.   _____     Decreased work of breathing
    2.   _____     Less effective cough
    3.   _____     Relaxed chest movement
    4.   _____     Diaphragm flattens
    5.   _____     Decreased ability to inhale and exhale

**D.  Diagnostic Procedures.** Match the description of the diagnostic tests and procedures in the numbered column with the most appropriate term in the lettered column. Answers may be used more than once.

1. _____  Detects pulmonary embolism and other obstructive conditions *(516)*

2. _____  Used to visualize abnormalities in the respiratory system *(517)*

3. _____  Aspiration of pleural fluid so that it can be examined for pathogens *(517)*

4. _____  Measures culture and sensitivity of sputum *(520)*

5. _____  Detects alterations in oxygenation status, including alkalosis or acidosis *(520)*

6. _____  Distinguishes malignant from benign cells and evaluates effectiveness of cancer treatment *(518)*

7. _____  Must remain NPO until gag reflex returns *(517)*

8. _____  Report dyspnea and asymmetric chest movement following procedure *(517)*

9. _____  Assure patient that radiation dose is small and that isotope is quickly eliminated *(516)*

10. _____  Apply pressure at the puncture site for 5–10 minutes *(520)*

11. _____  Collect the specimen early in the morning before breakfast *(518)*

A.  Ventilation-perfusion scan (lung scan)
B.  Fiberoptic bronchoscopy
C.  Sputum analysis examination
D.  Arterial blood gas analysis
E.  Thoracentesis
F.  Positive emission tomography (PET) scan

E. **Types of Breathing Patterns.** Refer to Table 30-1, Types of Breathing Patterns, p. 512 in the textbook. Match the descriptions of breathing patterns in the numbered columns with the most appropriate term in the lettered column. *(512)*

1. _____ Respiratory rate faster than 20 breaths/minute

2. _____ Periodic deep breaths (more than three sighs per minute)

3. _____ Regular deep breaths faster than 20 breaths per minute

4. _____ Regular even breaths 12–20 breaths per minute

5. _____ Varying, irregular breaths with sudden periods of apnea

6. _____ Breaths progressively deeper, becoming more shallow, followed by periods of apnea

7. _____ Gradual rise in end-expiratory level with each successive breath

8. _____ Associated with severe brain pathology

9. _____ Causes include fever and pain

10. _____ Associated with emphysema

11. _____ Related to the use of sedatives and narcotics

12. _____ Related to metabolic acidosis, diabetic ketoacidosis, and renal failure

A. Normal
B. Tachypnea
C. Bradypnea
D. Sighing respirations
E. Cheyne-Stokes respirations, apnea
F. Kussmaul's respirations (with hyperventilation)
G. Biot's respirations
H. Obstructive breathing

F.  **Rib Fractures.** List one nursing goal, three outcome criteria, and five nursing interventions for the following nursing diagnosis for the patient with fractured ribs.

*Nursing Diagnosis*

Ineffective breathing pattern related to pain that occurs with ventilation

*Nursing Goal (544)*

1.  _____

*Outcome Criteria (544)*

1.  _____

2.  _____

3.  _____

*Nursing Interventions (545)*

1.  _____

2.  _____

3.  _____

4.  _____

5.  _____

G.  **Pulmonary Embolus.** Which of the following are signs and symptoms of pulmonary embolus (PE)? Select all that apply. *(546)*

1.  _____     Fever and tachycardia

2.  _____     Skin cool and dry

3.  _____     Sudden chest pain

4.  _____     Cough and hemoptysis

5.  _____     Spontaneous onset of chest wall tenderness

H.  **Artificial Airways.** Match the definition or description in the numbered column with the most appropriate term in the lettered column. *(528)*

1.  _____     Tube used with a surgically          A.   Endotracheal tube
                    created opening through       B.   Nasal airway
                    the neck into the trachea     C.   Tracheostomy tube
                                                  D.   Oral airway
2.  _____     Curved tube used to main-
                    tain an airway temporarily

3.  _____     Soft rubber tube inserted
                    through the nose and
                    extended to the base of the
                    tongue

4.  _____     Long tube inserted
                    through the mouth or nose
                    into the trachea

I. **Drug Therapy.** Match the definition or description in the numbered column with the most appropriate term in the lettered column.

1. _____　Suppress cough reflex *(532)*
2. _____　Dry up nasal secretions *(532)*
3. _____　Relax smooth muscle in the bronchial airways and blood vessels *(532)*
4. _____　Kill or inhibit growth of bacteria, viruses, or fungi *(534)*
5. _____　Reduce frequency of acute asthma attacks (not used to stop them after they've started) *(533)*
6. _____　Inhibit allergic response; prevent asthmatic attacks *(533)*
7. _____　Cause constriction of nasal blood vessels and reduce swelling of mucous membranes *(532)*
8. _____　Anti-inflammatory drugs used to treat asthma *(533)*
9. _____　Thin respiratory secretions so that they are more readily mobilized and can be coughed up *(532)*
10. _____　Dissolve clots and used to treat pulmonary emboli *(533)*
11. _____　Reduce thickness of mucus and used to treat bronchitis and asthma *(534)*

A. Decongestants
B. Antitussives
C. Expectorants
D. Antihistamines
E. Mast cell stabilizers
F. Bronchodilators
G. Corticosteroids
H. Leukotriene inhibitors
I. Mucolytics
J. Antimicrobials
K. Thrombolytics

J. **Thoracic Surgery.** Match the definition or description in the numbered column with the most appropriate term in the lettered column.

1. _____　Surgical incision of the chest wall *(530)*
2. _____　Removal of entire lung *(530)*
3. _____　Stripping of the membrane that covers the visceral pleura *(530)*
4. _____　Performed by inserting an endoscope through a small thoracic incision *(531)*
5. _____　Removal of ribs *(530)*
6. _____　Preset amount of oxygenated air delivered during each ventilator breath *(528)*
7. _____　Collapsed alveoli *(519)*

A. Tidal volume
B. Thoracotomy
C. Pneumonectomy
D. Thoracoplasty
E. Atelectasis
F. Decortication of lung
G. Thoracoscopy

**K.  Bronchioles and Alveoli.** Label the structures in the figure below. Refer to Figure 31-1A, p. 551 in your textbook. *(551)*

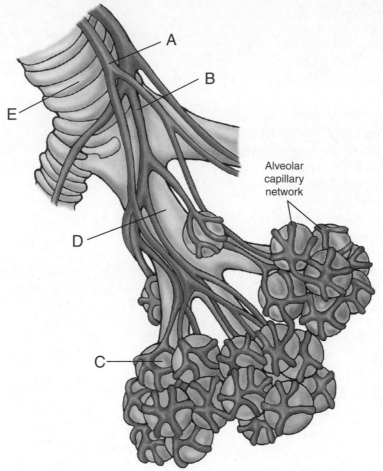

Alveolar
capillary
network

A. _____

B. _____

C. _____

D. _____

E. _____

## MULTIPLE-CHOICE QUESTIONS

**L.**  Choose the most appropriate answer.

1.  Who is at risk for having aspiration pneumonia? *(537)*
    1.  Chronically ill patients
    2.  Patients with tube feedings
    3.  Immunosuppressed patients
    4.  Smokers

2.  To prevent the spread of germs from person to person, a priority "respiratory etiquette" health promotion behavior which nurses should teach is: *(535)*
    1.  a common cold from a viral cause does not require antimicrobial therapy.
    2.  cover your mouth and nose when coughing or sneezing.
    3.  wash your hands with soap and warm water for at least 20 seconds.
    4.  adequate nutrition is available to reduce susceptibility to infectious organisms.

3. For a patient with influenza, which type of drugs must be started within 24–48 hours after the onset of symptoms and continued for 10 days? *(536)*
   1. Antimicrobials
   2. Antifungals
   3. Antivirals
   4. Corticosteroids

4. Which type of influenza vaccine is recommended for adults over the age of 50 and all health care workers? *(536)*
   1. Live vaccine (FluMist)
   2. Inactivated vaccine
   3. First-generation antiviral
   4. Second-generation antiviral

5. What is a common cause of thoracic surgery? *(530)*
   5. Emphysema
   6. Pneumonia
   7. Asthma
   8. Chest injury

6. Which of the following conditions indicates a medical emergency? *(514, 521)*
   1. Pneumothorax
   2. Acute bronchitis
   3. Pleurisy
   4. Pneumonia

7. Which abnormal breath sound is due to fluid accumulation in the alveoli and does not clear with coughing? *(514)*
   1. Wheezes
   2. Rhonchi
   3. Fine crackles
   4. Coarse crackles

8. Chest physiotherapy should be performed:
   1. eight times each day. *(523)*
   2. after meals.
   3. before meals.
   4. at bedtime.

9. The technique of positioning the patient to facilitate gravitational movement of respiratory secretions toward the bronchi and trachea for expectoration is: *(523)*
   1. postural drainage.
   2. chest percussion.
   3. chest vibration.
   4. clapping.

10. If excessive secretions that the patient cannot expectorate accumulate in the oral or nasal airway, what may be required? *(524)*
    1. Spirometry
    2. A lung scan
    3. An MRI
    4. Suctioning

11. What are risks associated with using intermittent positive-pressure breathing (IPPB) treatments? *(527)*
    1. Atelectasis
    2. Respiratory alkalosis
    3. Contamination of fluid reservoir
    4. Bronchospasm

12. With simple oxygen masks for patients, flow rates from the flowmeter should be adjusted to: *(527)*
    1. 1–6 liters/min.
    2. 6–10 liters/min.
    3. 10–12 liters/min.
    4. 15–20 liters/min.

13. Ventilators are most commonly required for patients with: *(528)*
    1. oxygen toxicity.
    2. tachycardia.
    3. hypoxemia.
    4. hyperventilation.

14. The preset amount of oxygenated air delivered during each ventilator breath is called the: *(528)*
    1. vital capacity.
    2. nebulizing dose.
    3. tidal volume.
    4. respiratory rate.

15. The total number of breaths delivered per minute with mechanical ventilation is called the: *(528)*
    1. oxygen level setting.
    2. tidal volume setting.
    3. pressure setting.
    4. respiratory rate setting.

16. What is prescribed to keep the pressure in the lungs above the atmospheric pressure at the end of expiration? *(528)*
    1. The oxygen level setting
    2. The tidal volume setting
    3. Positive end-expiratory pressure (PEEP)
    4. Negative inspiratory pressure

17. Which factor interferes with accurate measurement of the pulse oximeter? *(520)*
    1. Hypotension
    2. Hyperthermia
    3. Vasodilation
    4. Heart rate

18. Which group of people abstain from using tobacco? *(513)*
    1. Greek Orthodox
    2. Protestants
    3. Mormons
    4. Orthodox Jews

19. The primary nursing diagnosis for the patient who has fractured ribs is Ineffective breathing pattern related to: *(544)*
    1. increased sputum production.
    2. ineffective cough.
    3. pain.
    4. atelectasis.

20. Which herb is taken to decrease the duration and severity of a cold? *(537)*
    1. Ginkgo
    2. Ginseng
    3. Kava kava
    4. Echinacea

M. **Nursing Care Plan.** Refer to Nursing Care Plan, The Patient with Pneumonia, p. 539 in your textbook.

1. Which nursing diagnosis should the nurse plan to address first? *(539)*

2. Does this patient exhibit any signs of hypoxemia? *(539)*

3. What nursing action is indicated regarding this patient's temperature? *(539)*

# Chronic Respiratory Disorders

---

## OBJECTIVES

1. Identify examples of chronic inflammatory, obstructive, and restrictive pulmonary diseases.

2. Explain the relationship between cigarette smoking and chronic respiratory disorders.

3. For selected chronic respiratory disorders, describe the pathophysiology, signs and symptoms, complications, diagnostic measures, and medical treatment.

4. Assist in developing a nursing care plan for the patient who has a chronic respiratory disorder.

---

## LEARNING ACTIVITIES

A.  **Key Terms.** Match the definition in the numbered column with the most appropriate term in the lettered column.

1. _____ One of many occupational diseases caused by inhalation of particles of industrial substances *(566)*

2. _____ Permanent dilation of a portion of the bronchi or bronchioles *(561)*

3. _____ A collection of inflammatory cells commonly surrounded by fibrotic tissue that represents a chronic inflammatory response to infectious or noninfectious agents *(566)*

4. _____ A condition characterized by episodes of bronchospasm that causes wheezing and dyspnea; reactive airway disease *(550)*

5. _____ Abnormal accumulation of air in body tissues; in the lung, a disorder characterized by loss of lung elasticity with trapping of air, retained carbon dioxide, and dyspnea *(554)*

6. _____ Inflammation of the lung *(566)*

7. _____ Placement of a radiation source in the body to treat a malignancy *(567)*

8. _____ Bronchial inflammation *(553)*

9. _____ Interstitial fibrosis caused by inhalation of asbestos fibers *(566)*

A.  Granuloma
B.  Asthma
C.  Brachytherapy
D.  Pneumoconiosis
E.  Asbestosis
F.  Bronchiectasis
G.  Pneumonitis
H.  Bronchitis
I.  Emphysema

**B. COPD.** Complete the statement in the numbered column with the most appropriate term in the lettered column. Some terms may be used more than once, and some terms may not be used.

1. Chronic obstructive pulmonary disease (COPD) is characterized as varying combinations of asthma, chronic bronchitis, and _____. *(550)*

2. Constriction of the airways is called _____. *(550)*

3. Severe, persistent bronchospasm is called _____. *(551)*

4. Bronchial inflammation characterized by increased production of mucus and chronic cough that persist for at least 3 months of the year for 2 consecutive years is called _____. *(553)*

5. A degenerative, nonreversible disease characterized by the breakdown of the alveolar walls distal to the terminal bronchioles is _____. *(554)*

6. The term used to describe right-sided heart failure secondary to pulmonary disease is _____. *(554)*

A. Cor pulmonale
B. Acute bronchitis
C. Emphysema
D. Congestive heart failure
E. Bronchospasm
F. Status asthmaticus
G. Chronic bronchitis
H. Status epilepticus

**C. Pulmonary Disorders.** Match the definition or description in the numbered column with the most appropriate term in the lettered column. Some terms may be used more than once, and some terms may not be used.

1. _____ An abnormal dilation and distortion of the bronchi and bronchioles that is usually confined to one lung lobe or segment *(561)*

2. _____ A hereditary disorder that is characterized by dysfunction of the exocrine glands and the production of thick, tenacious mucus *(561)*

3. _____ An infection spread by droplets emitted by infected people during coughing, laughing, sneezing, and singing *(562)*

A. Chronic bronchitis
B. Cystic fibrosis
C. Sarcoidosis
D. Tuberculosis
E. Bronchiectasis

**D. Lung Cancer.** Complete the statements in the numbered column with the most appropriate term in the lettered column. Some terms may be used more than once, and some terms may not be used.

1. The leading cause of lung cancer is
   _____. *(566)*

2. Four types of lung surgery procedures include a wedge resection, segmental resection, pneumonectomy, and _____. *(567)*

3. The four warning signs of lung cancer are recurring pneumonia, chest pain, persistent cough, and _____. *(567)*

4. The four major types of lung cancer are small-cell (oat cell) carcinoma, adenocarcinoma, large-cell carcinoma, and _____. *(566)*

A. Hemoptysis
B. Squamous cell carcinoma
C. Fever
D. Lobectomy
E. Bronchitis
F. Cigarette smoking

**E. Impaired Gas Exchange.** What are signs and symptoms of impending respiratory failure to watch for with patients experiencing impaired gas exchange? Select all that apply. *(553)*

1. _____    Easy bruising

2. _____    Tachypnea

3. _____    Deep respirations

4. _____    Diaphoresis

5. _____    Bradycardia

6. _____    Loss of consciousness

**F. Hypoxemia.** Explain why the red blood cell count is typically elevated in patients with chronic hypoxemia. *(555)*

**G. Oxygen Therapy.** In the treatment of COPD, the initial flow of oxygen is usually 1–3 liters/min. Why are high levels of oxygen not administered to COPD patients? *(556)*

**H. Tuberculosis.** Tuberculosis was a leading cause of death in the United States until effective drugs became available in the 1940s and 1950s. The incidence declined until 1986, when the numbers of reported cases began to rise. Which of the following are reasons for this rise? Select all that apply. *(562)*

1. _____    Development of drug-resistant strains

2. _____    Increased population of people with HIV

3. _____    Increased cigarette smoking population

4. _____    Increased irritating substances in the environment

I.  **Diagnostic Tests for Tuberculosis.** Which diagnostic tests are done to confirm the diagnosis of tuberculosis? Select all that apply. *(562)*

1.  _____ Fiberoptic bronchoscopy

2.  _____ Sputum cultures

3.  _____ Acid-fast smears of body fluids

4.  _____ Tuberculin skin tests

5.  _____ Auscultation of the lungs

6.  _____ Pulmonary function tests

7.  _____ Chest radiographs

J.  **Occupational Lung Disease.** Which of the following are examples of offending substances that may lead to occupational lung diseases? Select all that apply. *(565)*

1.  _____ Bacteria

2.  _____ Fungi

3.  _____ Dust

4.  _____ Chlorine

5.  _____ Asbestos

6.  _____ Coal dust

7.  _____ Viruses

K.  Match the definition in the numbered column with the most appropriate term in the lettered column. Some terms may be used more than once, and some terms may not be used. *(550)*

1.  _____ The patient's ability to inhale or to exhale by force

2.  _____ Vital capacity, inspiratory capacity, expiratory reserve volume, residual volume, and total lung capacity

3.  _____ Measurement of the ability of gases to diffuse across the alveolar capillary membrane

A.  Air flow limitation
B.  Lung volumes
C.  Airway dynamics
D.  Diffusing capacity
E.  Osmosis

L.  Which of the following are increased by cigarette smoking? Select all that apply. *(557)*

1.  _____ Emphysema

2.  _____ Cardiovascular disease

3.  _____ Renal disease

4.  _____ Esophageal reflux

5.  _____ Chronic bronchitis

**M. Pulmonary Disorders.** Match the signs and symptoms in the numbered column with their respective conditions in the lettered column. Some conditions may be used more than once, and some may not be used.

1. _____   Productive cough, exertional dyspnea, and wheezing *(555)*

2. _____   Cough, night sweats, chest pain and tightness, fatigue, and anorexia *(562)*

3. _____   Dyspnea on exertion; may display use of accessory muscles of respiration; barrel chest *(555)*

A.   Emphysema
B.   Chronic bronchitis
C.   Tuberculosis

**N. Nursing Diagnoses/COPD.** Match the nursing diagnosis for the patient with COPD in the numbered column with the "related to" statement in the lettered column. *(558)*

1. _____   Impaired gas exchange
2. _____   Ineffective airway clearance
3. _____   Anxiety
4. _____   Altered nutrition: less than body requirements
5. _____   Risk for infection
6. _____   Activity intolerance
7. _____   Decreased cardiac output

A.   Decreased ciliary action, increased secretions, weak cough
B.   Alveolar destruction, bronchospasm, air trapping
C.   Anorexia, dyspnea
D.   Right-sided heart failure
E.   Increased secretions, weak cough
F.   Inability to meet oxygen needs
G.   Hypoxemia

## MULTIPLE-CHOICE QUESTIONS

**O.** Choose the most appropriate answer.

1.  The basic pathology with asthma is the narrowing of the bronchi or bronchioles as a result of: *(550)*
    1.  dilated smooth muscle around the airways.
    2.  contracted smooth muscle around the airways.
    3.  rapid, shallow respirations.
    4.  slow, deep respirations.

2.  The opening of the airways decreases in size in patients with asthma due to contracted smooth muscle and: *(551)*
    1.  redness.
    2.  increased temperature.
    3.  infection.
    4.  inflammation.

3.  A serious complication of bronchoconstriction is: *(551)*
    1.  hypoxemia.
    2.  hypotension.
    3.  drowsiness.
    4.  headache.

4.  Signs and symptoms of an asthma attack include dyspnea, productive cough, and: *(551)*
    1.  tachycardia.
    2.  bradycardia.
    3.  slow respirations.
    4.  apnea.

5.  The best position for patients with bronchial asthma is: *(552)*
    1.  supine.
    2.  prone.
    3.  side-lying.
    4.  Fowler's.

6. Arterial blood gas findings that should be reported to the physician if they occur in patients with impaired gas exchange include: *(553)*
   1. $PaO_2$ decreases, pH increases.
   2. $PaO_2$ increases, pH increases.
   3. $PaO_2$ decreases, $PaCO_2$ increases.
   4. $PaO_2$ increases, $PaCO_2$ increases.

7. A nasal cannula is preferred over a face mask because the mask may increase the patient's feeling of: *(553)*
   1. insecurity.
   2. safety.
   3. suffocation.
   4. self-esteem.

8. In patients with emphysema, the lungs often become hyperinflated, causing the diaphragm to flatten and increasing the reliance on: *(554)*
   1. coughing and deep-breathing exercises.
   2. accessory muscles for breathing.
   3. extra fluids to thin secretions.
   4. increased heart rate.

9. The most serious complications of COPD are respiratory failure and: *(554)*
   1. kidney failure.
   2. heart failure.
   3. brain hemorrhage.
   4. paralytic ileus.

10. The term *blue bloater* is used to describe patients with: *(555)*
    1. advanced emphysema.
    2. pneumonia.
    3. adult respiratory distress syndrome.
    4. advanced chronic bronchitis.

11. The term *pink puffer* is used to describe patients with emphysema because skin color is likely to be normal because of: *(555)*
    1. normal arterial blood gases.
    2. unlabored respirations.
    3. barrel-chest formation.
    4. normal body temperature.

12. The most reliable diagnostic test for COPD is: *(555)*
    1. the chest radiograph.
    2. an MRI.
    3. the pulmonary function test.
    4. the CBC (complete blood count).

13. Drugs that are ordered to decrease airway resistance and the work of breathing for patients with COPD are called: *(556)*
    1. vasoconstrictors.
    2. diuretics.
    3. calcium channel blockers.
    4. bronchodilators.

14. The preferred route of administration of bronchodilator drugs for patients with COPD is by: *(556)*
    1. mouth.
    2. inhalation.
    3. intramuscular injection.
    4. intravenous injection.

15. During the physical examination of patients with COPD, the nurse observes the neck for: *(555, 557)*
    1. edema.
    2. distended veins.
    3. enlarged lymph nodes.
    4. cyanosis.

16. Because good hydration helps to thin secretions in patients with impaired gas exchange, what is the recommended daily fluid intake? *(553)*
    1. 600–800 ml
    2. 1000–1500 ml
    3. 2500–3000 ml
    4. 4000–5000 ml

17. The feeling of not being able to breathe is frightening; in addition, feelings of restlessness and anxiety are increased in the asthma patient due to decreased: *(553)*
    1. arterial oxygen.
    2. arterial carbon dioxide.
    3. heart rate.
    4. respiratory rate.

18. During the physical examination of patients with COPD, the thorax is inspected for the classic: *(557)*
    1. pink color.
    2. blue tinge.
    3. pulmonary edema.
    4. barrel-chest shape.

19. The patient with COPD is monitored for signs and symptoms of airway obstruction, which include tachycardia, abnormal breath sounds, and: *(560)*
    1. headache.
    2. oliguria.
    3. constipation.
    4. dyspnea.

20. Patients with COPD are encouraged to drink extra fluids each day in order to: *(560)*
    1. improve urinary output.
    2. increase circulation.
    3. liquefy secretions.
    4. prevent kidney stones.

21. The work of breathing is increased with COPD, which in turn increases the patient's: *(560)*
    1. caloric requirements.
    2. requirements for calcium.
    3. requirements for sodium.
    4. dietary roughage requirements.

22. The recommended diet for the patient who is dyspneic is a soft diet with: *(560)*
    1. three large meals.
    2. a low-protein emphasis.
    3. a low-calorie emphasis.
    4. frequent, small meals.

23. If the COPD patient becomes excessively dyspneic or develops tachycardia during activity, the patient should: *(560)*
    1. increase the activity slowly.
    2. stop the activity.
    3. sit down briefly and then resume activity.
    4. drink a full glass of water.

24. Patients with chronic bronchitis and emphysema are at risk for heart failure and decreased cardiac output; the nurse monitors for signs of heart failure, which include increasing dyspnea, dependent edema, and: *(561)*
    1. bradycardia.
    2. tachycardia.
    3. increased urine output.
    4. dehydration.

25. A persistent, productive cough with bloody sputum (hemoptysis) is a common symptom of: *(562)*
    1. emphysema.
    2. cystic fibrosis.
    3. sinusitis.
    4. tuberculosis.

26. The most common preventive drug therapy for tuberculosis is: *(563)*
    1. prednisone.
    2. isoniazid.
    3. gamma globulin.
    4. aminophylline.

27. The patient who is thought to have active tuberculosis is isolated at first. Which of the following is *not* necessary related to the care of the patient? *(564)*
    1. good handwashing
    2. wearing masks
    3. wearing gowns
    4. standard precautions

## ALTERNATE FORMAT QUESTIONS

P. 1. Which of the following problems develop when status asthmaticus is not treated? Select all that apply. *(551)*
    1. Pneumothorax
    2. Acidosis
    3. Right-sided heart failure
    4. Renal failure
    5. Liver failure

2. Which complications occur when severe, persistent bronchospasm is not treated? Select all that apply. *(551)*
   1. Constriction of bronchial smooth muscle
   2. Thickening of airway tissues
   3. Air trapping in the alveoli
   4. Hypoinflation of the lungs

**Q. Nursing Care Plan.** Refer to the Nursing Care Plan, The Patient with Chronic Obstructive Pulmonary Disease, p. 558 in the textbook.

1. What is the most important risk factor of this patient for the development of chronic bronchitis and emphysema? *(558)*

2. What signs and symptoms of COPD does this patient exhibit? Select all that apply. *(558)*
   1. Fatigue
   2. Orthopnea
   3. Productive cough
   4. Clear sputum
   5. Normal respiratory rate
   6. Bluish skin color
   7. Pursed-lip breathing
   8. Barrel-shaped thorax

3. Why do you monitor this patient for peripheral edema? *(558)*

4. Which signs of heart failure would you be monitoring? Select all that apply. *(558)*
   1. Increasing dyspnea
   2. Increasing urine output
   3. Bradycardia
   4. Dependent edema

5. What are the most serious complications of COPD? Select all that apply. *(558)*
   1. Renal failure
   2. Liver failure
   3. Respiratory failure
   4. Heart failure

6. Which of the following are characteristics of emphysema? Select all that apply. *(558)*
   1. Bullae are formed between the alveolar spaces.
   2. Lungs becomes hypoinflated.
   3. Respiratory bronchiole walls break down.
   4. Alveolar walls enlarge and break down.
   5. Ruptured blebs cause the lung to collapse.

7. What is the priority nursing diagnosis for this patient? *(558)*

8. What tasks for this patient could be assigned to unlicensed assistive personnel? Select all that apply. *(558)*
   1. Monitor vital signs and arterial blood gases.
   2. Assist to comfortable high Fowler's position in bed.
   3. Observe respiratory status before and after use of bronchodilator.
   4. Encourage 2500–3000 mL of fluid daily.
   5. Provide comfort measures.
   6. Identify stressors in addition to hypoxemia.
   7. Provide pleasant environment for meals.
   8. Monitor sputum color and body temperature.
   9. Monitor for signs of heart failure, especially peripheral edema.
   10. Assist with oral hygiene.

# Hematologic Disorders

---

## OBJECTIVES

1.   List the components of the hematologic system and describe their role in oxygenation and hemostasis.

2.   Identify data to be collected when assessing a patient with a disorder of the hematologic system.

3.   Describe tests and procedures used to diagnose disorders of the hematologic system and nursing considerations for each.

4.   Describe nursing care for patients undergoing common therapeutic measures for disorders of the hematologic system.

5.   For selected disorders of the hematologic system, describe the pathophysiology, signs and symptoms, medical diagnosis, and medical treatment.

6.   Assist in planning nursing care for a patient with a disorder of the hematologic system.

---

## LEARNING ACTIVITIES

A.  **Key Terms.** Match the definition in the numbered column with the most appropriate term in the lettered column.

1. _____   Person with type AB-positive blood who can receive transfusions with any type of blood because all the common antigens (A, B, and Rh) are present in the blood *(578)*

2. _____   A purplish skin lesion resulting from blood leaking outside the blood vessels *(576)*

3. _____   A reduction in the number of red blood cells or in the quantity of hemoglobin *(581)*

4. _____   A small (1–3 mm) red or reddish-purple spot on the skin resulting from blood capillaries breaking and leaking small amounts of blood into the tissues *(575)*

5. _____   A primary function of the hematologic system *(571)*

6. _____   Person with type O-negative blood who can donate blood to anyone because none of the common antigens are present in the blood *(578)*

7. _____   Changes in blood pressure and pulse as person moves from lying to sitting to standing positions *(574)*

8. _____   Red or reddish-purple skin lesions 3 mm or more in size that result from blood leaking outside of the blood vessels *(576)*

9. _____   Control of bleeding *(571)*

A.   Anemia
B.   Oxygenation
C.   Ecchymosis
D.   Orthostatic vital sign changes
E.   Petechia
F.   Purpura
G.   Universal donor
H.   Universal recipient
I.   Hemostasis

B.  **Red Blood Cell Disorders.** Match the definition in the numbered column with the appropriate red blood cell disorder in the lettered column. Answers may be used more than once.

1.  _____  Results from complete failure of bone marrow *(582)*

2.  _____  Condition in which too many red blood cells are produced *(582)*

3.  _____  Occurs when a person does not absorb vitamin $B_{12}$ from the stomach *(583)*

4.  _____  A genetic disease carried on a recessive gene *(582)*

5.  _____  Person often has a ruddy (reddish) complexion *(582)*

6.  _____  Symptoms include headache, dizziness, ringing in the ears, and blurred vision *(582)*

7.  _____  Person has high bilirubin levels in the blood *(583)*

8.  _____  Symptoms include fatigue, severe pain, and cardiomegaly *(584)*

9.  _____  Blood becomes more viscous and does not circulate freely through the body *(582)*

10.  _____  May be caused by drugs (such as streptomycin and chloramphenicol) and exposure to toxic chemicals and radiation *(582, 583)*

11.  _____  Symptoms include weakness, sore tongue, and numbness of hands or feet *(583)*

12.  _____  Misshapen red blood cells become fragile and rupture easily *(583)*

13.  _____  Symptoms include fatigue, shortness of breath, hypotension, and jaundice *(583)*

14.  _____  Bone marrow makes adequate amounts of blood cells, but they are destroyed once they are released into the circulation *(583)*

15.  _____  Symptoms include pallor, extreme fatigue, tachycardia, shortness of breath, bleeding, and frequent infections *(582)*

16.  _____  Results from diet low in iron or inability of the body to absorb enough iron from GI tract *(583)*

A.  Autoimmune hemolytic anemia
B.  Aplastic anemia
C.  Polycythemia vera
D.  Pernicious anemia
E.  Sickle cell anemia
F.  Iron deficiency anemia

C.  **Anemia.** Which of the following are ways the body compensates when a person is anemic with chronic blood loss? Select all that apply. *(582)*

1. _____   Increased heart rate
2. _____   Decreased respiratory rate
3. _____   Blood redistributed toward the skin
4. _____   Increased production of erythropoietin

D.  **Thrombocytopenia.** Which of the following are signs and symptoms of thrombocytopenia? Select all that apply. *(587)*

1. _____   Petechiae
2. _____   Gingival bleeding
3. _____   Fever
4. _____   Orthostatic hypotension
5. _____   Epistaxis
6. _____   Purpura

E.  **Coagulation Disorders.** Match the descriptions in the numbered column with the appropriate type of coagulation disorder in the lettered column. Answers may be used more than once. *(587)*

1. _____   Diagnosis is made with blood tests and bone marrow biopsy

2. _____   Treatment may include platelet transfusions

3. _____   Causes include cancer chemotherapy and radiation

4. _____   Diagnosis is made with prothrombin time (PT) and partial thromboplastin time (PTT)

5. _____   Secondary disorder to another pathologic process, such as sepsis, shock, burns, or obstetric complications

6. _____   Treated with transfusion of fresh frozen plasma or cryoprecipitate

7. _____   Hypercoagulable state with thrombosis and hemorrhage

8. _____   Genetic disease in which a person lacks blood-clotting factors normally found in the plasma

9. _____   Diagnosis is made with factors VIII and IX

A.  Thrombocytopenia
B.  Disseminated intravascular coagulation (DIC)
C.  Hemophilia

**F.** **Commonly Transfused Blood Products.** Refer to Table 32-1, Commonly Transfused Blood Products, p. 579 in the textbook. Match the indications for use of blood components in the numbered column on the left with the actual drug component in the lettered column on the right. *(579)*

1. _____ Used for clotting deficiencies, hemophilia, for rapid reversal of warfarin (Coumadin) effects, and with massive red blood cell transfusions

2. _____ Used for symptoms related to low hematocrit or hemoglobin such as shortness of breath, tachycardia, decreased blood pressure, chest pain, lightheadedness, and fatigue

3. _____ Used for hemophilia A and DIC

4. _____ Used for bleeding from thrombocytopenia

A. Platelets
B. Cryoprecipitate
C. Packed red blood cells (PRBC)
D. Fresh frozen plasma (FFP)

**G. Drug Therapy.** Refer to Drug Therapy 32-1, Drugs Used to Treat Disorders of the Hematologic System, p. 582 in the textbook. Match the drug action and the appropriate nursing intervention in the numbered column with the name of the drug in the lettered column. Answers may be used more than one time. *(582)*

1. _____  Replaces iron
2. _____  Stimulates the bone marrow to produce red blood cells
3. _____  Intramuscular injection; must be given every month for the rest of the person's life
4. _____  Have the patient take the drug with food but not with milk, or caffeinated drinks because the milk and caffeine inhibit drug absorption; if the patient is taking a liquid form, dilute the drug and administer through a straw to prevent the drug from staining the teeth
5. _____  May be given by intravenous or subcutaneous injection; patient is usually treated three times per week until the hematocrit is 30–33
6. _____  Test dose before starting treatment; give intramuscular injections only in the upper outer quadrant of the buttock using the Z-track technique

A.   Vitamin B$_{12}$
B.   Ferrous sulfate
C.   Epoietin alfa
D.   Iron dextran

## MULTIPLE-CHOICE QUESTIONS

**H.** Choose the most appropriate answer.

1. A condition in which there are too many blood cells is called: *(582)*
   1. pernicious anemia.
   2. aplastic anemia.
   3. hemolytic anemia.
   4. polycythemia vera.

2. The treatment for autoimmune hemolytic anemia is: *(583)*
   1. vitamin B$_{12}$ injections.
   2. a ferrous sulfate and high-iron diet.
   3. an iron dextran and high-carbohydrate diet.
   4. corticosteroids and blood transfusions.

3. The treatment for aplastic anemia is: *(583)*
   1. vitamin B$_{12}$ injections.
   2. a ferrous sulfate and high-iron diet.
   3. an iron dextran and high-carbohydrate diet.
   4. transfusions, antibiotics, and corticosteroids.

4. Treatment for sickle cell crisis includes: *(584)*
   1. a ferrous sulfate and high-iron diet.
   2. an iron dextran and high-carbohydrate diet.
   3. aggressive intravenous hydration and IV morphine.
   4. corticosteroids and transfusions.

5. For each unit of packed RBCs transfused, the patient's hemoglobin should increase approximately: *(578)*
   1. 10 g/dL.
   2. 5 g/dL.
   3. 3 g/dL.
   4. 1 g/dL.

6. Red or reddish-purple spots 3 mm or larger that are the result of blood vessels breaking are: *(576)*
   1. petechiae.
   2. purpura.
   3. ecchymoses.
   4. nodes.

7. Patients with low red blood cell counts may have: *(576)*
   1. bradycardia.
   2. hypotension.
   3. bleeding problems.
   4. tachycardia.

8. If a patient with anemia is orthostatic and tilt-positive, which should be increased? *(575)*
   1. Carbohydrates
   2. Fiber
   3. Fluids
   4. Vitamins

9. Once blood is picked up from the blood bank, the transfusion should be started within: *(580)*
   1. 5 minutes.
   2. 20 minutes.
   3. 30 minutes.
   4. 2 hours.

10. Platelets are generally administered when a patient's platelet count drops below: *(580)*
    1. 10,000/mm³.
    2. 15,000/mm³.
    3. 20,000/mm³.
    4. 300,000/mm³.

11. If platelets are ordered before a procedure such as a lumbar puncture or endoscopy to prevent postprocedure bleeding, the platelets should be administered: *(580)*
    1. 1 week before the procedure.
    2. 1 day before the procedure.
    3. 6 hours before the procedure.
    4. immediately before the procedure.

12. The treatment for hemophilia is: *(587)*
    1. plasma and cryoprecipitate transfusions.
    2. red blood cell transfusions and antibiotics.
    3. white blood cell transfusions and potassium.
    4. platelet and anticoagulant transfusions.

13. Symptoms of thrombocytopenia include: *(587)*
    1. fatigue and pallor.
    2. petechiae and purpura.
    3. nausea and vomiting.
    4. tachycardia and palpitations.

14. Treatment for thrombocytopenia includes: *(587)*
    1. red blood cell transfusions and iron.
    2. white blood cell transfusions and antibiotics.
    3. platelet transfusions.
    4. cryoprecipitate transfusions and anticonvulsants.

15. The condition in which a person has too few platelets circulating in the blood is called: *(587)*
    1. leukemia.
    2. anemia.
    3. lymphoma.
    4. thrombocytopenia.

16. Four types of blood transfusion reactions include hemolytic, circulatory overload, febrile, and: *(581)*
    1. thrombocytopenic.
    2. anaphylactic.
    3. anemic.
    4. leukopenic.

17. Feverfew, garlic, and ginkgo are herbs that affect: *(575)*
    1. wound healing.
    2. blood clotting.
    3. resistance to infection.
    4. kidney function.

18. What is the role of the spleen related to the hematologic system? *(571)*
    1. Produces platelets
    2. Manufactures clotting factors
    3. Removes old blood cells from circulation
    4. Synthesizes vitamins

19. How many liters of blood circulating through the body does a healthy adult have? *(571)*
    1. 2 liters
    2. 6 liters
    3. 10 liters
    4. 24 liters

20. What is the most common site for a bone marrow biopsy? *(577)*
    1. Posterior iliac crest
    2. Sternum
    3. Femur
    4. Tibia

21. What is a term used to describe the series of events that occur in the process of blood clotting? *(572)*
    1. Anticoagulation
    2. Hemostasis
    3. Hemolysis
    4. Coagulation cascade

## ALTERNATE FORMAT QUESTIONS

I.  1. Which of the following bone marrow sites produce the majority of red blood cells and platelets? Select all that apply. *(571)*
       1. Humerus
       2. Sternum
       3. Pelvis

    2. Which of the following functions of the liver are related to hematologic functions? Select all that apply. *(571)*
       1. Manufactures red blood cells
       2. Manufactures clotting factors
       3. Clears red blood cells from the circulation
       4. Stores glucose in the form of glycogen
       5. Aids in phagocytosis of bacteria

    3. Which of the following are antigens found on the cell membranes of red blood cells? Select all that apply. *(572)*
       1. A antigens
       2. B antigens
       3. AB antigens
       4. O antigens
       5. Rhesus (Rh) antigens
       6. pH antigens

    4. Which of the following are types of blood transfusion reactions? Select all that apply. *(581)*
       1. Hemolytic
       2. Anaphylactic
       3. Febrile
       4. Circulatory overload
       5. Anemic

    5. Which of the following are nursing actions for the patient at risk for injury from low red blood cell counts? Select all that apply. *(578)*
       1. Allow for rest between periods of activity.
       2. Elevate the patient's head on pillows to reduce shortness of breath.
       3. Administer analgesics as prescribed.
       4. Decrease daily fluid intake.
       5. Increase food intake of iron.

6. Which of the following are nursing actions for the patient at risk for injury from bleeding? Select all that apply. *(579)*
   1. Avoid intramuscular injections.
   2. Use a soft-bristled toothbrush.
   3. Avoid foods high in vitamin D.
   4. Avoid the use of suppositories.

7. Which of the following foods are high in iron content? Select all that apply. *(575)*
   1. Fish
   2. Dark green vegetables
   3. Red meats
   4. Beans
   5. Pasta
   6. Rice

8. The nurse is collecting data from a patient with a hematologic disorder. What characteristics may be indicative of an underlying hematologic disorder? Select all that apply. *(573)*
   1. Kussmaul respirations
   2. Easy bruising
   3. Elevated temperature
   4. Chronic fatigue
   5. Periods of unusually long bleeding
   6. Hypertension

9. Which of the following manifestations might indicate a hematologic problem in a patient? Select all that apply. *(573)*
   1. Severe headache
   2. High fever
   3. Changes in vision
   4. Epistaxis
   5. Heart palpitations
   6. Chest pain
   7. Joint pain
   8. Kidney pain
   9. Cold intolerance
   10. Fatigue
   11. Dyspnea
   12. Bradypnea

J. **Nursing Care Plan.** Refer to the Nursing Care Plan, The Patient in Sickle Cell Crisis, p. 585 in the textbook.

1. What data has been collected about this patient that indicates sickle cell crisis? *(585)*

2. What patient problem should the nurse address first when she is admitted to the emergency department? *(585)*
   1. Acute pain
   2. Risk for injury related to orthostatic hypotension
   3. Risk for deficient fluid volume
   4. Anxiety related to hospitalization

3. What changes in the heart occur as her body tries to compensate for persistently low red blood cell counts? *(585)*

4. Which of the following are signs and symptoms related to stressors that can trigger a sickle cell crisis? Select all that apply. *(586)*
   1. Infection
   2. Dehydration
   3. Overexertion
   4. Edema
   5. Hot weather changes
   6. Smoking
   7. High-fat diet

5. What causes the pain in sickle cell anemia? *(584)*

6. What are probable causes of the fever this patient has? *(584)*

7. How long do sickle cell crises typically last? *(584)*

8. What is commonly prescribed for pain relief during a sickle cell crisis? *(584)*

9. Why is aggressive IV hydration indicated during sickle cell crisis? *(584)*

10. Why should you pay special attention to the temperature of this patient? *(585)*

11. What is a common fear in patients with sickle cell crisis? *(586)*

# Immunologic Disorders

---

## OBJECTIVES

1. List the components of the immune system and describe their role in innate immunity, acquired immunity, and tolerance.

2. List the data to be collected when assessing a patient with a disorder of the immune system.

3. Describe the tests and procedures used to diagnose disorders of the immune system and nursing considerations for each.

4. Describe the nursing care for patients undergoing common therapeutic measures for disorders of the immune system.

5. Describe the pathophysiology, signs and symptoms, medical diagnosis, and medical treatment for selected disorders of the immune system.

6. Assist in developing a nursing care plan for a patient with a disorder of the immune system.

---

## LEARNING ACTIVITIES

**A. Key Terms.** Match the definition or description in the numbered column with the most appropriate term in the lettered column.

1. _____    Resistance to or protection from a disease *(594)*

2. _____    Certain white blood cells (neutrophils, monocytes, and macrophages) that engulf and destroy invading pathogens, dead cells, and cellular debris *(594)*

3. _____    Class of fatty acids that regulates vasodilation, temperature elevation, white blood cell activation, and other physiologic processes *(594)*

4. _____    Freely circulating Y-shaped antigen-binding protein produced by B lymphocytes and plasma cells *(593)*

5. _____    Disease-causing microorganism *(591)*

6. _____    A substance, usually a protein, that is capable of stimulating a response from the immune system *(592)*

7. _____    Defensive system that is operational at all times, consisting of anatomic and physiologic barriers, the inflammatory response, and the ability of certain cells to phagocytose invaders *(594)*

8. _____    Defensive response by $T_C$ cells aimed at intracellular defects such as viruses and cancer *(594)*

9. _____    Antibody-mediated or cell-mediated response that is specific to a particular pathogen and is activated when needed *(594)*

A.   Acquired immunity
B.   Antibody
C.   Antibody-mediated immunity
D.   Antigen
E.   Cell-mediated immunity
F.   Compromised Host Precautions
G.   Eicosanoid
H.   Immunity
I.   Immunoglobulin
J.   Innate immunity
K.   Leukemia
L.   Pathogen
M.   Phagocytes

10. _____ Defensive response by B cells assisted by T$_H$ cells, aimed at invading microorganisms such as bacteria *(594)*

11. _____ Membrane-bound, Y-shaped binding protein produced by B lymphocytes; called *antibody* when released from the cell membrane *(593)*

12. _____ Actions taken to help protect patients with low white blood cell counts from infection *(603)*

13. _____ Cancer of the white blood cells in which the bone marrow produces too many immature white blood cells *(603)*

B. **Immune System.** Match the organ in the numbered column with its function in the lettered column.

1. _____ Lymph nodes *(591)*
2. _____ Bone marrow *(591)*
3. _____ Spleen *(592)*
4. _____ Thymus *(592)*

A. Participate(s) in the maturation of T lymphocytes
B. Act(s) as filter to remove microorganisms from the lymph fluid before it returns to the blood
C. Filter(s) and destroy(s) microorganisms in the blood
D. Produce(s) white blood cells

C. **White Blood Cells.** Match the type of white blood cell in the numbered column with its function in the lettered column. *(593)*

1. _____ Basophils
2. _____ B lymphocytes
3. _____ Neutrophils
4. _____ Monocytes
5. _____ Eosinophils
6. _____ Mast cells
7. _____ T lymphocytes

A. Called *macrophages* when they enter tissue; powerful phagocytes
B. Initiate inflammatory response; circulate in blood and release histamine
C. Fight bacterial infections; most numerous type of the white blood cells
D. Combat parasitic infections; associated with allergies
E. Manufacture immunoglobulins and stimulate the production of antibodies
F. Store histamine; located in body tissues
G. Secrete cytokines, facilitating body's immune system

**D. Immunoglobulins.** Match the definition or description in the numbered column with the appropriate type of immunoglobulin in the lettered column. *(593)*

1. _____    Present in secretions such as mucus and mother's milk

    A.   IgG
    B.   IgM
    C.   IgA
    D.   IgE

2. _____    First immunoglobulin to be secreted during the primary immune response to an antigen

3. _____    Secreted during secondary immune response and is specific to a particular antigen

4. _____    Attaches to cell membranes of basophils and mast cells, where it triggers the cell to release histamine

**E. Immunity.** Match the definition or description in the numbered column with the most appropriate term in the lettered column. *(594)*

1. _____    Process of ingesting and digesting invading pathogens, dead cells, and cellular debris

    A.   Acquired immunity
    B.   Innate immunity
    C.   Tolerance
    D.   Phagocytosis
    E.   Antibody-mediated immunity
    F.   Cell-mediated immunity

2. _____    Process of self-recognition that occurs as part of normal neonatal growth and development

3. _____    Response initiated when IgM immunoglobulins on the surface of B lymphocytes detect a foreign antigen

4. _____    System activated only when needed in response to a specific antigen; can be antibody-mediated or cell-mediated

5. _____    Response aimed at intracellular defects caused by viruses and cancer; responsible for delayed hypersensitivity reactions and transplant organ tissue rejection

6. _____    System that consists of anatomic and physiologic barriers, inflammatory response, and action of phagocytic cells

F. **Lines of Defense.** Explain how the following anatomic and physiologic barriers function as the body's first line of defense. *(594)*

1. Skin: _____

2. Sweat glands: _____

3. GI and GU mucosae: _____

4. Respiratory and gastrointestinal secretions: _____

G. **Immunity.** Match the definition or description in the numbered column with the appropriate immunity type in the lettered column. Some answers may be used more than once. *(594)*

1. _____ Defense systems present at birth

2. _____ Initiated when the IgM immunoglobulins on the surface of B lymphocytes detect a foreign antigen

3. _____ Defense systems specific to a particular pathogen

4. _____ Anatomic and physiologic barriers, inflammatory response, and phagocytic ability of certain cells

5. _____ Occurs when an antibody produced by a person is transferred to another person

6. _____ Occurs when a person produces his or her own antibodies in response to a pathogen

7. _____ Occurs when a person receives a vaccination

8. _____ Permanent type of immunity

9. _____ Primary component is $T_C$ cells, which recognize foreign antigens in cells

10. _____ Immunity responsible for delayed hypersensitivity reactions

11. _____ Immunity aimed at invading microorganisms such as bacteria

12. _____ Immunity lasts only 1–2 months after antibodies have been received

13. _____ Immunity responsible for rejection of transplanted tissue

14. _____ Occurs when a person has an infection and produces his or her own antibodies

15. _____ Immunity obtained by babies through breast milk

16. _____ Immunity aimed at intracellular defects caused by viruses and cancer

17. _____ Immunity obtained from gamma globulin injections given to people exposed to hepatitis

A. Innate immunity
B. Acquired immunity
C. Antibody-mediated immunity
D. Cell-mediated immunity
E. Active acquired antibody immunity
F. Passive acquired antibody immunity

**H. Systemic Lupus Erythematosus.** Which of the following are symptoms of systemic lupus erythematosus (SLE)? Select all that apply. *(607)*

1. _____   Characteristic rash
2. _____   Easy bruising
3. _____   Photosensitivity with exposure to sunlight
4. _____   Arthritis
5. _____   Proteinuria
6. _____   Petechiae
7. _____   Hematologic disorder, such as leukopenia

**I.   Shift to the Right.** List two conditions that may cause a "shift to the right" on a CBC. *(607)*

1. _____

2. _____

**J.   Diagnostic Procedures.** Match the diagnostic test in the numbered column with the disease or disorder it is used to diagnose in the lettered column. Answers may be used more than once.

1. _____   Serum protein electropho-          A.   Malignant lymphoid tissue
                 resis *(603)*                      B.   Hodgkin's disease
2. _____   Antinuclear antibody test          C.   Hypersensitivities
                 *(597)*                             D.   Leukemia
                                                     E.   Multiple myeloma
3. _____   Gallium scan *(600)*                F.   SLE
4. _____   Urine protein electropho-
                 resis *(603)*
5. _____   Bone marrow biopsy *(603)*
6. _____   Lymphangiography *(600)*
7. _____   Liver-spleen scan *(600)*
8. _____   Skin tests *(600, 601)*

**K.  Bone Marrow Transplants.** Which of the following are indications for bone marrow transplant? Select all that apply. *(599)*

1. _____   Thrombocytopenia
2. _____   High doses of chemotherapy
3. _____   High doses of radiation therapy
4. _____   Hypersensitivity reaction
5. _____   Aplastic anemia

**L. Bone Marrow Transplants.** Match the definition or description of bone marrow transplants in the numbered column with the appropriate type of transplant in the lettered column. Answers may be used more than once.

1. _____ Requires a matched donor *(599)*

2. _____ Procedure in which a patient's own bone marrow is returned to the patient *(599)*

3. _____ Procedure in which colony-stimulating factors are administered to the patient to stimulate the bone marrow to produce white blood cells *(600)*

4. _____ Procedure that reduces the duration of neutropenia *(601)*

5. _____ Best option for patients with a solid tumor that has not metastasized to the bone marrow, such as patients with breast cancer or lymphoma *(599)*

6. _____ Following harvesting of stem cells through apheresis, the patient is treated with chemotherapy and radiation therapy *(601)*

7. _____ Type of transplant that has been done the longest *(599)*

8. _____ Used to restore bone marrow function in patients with leukemia *(599)*

9. _____ Newest type of transplant, which is becoming the most common type *(599)*

10. _____ High doses of chemotherapy and radiation therapy are given to destroy bone marrow, followed by bone marrow transfusion from a human leukocyte antigen (HLA) donor to restore bone marrow function *(599)*

11. _____ Procedure in which a patient's own bone marrow is harvested before chemotherapy and radiation therapy *(600)*

A. Allogeneic bone marrow transplant
B. Autologous bone marrow transplant
C. Peripheral blood stem cell transplant

**M. Complications.** Which of the following are major complications of bone marrow and peripheral blood stem cell transplants? Select all that apply. *(601)*

1. _____    Hemorrhage
2. _____    Infection
3. _____    Shock
4. _____    Thrombocytopenia
5. _____    Graft-versus-host disease

**N. Neutropenia.** Which are causes of neutropenia? Select all that apply. *(602)*

1. _____    Decreased bone marrow production
2. _____    Chemotherapy
3. _____    Hypersensitivity reactions
4. _____    Radiation therapy
5. _____    Autoimmune reactions

**O. Leukemia.** Explain why a patient with leukemia may have signs of anemia, such as fatigue, paleness, tachycardia, and tachypnea. *(607)*

**P. Nursing Diagnoses/Leukemia.** Which are common nursing diagnoses for patients with acute leukemia? Select all that apply. *(604)*

1. _____    Risk for injury
2. _____    Risk for acute confusion
3. _____    Impaired oral mucous membrane
4. _____    Urinary retention
5. _____    Imbalanced nutrition
6. _____    Fatigue

**Q.** Match the definition or description in the numbered column with the appropriate immune system disorder in the lettered column.

1. _____    Cancer of the white blood cells *(603)*
2. _____    Cancer of the lymph system staged as low-, intermediate-, or high-grade *(599)*
3. _____    Cancer of the lymph system characterized by the presence of Reed-Sternberg cells in the lymph nodes *(592)*
4. _____    Cancer of the plasma cells in the bone marrow *(603)*
5. _____    Autoimmune disease that affects multiple organs *(606)*
6. _____    Retrovirus *(608)*

A.   HIV infection
B.   Hodgkin's disease
C.   Leukemia
D.   Non-Hodgkin's lymphoma
E.   Multiple myeloma
F.   SLE

**R.** Match the example of an antigen in the numbered column with the appropriate classification of hypersensitivity reaction in the lettered column. Answers may be used more than once. *(605-606)*

1. _____ Autoimmune reactions
2. _____ Contact dermatitis
3. _____ Tuberculin skin testing
4. _____ SLE
5. _____ Insect stings
6. _____ Pollen
7. _____ Organ transplant cells; transplanted graft rejection
8. _____ Blood transfusion cells; mismatched blood transfusion
9. _____ Dust

A. Type I immediate hypersensitivity reaction mediated by IgE
B. Type II immediate hypersensitivity reaction mediated by antibodies
C. Type III immediate hypersensitivity reaction resulting in tissue damage
D. Type IV delayed hypersensitivity reaction

**S. HIV Infection.** Explain why patients with HIV infection are at increased risk for cancer. *(607)*




**T. Compromised Host Precautions.** Refer to GB 33-2 in the textbook. List 16 nursing actions for the patient at risk for injury from infection related to compromised host precautions in the following areas. *(607)*

1. Handwashing: _____

2. Hematopoietic growth factors: _____

3. Vital signs: _____

4. Invasive procedures: _____

5. Aseptic technique: _____

6. Stethoscope and thermometer use: _____

7. Staff use of masks: _____

8. Cleaning tabletops, equipment, and floor: _____

9. Personal hygiene of patient: _____

10. Cough and deep-breathe: _____

11. Dietary concerns: _____

12. Scheduling of patient appointments: _____

13. Patient's use of masks: _____

14. Flowers and plants: _____

15. Use of humidifiers: _____

16. Patient teaching: _____

**U.  Lymphatic System.** Using the figure below (Figure 33-1, p. 592), label the parts of the lymphatic system. *(592)*

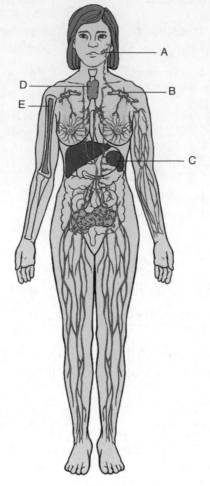

A.  _____

B.  _____

C.  _____

D.  _____

E.  _____

## MULTIPLE-CHOICE QUESTIONS

**V.**  Choose the most appropriate answer.

1.  The body's defense network against infection is the: *(591)*
    1.  cardiovascular system.
    2.  respiratory system.
    3.  immune system.
    4.  circulatory system.

2.  Which filters microorganisms from the lymph fluid before it is returned to the bloodstream? *(591)*
    1.  Thymus
    2.  Bone marrow
    3.  Spleen
    4.  Lymph node

3.  The body's first line of defense is: *(594)*
    1.  skin and inflammation.
    2.  phagocytosis and kidney.
    3.  blood vessels and kidney.
    4.  skin and mucous membranes.

4. Which is responsible for delayed hypersensitivity reactions and rejection of transplanted tissue? *(594)*
   1. Humoral immunity
   2. Interferon immunity
   3. Cell-mediated immunity
   4. Antibody-mediated immunity

5. What is the priority nursing diagnosis for a patient with acute leukemia? *(604)*
   1. Fatigue
   2. Imbalanced nutrition
   3. Risk for injury
   4. Ineffective therapeutic regimen management

6. The most numerous white blood cells are the: *(592)*
   1. neutrophils.
   2. basophils.
   3. lymphocytes.
   4. eosinophils.

7. Interferon, interleukin, and erythropoietin are examples of: *(593)*
   1. lymphocytes.
   2. immunoglobulins.
   3. cytokines.
   4. eicosanoids.

8. A class of fatty acids that regulates vasodilation, temperature elevation, white blood cell activation, and other immune processes includes: *(594)*
   1. cytokines.
   2. eicosanoids.
   3. lymphocytes.
   4. neutrophils.

9. Substances that make the antigen more recognizable to neutrophils, monocytes, and macrophages are: *(593)*
   1. eicosanoids.
   2. eosinophils.
   3. antibodies.
   4. cytokines.

10. When there is a breakdown of tolerance, what types of diseases occur? *(594)*
    1. Autoimmune
    2. Viral
    3. Bacterial
    4. Cancers

11. Rheumatoid arthritis, SLE, Graves' disease, ITP, and type 1 diabetes mellitus are examples of what type of disease? *(594, 595)*
    1. Lymphoma
    2. Pyrogenic
    3. Allergic
    4. Autoimmune

12. The body's ability to determine self from nonself is called: *(594)*
    1. tolerance.
    2. phagocytosis.
    3. immunity.
    4. inflammation.

13. A "shift to the left" on a CBC indicates that more than 60% of white blood cells are: *(597)*
    1. lymphocytes.
    2. basophils.
    3. eosinophils.
    4. neutrophils.

14. A blood test that detects antibodies present in the blood that may indicate autoimmune disorders is: *(597)*
    1. complete blood count (CBC).
    2. Western blot test.
    3. antinuclear antibody test.
    4. T cell counts.

15. Which diagnostic procedure is done to detect and identify microorganisms in blood? *(598)*
    1. Western blot
    2. Viral load
    3. Complete blood count (CBC)
    4. Blood culture

16. The function of colony-stimulating factors (CSFs) is to stimulate the: *(593)*
    1. bone marrow to produce more blood cells.
    2. heart to increase the force of contraction.
    3. kidney to promote the reabsorption of water.
    4. bronchi of the lung to dilate.

17. A complication of allogeneic bone marrow transplants in which T lymphocytes in the transplanted bone marrow identify the patient's tissue as foreign and try to destroy the patient's tissues is: *(601)*
    1. hepatic veno-occlusive disease.
    2. graft-versus-host disease.
    3. renal insufficiency.
    4. thrombocytopenia.

18. A condition that puts a patient at increased risk of infection is: *(602)*
    1. anemia.
    2. thrombocytopenia.
    3. eosinophilia.
    4. neutropenia.

19. A cancer of the white blood cells in which the bone marrow produces too many immature WBCs is: *(603)*
    1. Hodgkin's disease.
    2. non-Hodgkin's lymphoma.
    3. leukemia.
    4. multiple myeloma.

20. Which disease is related to myelogenous and lymphocytic types? *(603)*
    1. Leukemia
    2. SLE
    3. HIV infection
    4. Hodgkin's disease

21. The leading cause of death in people with leukemia is: *(604)*
    1. cardiac arrest.
    2. infection.
    3. hemorrhage.
    4. shock.

22. Which change in vital signs may indicate sepsis, a common complication of leukemia? *(604)*
    1. Tachycardia
    2. Dyspnea
    3. Hypertension
    4. Decreased temperature

23. The reason pus may not be seen even though infection is present in a patient with leukemia is that patients with leukemia do not have normal: *(604)*
    1. platelets.
    2. red blood cells.
    3. white blood cells.
    4. cytokines.

24. When a patient's absolute neutrophil count falls below 1000/mm$^3$, what precautions are instituted? *(603)*
    1. Enteric precautions
    2. Droplet precautions
    3. Compromised Host Precautions
    4. Transmission-based precautions

25. A common finding in patients with leukemia is a hematocrit below 30 and hemoglobin below 10 g/dL, indicating the condition of: *(605)*
    1. anemia.
    2. thrombocytopenia.
    3. leukopenia.
    4. sepsis.

26. What minimizes the chance of the recipient's immune system attacking the transplanted organ? *(608)*
    1. Administration of steroids
    2. Tissue matching of donor to recipient
    3. Administration of antibiotics
    4. Administration of platelets

27. Exaggerated immune responses that are uncomfortable and potentially harmful are: *(605)*
    1. hypersensitivity reactions.
    2. bacterial lung infections.
    3. tachycardiac reactions.
    4. peripheral neuropathy reactions.

28. What presents the greatest risk to patients with leukemia? *(603)*
    1. Hemorrhage
    2. Anemia
    3. Infection
    4. Fatigue

## OBJECTIVES

1. Describe the history of HIV/AIDS.

2. Explain the pathophysiology and etiology of HIV infection.

3. List risk factors associated with HIV infection.

4. Identify complications associated with HIV infection.

5. Identify criteria for diagnosis of AIDS.

6. Name the major HIV drugs, indications, side effects, and nursing considerations.

7. Describe appropriate nursing care of the HIV/AIDS patient.

## LEARNING ACTIVITIES

A.  **Stages of HIV Infection.** Match the description in the numbered column with the stage of HIV infection in the lettered column. Answers may be used more than once. *(614)*

1. _____    Stage in which the virus begins to replicate

2. _____    Stage which ends in death, usually within 1 year

3. _____    Patient experiences generalized flu-like symptoms

4. _____    Patient experiences opportunistic infections

5. _____    Stage in which virus is inactive in host cells

6. _____    Patient is asymptomatic

7. _____    Stage which lasts 4 to 8 weeks

8. _____    Stage which lasts up to 1 year

9. _____    Stage which lasts 2–12 years

10. _____   Stage which lasts 2–3 years

11. _____   Stage in which virus levels are high in the lymph nodes but low in the blood

12. _____   Stage in which the patient is considered to have AIDS

A.  First stage (initial stage)
B.  Second stage (latent stage)
C.  Third stage
D.  Fourth stage

B.  **Signs and Symptoms.** Which are common signs and symptoms of HIV infection? Select all that apply. *(615)*

1. _____    Heart palpitations

2. _____    Abdominal pain

3. _____    Fever

4. _____    Night sweats

5. _____    Swollen lymph nodes

C.  **Major Complications.** Which of the following are major complications of HIV infection? Select all that apply. *(615)*

1. _____    Hemorrhage

2. _____    Opportunistic infections

3. _____    Weight loss

4. _____    Edema

5. _____    Dementia

6. _____    Malnutrition

D. **Wasting Syndrome.** Which factors contribute to the wasting syndrome experienced by patients with HIV infection? Select all that apply. *(615)*

1. _____ Liver disorder

2. _____ Kidney failure

3. _____ Malabsorption of nutrients

4. _____ Reduced food intake

E. **Cancers with HIV Infection.** List four types of cancers that may occur in 40% of patients with HIV infection. *(615)*

1. _____

2. _____

3. _____

4. _____

F. **Transmission of HIV.** How is HIV transmitted? Select all that apply. *(611)*

1. _____ Saliva

2. _____ Breast milk

3. _____ Semen

4. _____ Urine

5. _____ Blood

6. _____ Vaginal fluids

7. _____ Tears

8. _____ Sweat

G. **Toxoplasmosis.** Which of the following are teaching points for patients with toxoplasmosis? Select all that apply. *(616)*

1. _____ Avoid dark green vegetables

2. _____ Avoid undercooked raw meats

3. _____ Practice good handwashing

4. _____ Prevent dehydration

5. _____ Avoid cat litter boxes

6. _____ Avoid ingestion of potentially contaminated water

**H. Opportunistic Infections.** Match the description in the numbered column with the opportunistic infection complication in the lettered column. Answers may be used more than once.

1. _____ People become infected by ingesting contaminated, undercooked meats or vegetables *(616)*

2. _____ Main symptom is severe, persistent, watery diarrhea *(616)*

3. _____ Second leading cause of death among AIDS patients *(616)*

4. _____ Occurs in about 80% of HIV patients *(617)*

5. _____ Mainly transmitted by blood and body fluids through unprotected sex *(618)*

6. _____ Infection starts with primary outbreak, then latency and possible reactivation later *(618)*

7. _____ Fungal infection with symptom of thrush *(617)*

8. _____ Symptoms include shortness of breath upon exertion, fever, and a nonproductive cough *(616)*

A. Candidiasis
B. *Pneumocystis carinii* pneumonia
C. Herpes simplex
D. Cytomegalovirus
E. Toxoplasmosis
F. Cryptosporidiosis

**I. Oncologic Conditions.** Match the description in the numbered column with the oncological condition in the lettered column. Answers may be used more than once. *(619)*

1. _____ Appears as a macular, painless, nonpruritic skin lesion

2. _____ Hypoxia may occur when respiratory system is affected

3. _____ A fever for more than 2 weeks is a symptom

4. _____ Protected sex is the only means of prevention

5. _____ Diagnosis by CT scan and lumbar puncture

A. Kaposi's sarcoma
B. Lymphoma

**J.  Drug Therapy.** Which are common side effects of highly active antiretroviral therapy (HAART) therapy? Select all that apply. *(620)*

1. _____  Decreased triglycerides

2. _____  Increased cholesterol

3. _____  Nausea and vomiting

4. _____  Peripheral neuropathy

5. _____  Easy bruising

**K.  Drug Therapy.** Match the description in the numbered column with the correct drug(s) used to treat patients with HIV infection in the lettered column. Refer to Drug Therapy, p. 621 in the textbook. *(621)*

1. _____  Used in patients with HIV to slow the replication and progression of HIV by interfering with HIVE replication inside the CD4 cell.

2. _____  Used in patients with HIV to slow the replication and progression of HIV by blocking an enzyme so that the infected cell cannot produce any more HIV proteins.

A.  Nucleoside reverse transcriptase inhibitors (AZT, Retrovir)

B.  Protease inhibitors (Invirase, Norvir)

C.  Non-nucleoside reverse-transcriptase inhibitors (Viramune)

**L.  Diagnostic Procedures.** Which of the following diagnostic tools are included in the examination of patients with HIV? Select all that apply. *(624)*

1. _____  CD4 count

2. _____  HIV viral load

3. _____  CBC

4. _____  Lipid profile

5. _____  Electrolyte screen

6. _____  BUN

7. _____  Toxoplasmosis antibody titers

**M.  Nutrition.** Which are nutrition teaching points for the patient with HIV? Select all that apply. *(624)*

1. _____  Thoroughly cook meats and poultry

2. _____  Thaw frozen foods at room temperature

3. _____  Eat small frequent meals high in lactose

4. _____  Eat meals low in fat

**N.**  Explain why patients with HIV infection are at increased risk for cancer. *(608)*

**O. Diagnostic Bloodwork.** List four types of diagnostic bloodwork that may aid in the diagnosis of HIV infection. Select all that apply. *(614, 619, 623)*

1. _____     ELISA

2. _____     Western blot

3. _____     PTT

4. _____     T cell count

5. _____     Viral load count

6. _____     Lipid profile

**P. Nursing Diagnoses.** Which are common nursing diagnoses for patients with HIV infection? Select all that apply. *(622)*

1. _____     Risk for aspiration

2. _____     Anxiety

3. _____     Risk for injury

4. _____     Fluid volume excess

5. _____     Imbalanced nutrition

6. _____     Urinary stress incontinence

7. _____     Impaired oral mucous membranes

## MULTIPLE-CHOICE QUESTIONS

**Q.** Choose the most appropriate answer.

1. What is the leading cause of death in people with AIDS? *(622)*
   1. Kaposi's sarcoma
   2. Malnutrition
   3. Pneumonia
   4. Encephalopathy

2. About how long after infection does the body produce enough antibodies to be detected by standard HIV testing? *(614)*
   1. 2–3 days
   2. 1 week
   3. 12 weeks
   4. 6 months

3. Which substances remain at high levels throughout the course of HIV infection? *(614)*
   1. HIV antibodies
   2. CD8 cells
   3. CD4 cells
   4. Red blood cells

4. What is one of the major reasons for noncompliance among patients receiving HAART therapy? *(622)*
   1. Muscle weakness
   2. Nightmares
   3. Gastrointestinal upset
   4. Hypersensitivity reactions

5. Antiviral medications are given to patients with HIV infection to: *(618)*
   1. prevent viral replication and destroy infected cells.
   2. destroy viral cells that are infected.
   3. slow viral replication and progression.
   4. destroy bacteria and prevent infection.

6. Which test for HIV infection is the most reliable diagnostic test? *(619)*
   1. ELISA
   2. Western Blot
   3. CD4 count
   4. CD8 count

7. How many newly diagnosed HIV infections occur annually in the United States? *(611)*
   1. 20,000
   2. 42,000
   3. 100,000
   4. 540,000

8. Which drug is used to treat opportunistic fungal infections in people with HIV infection? *(616)*
   1. AZT
   2. Retrovir
   3. Amphotericin B
   4. Bactrim

9. Which opportunistic infection is treated with Bactrim and Pentamidine? *(616)*
   1. *Pneumocystis carinii* pneumonia
   2. Candidiasis
   3. Histoplasmosis
   4. Cytomegalovirus

10. What is the usual combination of drugs for HIV patients who are started on the medication regimen called HAART? *(620)*
    1. Antimicrobials and protease inhibitor
    2. Nucleoside reverse transcriptase inhibitors (NRTIs) and protease inhibitor
    3. NRTIs and non-nucleoside reverse transcriptase inhibitors (NNRTs)
    4. Antimycotics and NNRTs

11. What is the most serious problem with HAART therapy? *(620)*
    1. Resistance
    2. Hypolipidemia
    3. Renal failure
    4. Infection

12. HIV gradually destroys cells that are essential for resisting pathogens; these cells are called: *(614)*
    1. neutrophils.
    2. T4 cells.
    3. B cells
    4. eosinophils

13. HIV is passed from person to person primarily through: *(611)*
    1. air droplet contact.
    2. hand-to-mouth contact.
    3. exposure to boldily fluids.
    4. mouth-to-mouth contact.

14. During the later stages, symptoms of HIV include fever, night sweats, anorexia, and: *(615)*
    1. edema.
    2. hypertension.
    3. confusion.
    4. weight loss.

15. The leading cause of death in people with AIDS is: *(616)*
    1. herpes zoster.
    2. dermatitis.
    3. pneumonia.
    4. Kaposi's sarcoma.

16. For many women, one of the first symptoms of HIV infection is: *(617)*
    1. vaginal candidiasis.
    2. burning on urination.
    3. menstrual irregularities.
    4. hemorrhoids.

17. A type of skin cancer that has dramatically increased as a result of AIDS is: *(619)*
    1. *Pneumocystis carinii* pneumonia.
    2. melanoma.
    3. Kaposi's sarcoma
    4. venereal warts.

18. The medical treatment of HIV infection includes the use of zidovudine (AZT, Retrovir), which is given to: *(621)*
    1. cure AIDS.
    2. prevent transmission to sexual partners.
    3. treat the secondary infections of AIDS.
    4. slow the progress of AIDS.

19. Drugs such as clindamycin, Pentamidine, and Bactrim are used to: *(616)*
    1. prevent or treat opportunistic infections.
    2. slow the progress of AIDS.
    3. decrease the dermatitis associated with AIDS.
    4. increase T4 lymphocytes.

20. The best way to prevent transmission of HIV is to: *(625)*
    1. use condoms during all sexual contact.
    2. wash hands thoroughly following contact with HIV-positive people.
    3. avoid risk behaviors.
    4. get plenty of rest and eat a nutritious diet.

21. The risk of transmission of HIV increases with: *(614)*
    1. donating blood.
    2. unprotected sex.
    3. hugging and kissing.
    4. using restrooms.

22. The transmission of HIV can occur through: *(611)*
    1. saliva.
    2. sweat.
    3. urine.
    4. blood.

23. The patient with AIDS is at high risk for opportunistic infections because of: *(616)*
    1. altered skin integrity.
    2. increased HIV antibodies.
    3. decreased CD4 cells.
    4. fatigue.

24. Patients with AIDS may have disturbed thought processes due to: *(622)*
    1. anxiety.
    2. dementia.
    3. anemia.
    4. brain damage.

25. The nurse can show support for patients with HIV infection by being sensitive, courteous, and: *(625)*
    1. reassuring.
    2. positive.
    3. accepting.
    4. authoritarian.

26. As the number of CD4 cell counts decreases, the patient becomes increasingly susceptible to: *(619)*
    1. myelosuppression.
    2. anemia.
    3. tuberculosis.
    4. opportunistic infections.

27. Which are tissues that can be infected by HIV? *(617)*
    1. Pancreas
    2. Stomach
    3. Kidney
    4. Lymph nodes

**R.  Nursing Care Plan.** Refer to Nursing Care Plan, The Patient with HIV Infection, p. 623 in the textbook.

1. What is the priority nursing diagnosis for this patient with HIV infection? *(623)*

2. Which nursing interventions for this patient could be assigned to unlicensed assistive personnel? Select all that apply. *(623)*
    1. Advise patient of the kinds of side and adverse effects that she might experience.
    2. Explain the importance of continuing the drugs under medical supervision.
    3. Discuss ways to conserve energy.
    4. Assist patient with ambulation.
    5. Weigh weekly.
    6. Assist with oral hygiene.

# Cardiac Disorders

---

## OBJECTIVES

1. Label the major parts of the heart.

2. Describe the flow of blood through the heart and coronary vessels.

3. Name the elements of the heart's conduction system.

4. State the order in which normal impulses are conducted through the heart.

5. Explain the nursing considerations for patients having procedures to detect or evaluate cardiac disorders.

6. Identify nursing implications for common therapeutic measures, including drug, diet, or oxygen therapy; pacemakers and cardioverters; cardiac surgery; and cardiopulmonary resuscitation.

7. For selected cardiac disorders, explain the pathophysiology, risk factors, signs and symptoms, complications, and treatment.

8. List the data to be obtained in assessing the patient with a cardiac disorder.

9. Assist in developing nursing care plans for patients with cardiac disorders.

---

## LEARNING ACTIVITIES

**A. Key Terms.** Match the definition or description in the numbered column with the most appropriate term in the lettered column.

1. _____ Slow heart rate, usually defined as fewer than 60 beats per minute (bpm) *(633)*

2. _____ Rapid heart rate, usually defined as greater than 100 bpm *(633)*

3. _____ Abnormal thickening and hardening of the arterial walls caused by fat and fibrin deposits *(653)*

4. _____ Obstruction of a blood vessel with a blood clot transported through the bloodstream *(655)*

5. _____ A sound heard on auscultation of the heart that usually indicates turbulent blood flow across heart valves *(633)*

6. _____ Abnormal thickening, hardening, and loss of elasticity of the arterial walls *(652)*

7. _____ The amount of blood in a ventricle at the end of diastole; the pressure generated at the end of diastole *(631)*

8. _____ Disturbance of rhythm; arrhythmia *(655)*

9. _____ Study of the movement of blood and the forces that affect it *(661)*

10. _____ A heartbeat that is strong, rapid, or irregular enough that the person is aware of it *(632)*

11. _____ Fainting *(632)*

12. _____ The amount of resistance the ventricles must overcome to eject the blood volume *(631)*

13. _____ Backward flow *(670)*

14. _____ Death of myocardial tissue caused by prolonged lack of blood and oxygen supply *(654)*

15. _____ Passage of blood through the vessels of an organ *(648)*

A.   Murmur
B.   Thromboembolism
C.   Hemodynamics
D.   Regurgitation
E.   Syncope
F.   Atherosclerosis
G.   Bradycardia
H.   Perfusion
I.   Preload
J.   Myocardial infarction
K.   Palpitation
L.   Tachycardia
M.   Afterload
N.   Arteriosclerosis
O.   Dysrhythmia

B. **Cardiac Function.** Match the definition or description in the numbered column with the most appropriate term in the lettered column.

1. _____ The delivery of a synchronized electric shock to the myocardium to restore normal sinus rhythm *(650)*

2. _____ Place where electrical impulse is initiated in heart *(629)*

3. _____ Terminal ends of bundle branches that cause ventricles to contract *(629)*

4. _____ The amount of blood (measured in liters) ejected by each ventricle per minute *(631)*

5. _____ Adaptations made by the heart and circulation to maintain normal cardiac output *(660)*

6. _____ The ability of a cell to generate an impulse without external stimulation *(641)*

7. _____ The ability of cardiac muscle to shorten and contract *(631)*

8. _____ Enlargement of existing cells, resulting in increased size of an organ or tissue *(661)*

9. _____ A wall that divides a body cavity *(627)*

10. _____ Termination of fibrillation, usually by electric shock *(670)*

11. _____ Contraction phase of the cardiac cycle *(631)*

12. _____ The ability of the cell to transmit electrical impulses rapidly and efficiently to distant regions of the heart *(629)*

13. _____ Formation of a blood clot *(655)*

14. _____ Relaxation phase of the cardiac cycle *(631)*

A. Cardiac output
B. Systole
C. Conductivity
D. SA node
E. Compensation
F. Defibrillation
G. Contractility
H. Cardioversion
I. Diastole
J. Hypertrophy
K. Purkinje fibers
L. Thrombosis
M. Septum
N. Automaticity

C. **Cardiac Innervation.** Indicate whether each of the following functions of the heart are (A) increased or (B) decreased by the sympathetic and parasympathetic nervous systems. *(631)*

1. Heart rate

    _____    Sympathetic

    _____    Parasympathetic

2. Speed of conduction through the AV node

    _____    Sympathetic

    _____    Parasympathetic

3. Force of contractions

    _____    Sympathetic

    _____    Parasympathetic

D. **Preload.** List two factors that increase preload and three factors that decrease preload. *(631)*

1. Increase preload: _____

2. Decrease preload: _____

E. **Age-Related Changes.** Indicate the age-related changes in:

1. Density of heart muscle connective tissue: *(631)* _____

2. Elasticity of myocardium: *(631)* _____

3. Cardiac contractility: *(631)* _____

4. Valves: *(631)* _____

5. Emptying of chambers: *(631)* _____

6. Number of pacemaker cells in the SA node: *(631)* _____

7. Number of nerve fibers in ventricles: *(631)* _____

8. Cardiac response to stress: *(632)* _____

F. **Age-Related Changes.** Indicate age-related changes to blood vessels for the areas listed below. *(632)*

1. Elastic fibers: _____

2. Systolic blood pressure: _____

3. Pulse pressure: _____

4. Veins: _____

**G. Diagnostic Blood Tests.** Match the characteristic of laboratory tests in the numbered column with the appropriate test in the lettered column. Some terms may be used more than once, and some may not be used.

1. _____ Indicates the body's ability to defend itself against infection and inflammation; elevated with acute myocardial infarction (AMI) *(640)*

2. _____ Determines ability of the blood to carry oxygen from the lungs to the tissues and carbon dioxide from the tissues to the lung *(640)*

3. _____ Percentage of packed RBCs in the total sample of whole blood *(640)*

4. _____ Measurement of main component of the RBCs whose function is to transport oxygen to the cells *(640)*

5. _____ Measurement of formed elements in the blood needed for coagulation *(640)*

6. _____ Indicates damage to myocardial cells *(639)*

7. _____ Protein found in cardiac muscle *(640)*

8. _____ Determination of body's ability to maintain acid-base balance *(638)*

A. Lipid profile
B. Erythrocyte sedimentation rate
C. Hematocrit
D. WBC
E. Arterial blood gas
F. RBC
G. Hemoglobin
H. Platelet
I. Creatine phosphokinase (CPK)
J. Myoglobin

**H. Referred Pain.** The pain of heart problems may radiate or may be referred to other areas. List three areas to which pain may radiate. *(655)*

1. _____

2. _____

3. _____

**I. Drug Therapy.** Match the drug classification in the numbered column with its use and action in the lettered column.

1. _____ Diuretics *(647)*

2. _____ Antianginals *(641)*

3. _____ Antiplatelets *(647)*

4. _____ Cardiac glycosides *(641)*

5. _____ Thrombolytics *(647)*

A. Increase cardiac output
B. Dissolve clots
C. Prevent strokes
D. Decrease fluid retention
E. Relieve pain

**J.   Drug Therapy.** Which of the following drugs are used to treat angina? Select all that apply. *(654)*

1. _____    Antidysrhythmics
2. _____    Nitrates
3. _____    Beta-adrenergic blockers
4. _____    Antiplatelets
5. _____    Calcium channel blockers
6. _____    Diuretics

**K.   Anginal Pain.** Which of the following are words that patients with stable angina use to describe anginal pain? Select all that apply. *(653)*

1. _____    Burning
2. _____    Squeezing
3. _____    Aching
4. _____    Dull
5. _____    Vise-like
6. _____    Smothering

**L.   Treatment/PTCA.** What are reasons that percutaneous transluminal coronary angioplasty (PTCA) may be a preferred treatment over bypass surgery? Select all that apply. *(657)*

1. _____    Done under local anesthesia instead of general anesthesia
2. _____    Less invasive than bypass surgery
3. _____    Faster recovery time
4. _____    Tiny holes are drilled in the myocardium using a laser

**M.   Mitral Stenosis.** Which findings would the nurse expect to observe in patients with mitral stenosis? Select all that apply. *(671)*

1. _____    Bradycardia
2. _____    Tachypnea
3. _____    Increasing pulse pressure
4. _____    Jugular vein distention
5. _____    Wheezing lung sounds
6. _____    Rumbling, low-pitched murmur sounds

N.  **Heart Chambers.** Match the characteristic in the numbered column with the appropriate heart chamber in the lettered column. Some chambers may be used more than once, and some chambers may not be used.

1.  _____ Contains the highest pressure in the heart *(628)*

2.  _____ Receives blood through the tricuspid valve *(627)*

3.  _____ Cone-shaped, has the thickest muscle mass of the four chambers *(628)*

4.  _____ Receives blood saturated with oxygen from the four pulmonary veins *(628)*

5.  _____ Receives blood from the inferior and superior vena cava *(627)*

A.  Right atrium (RA)
B.  Right ventricle (RV)
C.  Left atrium (LA)
D.  Left ventricle (LV)

O.  **Cardiac Function.** Indicate whether each of the following factor(s) (A) increases or (B) decreases preload, contractility, or afterload. *(631)*

1.  Dehydration, hemorrhage, and venous vasodilation _____ preload.

2.  Increased venous return to the heart and overhydration _____ preload.

3.  Catecholamines _____ contractility.

4.  Beta blockers _____ contractility.

5.  Vasodilation _____ afterload.

6.  Hypertension, vasoconstriction, and aortic stenosis _____ afterload.

**P.  Diagnostic Procedures.** Match the definition or description in the numbered column with the appropriate diagnostic test or procedure in the lettered column. Some answers may be used more than once, and some answers may not be used.

1. _____  An ambulatory ECG that provides continuous monitoring *(634)*

2. _____  A transducer is used that picks up sound waves and converts them to electrical impulses *(637)*

3. _____  A high-resolution, three-dimensional image of the heart; cardiac tissue is imaged without lung or bone interference *(637)*

4. _____  An exercise tolerance test that is a recording of an individual's cardiovascular response during a measured exercise challenge *(637)*

5. _____  Study of electrical activity of the heart *(634)*

6. _____  A procedure in which a catheter is advanced into the heart chambers or coronary arteries under fluoroscopy *(638)*

7. _____  Images of the heart obtained with a probe in the esophagus *(637)*

8. _____  Test that may determine pressures in the RA, RV, and pulmonary artery *(638)*

9. _____  Electrodes placed on the surface of the skin pick up the electrical impulses of the heart *(638)*

10. _____  The patient ambulates on a treadmill or a stationary bicycle while connected to a monitor *(635, 637)*

11. _____  Heart sonogram that is a visualization and recording of the size, shape, position, and behavior of the heart's internal structures *(637)*

A.  Stress test
B.  Cardiac catheterization
C.  ECG
D.  Echocardiogram
E.  Electrophysiology study (EPS)
F.  MRI
G.  Holter monitor
H.  Transesophageal echocardiogram (TEE)
I.  Multiple-gated acquisition scan (MUGA)
J.  Thallium imaging
K.  Pulse oximetry
L.  Implantable loop monitor/recorder (ILR)
M.  Ultrafast computed tomography (electron-beam CT or EBCT)

12. _____ Injection of technetium 99m that concentrates in necrotic myocardial tissue to measure ventricular failure *(637)*

13. _____ Noninvasive measurement of oxygen saturation *(638)*

14. _____ Evaluates patency of coronary artery bypass grafts *(638)*

15. _____ Use of catheters with multiple electrodes inserted through the femoral vein to record the heart's electrical activity *(638)*

16. _____ Fast form of imaging technology that allows for high-quality images of the heart as it contracts and relaxes *(638)*

**Q. Complications of CAD.** Match the description of complications of coronary artery disease in the numbered column with the most appropriate term in the lettered column. Some terms may be used more than once, and some terms may not be used. *(655)*

1. _____ Disturbances in heart rhythm

2. _____ When the injured left ventricle is unable to meet the body's circulatory demands

3. _____ The most frequent cause of death after an AMI; marked by hypotension and decreasing alertness

4. _____ When clots form in the injured heart chambers, they may break loose and travel to the lung

5. _____ A fatal complication in which weakened areas of the ventricular wall bulge and burst

A. Ventricular aneurysm/rupture
B. Mitral stenosis
C. Dysrhythmias
D. Hemorrhage
E. Cardiogenic shock
F. Thromboembolism
G. Heart failure

**R.  Mitral Stenosis.** Complete the statement in the numbered column with the most appropriate term in the lettered column. Some terms may be used more than once, and some terms may not be used.

1.  The narrowing of the opening in the valve that impedes blood flow from the left atrium into the left ventricle is called _____. *(670)*

2.  The leading cause of mitral stenosis is _____. *(670)*

3.  In patients with mitral stenosis, the chamber of the heart that dilates to accommodate the amount of blood not ejected is the _____. *(670)*

4.  Excision of parts of the leaflets of the mitral valve to enlarge the opening is called _____. *(671)*

5.  When collecting data for the assessment of the patient with mitral stenosis, the nurse takes the vital signs and auscultates for _____. *(671)*

A.  Tricuspid stenosis
B.  Commissurotomy
C.  Angioplasty
D.  Mitral stenosis
E.  Heart murmur
F.  Rheumatic heart disease
G.  Left ventricle
H.  Left atrium
I.  Right ventricle

**S.  Drug Therapy.** Match the drug used for cardiac disorders in the numbered column with its classification in the lettered column. Some classifications may be used more than once, and some may not be used.

1.  _____  Nitroglycerin *(642)*

2.  _____  Aspirin, dipyridamole (Persantine), and clopidogrel (Plavix) *(645)*

3.  _____  Heparin and warfarin (Coumadin) *(647)*

4.  _____  Morphine and meperidine hydrochloride (Demerol) *(648)*

5.  _____  Furosemide (Lasix) and hydrochlorothiazide (Esidrix, HCTZ, and Oretic) *(647)*

6.  _____  Streptokinase, sotalol hydrochloride (Betapacc), and tissue plasminogen activator *(647)*

7.  _____  Digoxin (Lanoxin) and digitoxin *(641)*

A.  Anticholinergics
B.  Antianginals
C.  Analgesics
D.  Antiplatelet agents
E.  Antidysrhythmics
F.  Diuretics
G.  Fibrinolytics (antithrombolytics)
H.  Anticoagulants
I.  Cardiac glycosides
J.  ACE inhibitors

**T. Cardiac Surgery.** Match the nursing diagnosis for the postoperative cardiac surgery patient in the numbered column with the most appropriate "related to" statement in the lettered column. *(651)*

1. _____ Ineffective thermoregula-tion

2. _____ Decreased cardiac output

3. _____ Risk for infection

A. Altered skin integrity
B. Cooling during surgery
C. Fluid loss or decreased fluid intake

**U. ECG.** Match the ECG change in the numbered column with the feature of AMI in the lettered column. *(656)*

1. _____ The T wave is inverted.

2. _____ There is ST segment eleva-tion.

3. _____ A significant Q wave is present; the Q wave is greater than one-third the height of the R wave.

A. Ischemia
B. Infarction
C. Injury

**V. Drug Therapy.** Match the use(s) of AMI drug therapy in the numbered column with the specific drug in the lettered column. Some drugs may be used more than once, and some may not be used.

1. _____ Used for chest pain *(656)*

2. _____ Administered through an IV or into the coronary arteries to dissolve thrombi *(656)*

3. _____ Following the administra-tion of antithrombolytics, this drug is administered to prevent further clot formation *(647)*

4. _____ Administered for ventricu-lar tachycardia *(644)*

5. _____ Increases myocardial con-tractility and decreases the heart rate *(642)*

A. Furosemide (Lasix)
B. Streptokinase
C. Digitalis
D. Morphine sulfate
E. Atropine sulfate
F. Lidocaine
G. Heparin

**W. Acute Myocardial Infarction.** Match the nursing diagnosis for a patient with AMI in the numbered column with the "related to" statement in the lettered column. *(658)*

1. _____ Anxiety

2. _____ Pain

3. _____ Decreased cardiac output

A. Dysrhythmia
B. Feeling of impending doom
C. Lack of oxygen to the myocardium

**X. Heart Failure.** For the following signs and symptoms of heart failure (HF), indicate whether they are indicative of (A) right-sided or (B) left-sided failure. *(661)*

1. _____    Dependent edema
2. _____    Decreasing BP readings
3. _____    Increased central venous pressure
4. _____    Anxious, pale, and tachycardiac
5. _____    Jugular vein distention
6. _____    Abdominal engorgement
7. _____    Crackles, wheezes, dyspnea, and cough
8. _____    Pulmonary edema
9. _____    Decreased urinary output

**Y. Drug Therapy.** Match the actions of drugs used to treat heart failure in the numbered column with the drug or drug classification in the lettered column. Some answers may be used more than once, and some answers may not be used. *(662)*

1. _____    Improve(s) pump function by increasing contractility and decreasing heart rate

2. _____    Decrease(s) circulating fluid volume and decrease(s) preload

3. _____    Decrease(s) anxiety, dilate(s) the vasculature, and reduce(s) myocardial consumption in the acute stage

A. Heparin
B. Morphine
C. Diuretics
D. Streptokinase
E. Cardiac glycosides or inotropic agents such as digoxin

**Z. Heart Failure.** Match the nursing diagnosis for the patient with heart failure in the numbered column with the "related to" statement in the lettered column. *(662)*

1. _____    Fluid volume excess
2. _____    Impaired gas exchange
3. _____    Anxiety
4. _____    Decreased cardiac output
5. _____    Activity intolerance

A. Inability to perform activities
B. Decreased pulmonary perfusion
C. Mechanical failure
D. Ineffective cardiac pumping
E. Edema and inability to breathe

**AA. Heart Circulation.** In the Figure 35-2 (p. 629) below, label the parts (A–M) of the heart. *(629)*

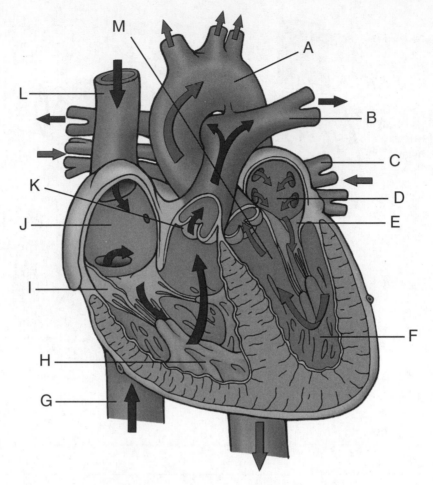

A. _____

B. _____

C. _____

D. _____

E. _____

F. _____

G. _____

H. _____

I. _____

J. _____

K. _____

L. _____

M. _____

**BB. Circulation System.** In the Figure 35-4 below (p. 630), label the parts (A–E) of the conduction system of the heart. *(630)*

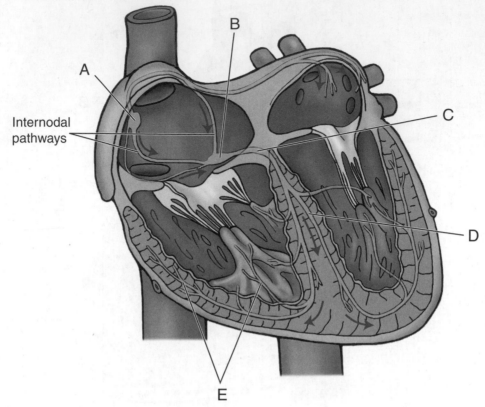

Internodal pathways

A. _____

B. _____

C. _____

D. _____

E. _____

## MULTIPLE-CHOICE QUESTIONS

**CC.** Choose the most appropriate answer.

1. The pressure is highest in which heart chamber? *(628)*
   1. Right atrium
   2. Left atrium
   3. Right ventricle
   4. Left ventricle

2. Afterload is decreased by: *(631)*
   1. vasodilation.
   2. overhydration.
   3. vasoconstriction.
   4. increased venous return to heart.

3. The first branches of the systemic circulation are the: *(629)*
   1. subclavian arteries.
   2. coronary arteries.
   3. carotid arteries.
   4. brachial arteries.

4. The ventricles contract when the electrical impulse reaches the: *(629)*
   1. SA node.
   2. AV node.
   3. Purkinje fibers.
   4. bundle of His.

5. Stroke volume, the amount of blood ejected with each ventricular contraction, depends on myocardial: *(631)*
   1. contractility.
   2. excitability.
   3. conductivity.
   4. automaticity.

6. If the valves of the heart do not close properly, the patient is said to have: *(633)*
   1. infarction.
   2. murmur.
   3. necrosis.
   4. tachycardia.

7. Ways to increase oxygen supply to the myocardium are to administer supplemental oxygen and to increase coronary blood flow by: *(631)*
   1. coronary artery vasoconstriction.
   2. increased myocardial contraction.
   3. coronary artery vasodilation.
   4. decreased myocardial contraction.

8. Thrombophlebitis and varicosities are more common in: *(632)*
   1. adolescents.
   2. young adults.
   3. middle-aged people.
   4. older people.

9. Which of the following is more likely to occur in older adults as the cardiovascular system adapts more slowly to changes in position? *(632)*
   1. Tachycardia
   2. Bradycardia
   3. Postural hypotension
   4. Headache

10. In asking cardiac patients about their diets, the nurse should especially record information about which two areas of intake? *(648)*
    1. Calcium and vitamin D
    2. Salt and fat
    3. Protein and iron
    4. Vitamin C and vitamin E

11. A noninvasive measure of cardiac output is: *(632)*
    1. cardiac catheterization.
    2. pulse pressure.
    3. angioplasty.
    4. blood gas measurement.

12. The sound produced by turbulent blood flow across the valves is called a(n): *(633)*
    1. heart murmur.
    2. ventricular gallop.
    3. atrial gallop.
    4. orthopnea.

13. A common diagnostic test that measures the electrical activity of the heart is the: *(634)*
    1. CT scan.
    2. echocardiogram.
    3. ECG.
    4. stress test.

14. A normal ECG finding is documented as a normal: *(634)*
    1. tachycardia.
    2. sinus rhythm.
    3. bradycardia.
    4. ventricular gallop.

15. The stress test must be stopped immediately if which of the following symptoms occur? *(637)*
    1. Angina and falling blood pressure
    2. Increased heart rate and increasing respirations
    3. Diaphoresis and thirst
    4. Slower respirations and hunger

16. The normal cardiac output is: *(631)*
    1. 1–3 liters/min.
    2. 4–8 liters/min.
    3. 10–13 liters/min.
    4. 15–20 liters/hour.

17. Patients with AMI often exhibit: *(640)*
    1. respiratory acidosis.
    2. respiratory alkalosis.
    3. elevated cholesterol levels.
    4. decreased WBC count.

18. A noninvasive measurement of arterial oxygen saturation is: *(638)*
    1. blood pressure.
    2. blood gases.
    3. pulse pressure.
    4. pulse oximetry.

19. What type of diet is generally recommended for cardiac patients? *(648)*
    1. Low-fat, high-calcium
    2. Low-fat, high-fiber
    3. Low-sodium, low-protein
    4. High-sodium, low-potassium

20. If fluid retention accompanies the cardiac problem, the physician may order restriction of: *(648)*
    1. potassium.
    2. sodium.
    3. fat.
    4. calcium.

21. Diuretics, such as furosemide, may cause a deficiency of: *(648)*
    1. sodium.
    2. calcium.
    3. fiber.
    4. potassium.

22. The purpose of temporary and permanent pacemakers is to improve cardiac output and tissue perfusion by restoring regular: *(648)*
    1. blood volume.
    2. blood pressure.
    3. impulse conduction.
    4. myocardial contractility.

23. The delivery of a synchronized shock to terminate atrial or ventricular tachyarrhythmias is called: *(650)*
    1. a pacemaker.
    2. cardiac catheterization.
    3. angioplasty.
    4. cardioversion.

24. During open-heart surgery, the patient's core temperature is reduced to decrease the body's need for: *(650)*
    1. oxygen.
    2. sodium.
    3. potassium.
    4. ATP.

25. Smoking, high blood pressure, and obesity are risk factors for: *(653)*
    1. mitral valve stenosis.
    2. atherosclerosis.
    3. pericarditis.
    4. endocarditis.

26. The most frequent symptom of coronary artery disease, which represents lack of oxygen to tissues, is: *(653)*
    1. fever.
    2. cyanosis.
    3. indigestion.
    4. pain.

27. The substernal pain resulting from lack of oxygen to the myocardium is called: *(653)*
    1. heartburn.
    2 dyspnea.
    3. pleurisy.
    4. angina pectoris.

28. Modifiable risk factors for AMI include hypertension, obesity, and: *(654)*
    1. diabetes mellitus.
    2. male gender.
    3. smoking.
    4. family history.

29. What drugs are used to prevent angina in patients with coronary artery disease? *(641)*
    1. Diuretics
    2. Analgesics
    3. Calcium channel blockers
    4. Antiplatelet agents

30. Nurses should be alert to complaints of decreased exercise tolerance and dyspnea in African-American males because they are at risk for: *(667)*
    1. hypertension.
    2. cardiomyopathy.
    3. endocarditis.
    4. mitral valve stenosis.

31. Cardiogenic shock is marked by hypotension, cool moist skin, oliguria, and: *(655)*
    1. decreasing alertness.
    2. restlessness.
    3. headache.
    4. cyanosis.

32. Which drug is administered to dilate coronary arteries and increase blood flow to the damaged area of a patient with AMI? *(655)*
    1. Nitroglycerin
    2. Furosemide
    3. Dipyridamole (Persantine)
    4. Streptokinase

33. Veins generally used in coronary artery bypass surgery as grafts to the coronary arteries include the internal mammary and _____ veins. *(657)*
    1. subclavian
    2. femoral
    3. jugular
    4. saphenous

34. In order to decrease cardiac workload and increase oxygenation to the myocardium, the recommended position for patients with HF is: *(664)*
    1. prone.
    2. supine.
    3. side-lying.
    4. semi-Fowler's or high-Fowler's.

35. The most common adverse effects of diuretic therapy for patients with HF are: *(664)*
    1. hypertension and tachycardia.
    2. fluid and electrolyte imbalances.
    3. headache and oliguria.
    4. confusion and weakness.

36. A common finding in patients with right-sided heart failure is: *(661)*
    1. increased urinary output.
    2. dependent edema.
    3. weight loss.
    4. cough.

37. Drugs that may be given to patients with HF include diuretics, vasodilators, and: *(661)*
    1. inotropics.
    2. anticonvulsants.
    3. antihistamines.
    4. cholinergics.

38. The most common site for organisms to accumulate in patients with infective endocarditis is the: *(665)*
    1. mitral valve.
    2. tricuspid valve.
    3. aortic valve.
    4. pulmonary valve.

39. Symptoms of endocarditis include weight loss, malaise, and: *(665)*
    1. oliguria.
    2. hypertension.
    3. fever.
    4. convulsions.

40. An important diagnostic test for patients with endocarditis is the: *(666)*
    1. RBC count.
    2. WBC count.
    3. hematocrit.
    4. hemoglobin.

41. The main drugs used for endocarditis are: *(666)*
    1. cardiac glycosides.
    2. diuretics.
    3. calcium channel blockers.
    4. antimicrobials.

42. The hallmark symptom of pericarditis is: *(666)*
    1. chest pain.
    2. headache.
    3. hypertension.
    4. indigestion.

43. The patient with pericarditis is treated with analgesics, anti-inflammatory agents, antibiotics, and: *(666)*
    1. diuretics.
    2. anticonvulsants.
    3. antipyretics.
    4. anticholinergics.

44. A procedure in which a peripherally inserted catheter is passed into an occluded artery and a balloon inflated to dilate the artery is: *(657)*
    1. percutaneous transluminal angioplasty.
    2. coronary atherectomy.
    3. intracoronary stent placement.
    4. laser angioplasty.

45. Disease of the heart muscle that generally has an unknown cause and leads to heart failure is called: *(667)*
    1. myocardial infarction.
    2. CHF.
    3. cardiomyopathy.
    4. pericarditis.

46. Which type of cardiomyopathy is associated with a high incidence of sudden death? *(667)*
    1. Hypertrophic
    2. Dilated
    3. Restrictive
    4. CHF

47. Lifelong medications that must be given to patients with heart transplants include: *(669)*
    1. antihistamines.
    2. analgesics.
    3. antimicrobials.
    4. immunosuppressives.

48. The two major valve problems of the heart are stenosis and: *(670)*
    1. inflammation.
    2. regurgitation.
    3. emboli.
    4. hemorrhage.

49. Heparin dosage for the patient with a cardiac disorder is adjusted according to the patient's: *(647)*
    1. hemoglobin.
    2. prothrombin time.
    3. partial thromboplastin time.
    4. hematocrit.

50. Diuretics such as furosemide and hydrochlorothiazide are used with cardiac conditions to treat: *(647)*
    1. hypokalemia.
    2. fluid retention.
    3. dehydration.
    4. dysrhythmias.

51. Before each dose of digitalis, the apical pulse is counted for 1 full minute; the drug is withheld and the physician notified if the pulse is below: *(641)*
    1. 60 bpm.
    2. 70 bpm.
    3. 72 bpm.
    4. 80 bpm.

52. Older people are more susceptible to adverse drug effects because they: *(632)*
    1. metabolize drugs more quickly.
    2. have decreased elasticity of vessels.
    3. excrete drugs more slowly.
    4. are hypersensitive to more drugs.

53. Patients taking immunosuppressive drugs to prevent rejection of transplanted tissue have reduced: *(669)*
    1. circulation.
    2. resistance to infection.
    3. metabolism of drugs.
    4. red blood cell counts.

54. Antidysrhythmic drugs work by slowing impulse conduction, increasing resistance to premature contraction, or: *(641)*
    1. increasing contractility.
    2. enhancing inotropism.
    3. depressing automaticity.
    4. stimulating the SA node.

55. A major part of treatment for people with heart disease is the reduction of dietary fat and: *(648)*
    1. sugar.
    2. protein.
    3. cholesterol.
    4. vitamin E.

56. An automatic implantable cardioverter-defibrillator is used to: *(670)*
    1. improve contractility in people with cardiomyopathy.
    2. decrease the risk of sudden cardiac death in people with recurrent life-threatening dysrhythmias.
    3. convert patients in cardiac arrest to normal sinus rhythm.
    4. support cardiac function in patients awaiting heart transplants.

57. The internal cardiac defibrillator is used to treat patients with life-threatening, recurrent: *(670)*
    1. hypertension.
    2. aortic stenosis.
    3. ventricular fibrillation.
    4. endocarditis.

58. A Swan-Ganz catheter is inserted into the pulmonary artery to measure: *(676, 677)*
    1. tricuspid valve function.
    2. right-sided heart pressure.
    3. mitral valve stenosis.
    4. aortic stenosis.

59. Measurements below normal from a central venous catheter threaded into the right atrium indicates: *(676)*
    1. hypovolemia.
    2. hypervolemia.
    3. hypotension.
    4. low cardiac output.

60. How should you document a pulse that is easily obliterated by slight finger pressure, which returns as the pressure is released? *(633)*
    1. Absent
    2. Nonpalpable
    3. Weak or thready
    4. Bounding

61. Which heart sound is normal in children and young adults but is pathologic if it is heard after the age of 30? *(633)*
    1. $S_1$
    2. $S_2$
    3. $S_3$, ventricular gallop
    4. $S_4$, atrial gallop

62. What type of drug therapy is used after an AMI to prevent strokes? *(645)*
    1. Cardiac glycosides
    2. Antidysrhythmics
    3. Antiplatelets
    4. Nitrates

63. Calcium channel blockers, vasodilators, and beta-adrenergic blockers are used to treat: *(641)*
    1. CHF.
    2. angina.
    3. AMI.
    4. heart murmurs.

64. Drugs that slow down the rate of impulse conduction in the heart are: *(641)*
    1. antidysrhythmics.
    2. nitrates.
    3. calcium channel blockers.
    4. antiplatelets.

65. The dosage of heparin is based on measurements of the patient's: *(647)*
    1. aPTT.
    2. INR.
    3. PT.
    4. CBC.

66. When the pericardium is inflamed, a sound heard along the left sternal border is the: *(633, 666)*
    1. heart murmur.
    2. friction rub.
    3. atrial gallop.
    4. ventricular gallop.

67. The most widely used drugs in the treatment of HF are: *(641)*
    1. cardiac glycosides.
    2. antianginals.
    3. antidysrhythmics.
    4. adrenergic beta-blockers.

68. The first medication given to patients with chest pain is: *(653)*
    1. morphine.
    2. aspirin.
    3. Demerol.
    4. nitroglycerin.

69. Which herb taken to lower plasma lipids may increase the effects of anticoagulants and insulin? *(648)*
    1. Kava kava
    2. Ephedra
    3. Garlic
    4. Aloe

70. Chambers paced, chambers sensed, and mode of response are three settings for a: *(649)*
    1. defibrillator.
    2. pacemaker.
    3. Holter monitor.
    4. cardioverter.

71. Patient teaching for patients with permanent pacemakers includes: *(650)*
    1. teaching patients how to count their pulse for 1 full minute daily.
    2. showing patients how to take and document weekly weights.
    3. encouraging patients to avoid foods high in vitamin K.
    4. limiting exercise to walking twice a week.

72. The leading cause of mitral stenosis is: *(670)*
    1. hypertension.
    2. AMI.
    3. infective endocarditis.
    4. rheumatic heart disease.

73. As left atrial pressure increases in mitral stenosis, this change leads to: *(671)*
    1. right ventricular hypertrophy.
    2. decreased pulmonary pressure.
    3. decreased workload on the right side of the heart.
    4. increased peripheral edema.

74. If dietary control does not reduce cholesterol sufficiently, treatment may include: *(645)*
    1. antihypertensives.
    2. antidysrhythmics.
    3. antianginals.
    4. lipid-lowering agents.

75. Questran, Lopid, and niacin are drugs classified as: *(645)*
    1. cardiac glycosides.
    2. nitrates.
    3. lipid-lowering drugs.
    4. antiplatelets.

**DD.** *Nursing Care Plan.* Refer to Nursing Care Plan, The Patient with Heart Failure, p. 663 in the textbook.

1. Which abnormal findings were found on physical examination for this patient related to heart failure? *(663)*
   1.              6.
   2.              7.
   3.              8.
   4.              9.
   5.              10.

2. What is the priority nursing diagnosis for this patient? *(663)*

3. Why is this patient more susceptible to adverse drug effects? *(663)*

4. If she is started on digitalis, what are early signs of digitalis toxicity you would be watching for? *(642)*

5. Why is it important for her to remain on bed rest? *(662)*

6. Which tasks can be assigned to unlicensed assistive personnel? *(663)*

# CHAPTER 36

# Vascular Disorders

---

## OBJECTIVES

1. Identify specific anatomic and physiologic factors that affect the vascular system and tissue oxygenation.

2. Indicate appropriate parameters for assessing a patient with peripheral vascular disease, aneurysm, and aortic dissection.

3. Discuss tests and procedures used to diagnose selected vascular disorders and the nursing considerations for each.

4. State the pathophysiology, signs and symptoms, complications, and medical or surgical treatments for selected vascular disorders.

5. Assist in developing a plan of care for patients with selected vascular disorders.

---

## LEARNING ACTIVITIES

**A. Key Terms.** Match the definition in the numbered column with the most appropriate term in the lettered column.

1. _____ Sudden obstruction of an artery by a floating clot or foreign material *(699)*

2. _____ An abnormal sensation *(688)*

3. _____ Concentration of the blood *(688)*

4. _____ Development of a clot in the presence of venous inflammation *(708)*

5. _____ Deficient blood flow due to obstruction or constriction of blood vessels *(689)*

6. _____ Increase in blood vessel diameter *(688)*

7. _____ Development of venous thrombi without venous inflammation *(708)*

8. _____ Decrease in blood vessel diameter *(687)*

9. _____ Coolness in an area of the body due to decreased blood flow *(689)*

10. _____ Thickness of the blood *(688)*

11. _____ Development or presence of a thrombus *(708)*

12. _____ Dilated segment of an artery caused by weakness and stretching of the vessel wall *(705)*

13. _____ Murmur detected by auscultation *(691)*

A. Thrombophlebitis
B. Thrombosis
C. Phlebothrombosis
D. Embolism
E. Vasoconstriction
F. Paresthesia
G. Bruit
H. Ischemia
I. Aneurysm
J. Hemoconcentration
K. Poikilothermy
L. Vasodilation
M. Viscosity

B. **Vascular System.** Match the definition or description in the numbered column with the most appropriate term in the lettered column. Some terms may be used more than once, and some may not be used.

1. _____ Vessels that return blood to the heart *(687)*

2. _____ The two main trunks of these vessels are the thoracic duct and the right lymphatic duct *(687)*

3. _____ Thick-walled, elastic structures *(685)*

4. _____ Equipped with valves that aid in the transportation of blood against gravity *(687)*

5. _____ Formed by a single layer of endothelial cells *(687)*

6. _____ Vessels that carry blood away from the heart *(685)*

7. _____ Transfer of oxygen and nutrients between the blood and the tissue cells occurs here *(686)*

8. _____ Thin-walled vessels that collect and drain fluid from the peripheral tissues and transport the fluid to the venous system *(687)*

A. Veins
B. Valves
C. Leaflets
D. Capillaries
E. Lymph vessels
F. Arteries
G. Lymph nodes

C. **Peripheral Resistance.** Indicate for each factor in the numbered column whether it (A) increases or (B) decreases peripheral resistance.

1. _____ Sympathetic nervous system stimulation *(687)*

2. _____ Epinephrine *(687)*

3. _____ Angiotensin *(687)*

4. _____ Vasoconstriction *(688)*

5. _____ Viscous blood *(688)*

6. _____ Vasodilation *(688)*

7. _____ Histamine *(688)*

8. _____ Prostaglandins *(688)*

**D. Peripheral Vascular Disease.** Match the description in the numbered column with the 6 Ps—characteristics of peripheral vascular disease in the lettered column. Answers may be used more than once.

1. _____ Decreased temperature at an ischemic site *(688)*

2. _____ Paleness apparent over an area of reduced blood supply *(689)*

3. _____ Associated with intermittent claudication *(688)*

4. _____ Detected by palpating the affected and surrounding areas *(688)*

5. _____ Determined by palpating peripheral pulses for rate, rhythm, and quality *(689)*

6. _____ Abnormal sensation such as numbness, tingling, or crawling sensation *(689)*

7. _____ Impairment of motor function *(689)*

8. _____ Characterized by "pins and needles" sensation *(689)*

9. _____ Described by patients as tenderness, heaviness, or fullness in the extremity *(689)*

A. Pain
B. Pulselessness
C. Poikilothermy
D. Pallor
E. Paresthesia
F. Paralysis

**E. Physical Examination.** Complete the statement in the numbered column with the most appropriate term in the lettered column. Some terms may be used more than once, and some may not be used.

1. A test to evaluate the pain response in the calf area to determine venous thrombosis is called _____. *(690)*

2. A test used to determine the patency of the ulnar and radial artery is called _____. *(690)*

3. When blood flowing through the arteries sounds like turbulent, fast-moving fluid, these sounds are called _____. *(691)*

4. Brown pigmentation sites with flaky skin over the edematous areas of the ankles are described as _____. *(689)*

A. Bruits
B. Babinski's reflex
C. Allen's test
D. Moro's reflex
E. Homans' sign
F. Stasis dermatitis

**F. Diagnostic Procedures.** Complete the statements in the numbered column with the most appropriate term in the lettered column. Some terms may be used more than once, and some terms may not be used.

1. A noninvasive, inexpensive diagnostic tool in which sound waves are directed toward the artery or vein being tested is _____. *(692)*

2. A noninvasive examination that measures the blood volume and graphs changes in the flow of blood and is often used for patients too ill to undergo arteriography is _____. *(692)*

3. The segmental limb pressure test and pulse volume measurement test are examples of _____. *(692)*

4. An invasive procedure that requires the injection of dye into the vascular system is called _____. *(692)*

5. A test that measures pulse volumes before and after exercise is _____. *(692)*

6. A test that evaluates blood flow by providing a two-dimensional image of blood vessels and blood flow is _____. *(691)*

A. MRI
B. Pressure measurement
C. Treadmill test
D. Angiography
E. Doppler ultrasound
F. Plethysmography
G. Duplex scanning
H. ECG

**G. Surgical Procedures.**

1. Match the description or definition in the numbered column with the most appropriate term in the lettered column. Some terms may be used more than once, and some terms may not be used. *(696)*

1. _____ The injection of a chemical that irritates the venous endothelium for patients with varicose veins

2. _____ A procedure that is done to relieve arterial stenosis in people who are poor surgical risks

3. _____ A procedure used to remove varicose veins

4. _____ An incision into the obstructed vessel to strip away emboli and atherosclerotic plaque followed by surgical closure of the vessel

5. _____ The excision of the sympathetic ganglia; used for patients with intermittent claudication

6. _____ The removal of a blood clot located in a large vessel

A. Sympathectomy
B. Percutaneous transluminal angioplasty
C. Thermotherapy
D. Embolectomy
E. Sclerotherapy
F. Intermittent pneumatic compression
G. Vein ligation and stripping
H. Endarterectomy

2. **Laboratory Tests/Cardiac Disease.** Match the description in the numbered column with the laboratory test in the lettered column. (Answers to G2 are in Chapter 35, p. 640.)

1. _____ Protein levels increase in cardiac disease as well as in skeletal muscle disorders. *(640)*

2. _____ Protein is elevated in serum inflammation. Elevated levels with cardiac disease. *(641)*

3. _____ Helps differentiate dyspnea related to cardiac problems from noncardiac -related dyspnea. Elevated in heart failure. *(641)*

4. _____ Measures protein released after myocardial injury. *(640)*

A. Troponin
B. Myoglobin
C. B-type natriuretic peptide (BNP)
D. C-reactive protein (CRP)

**H. Deep Vein Thrombosis.** Complete the statements relating to signs and symptoms of deep vein thrombosis in the numbered column with the most appropriate term in the lettered column. Some terms may be used more than once, and some terms may not be used. *(708)*

1. The affected extremity appears _____.

2. Superficial veins are _____.

3. The affected area of compromise may be _____.

4. Homans' sign is _____.

A. Warm and tender
B. Negative
C. Cool
D. Prominent
E. Positive
F. Edematous
G. Lack of sensation

**I. Venous Thrombosis.** Match the nursing diagnosis in the numbered column for a patient with venous thrombosis with the appropriate "related to" statement in the lettered column. *(709)*

1. _____ Impaired skin integrity
2. _____ Acute pain
3. _____ Activity intolerance
4. _____ Ineffective tissue perfusion

A. Impaired circulation and tissue ischemia
B. Venous stasis
C. Ineffective peripheral circulation
D. Leg pain or swelling

**J. Deep Vein Thrombosis.** What are risk factors for the development of deep vein thrombosis? Select all that apply. *(708)*

1. _____ Prescribed bed rest
2. _____ Obesity
3. _____ Malnourishment
4. _____ Use of oral contraceptives
5. _____ Use of anticoagulants
6. _____ Prescribed cast for fractures
7. _____ Surgery under general anesthesia for patients over 40
8. _____ Use of alcohol

K. **Deep Vein Thrombosis.** What is the treatment for deep vein thrombosis? Select all that apply. *(708)*
   1. _____ Frequent ambulation initially
   2. _____ Elevate extremity
   3. _____ Apply warm compresses
   4. _____ Anticoagulant therapy
   5. _____ Antiembolism hose

L. **Venous Thrombus.** What factors (called *Virchow's triad*) contribute to venous thrombus formation? Select all that apply. *(708)*
   1. _____ Stasis of the blood
   2. _____ Damage to the vessel walls
   3. _____ Hypertension
   4. _____ Hypercoagulability

M. **Deep Vein Thrombosis.** What are symptoms of a deep vein thrombosis in the lower leg? Select all that apply. *(708)*
   1. _____ Area is edematous.
   2. _____ Area is cool.
   3. _____ Area is dry.
   4. _____ Area is tender to touch.

N. **Deep Vein Thrombosis.** What percentage of patients with deep vein thrombosis have no visible signs or symptoms? *(708)*
   1. 10%
   2. 20%
   3. 45%
   4. 50%

O. **Deep Vein Thrombosis.** What is the most serious complication of deep vein thrombosis? *(708)*
   1. Hemorrhage
   2. Venous stasis
   3. Pulmonary embolism
   4. Hypvolemic shock

P. **Peripheral Vascular Disease.** Explain why care must be taken when using heat on patients with peripheral vascular disease. *(695)*

Q. **Drug Therapy.** Which are classifications of drugs that are used in the general management of peripheral vascular disease to improve peripheral circulation? Select all that apply. *(697)*
   1. _____ Antimicrobials
   2. _____ Diuretics
   3. _____ Anticoagulants
   4. _____ Thrombolytics

R. **Drug Therapy.** Which drugs are used to treat Raynaud's disease? Select all that apply. *(704)*

1. _____    Thrombolytics
2. _____    Calcium channel blockers
3. _____    Anticoagulants
4. _____    Bosentan (endothelin receptor antagonist)
5. _____    Sildenafil (phosphodiesterase inhibitor)
6. _____    Vasodilators
7. _____    Analgesics
8. _____    Antidysrhythmics
9. _____    Beta adrenergic blockers

S. **Anticoagulants.** List two primary anticoagulants and their antidotes. *(697)*

1. Oral drug and antidote: _____

2. Parenteral drug and antidote: _____

T. **Anticoagulants.** When are anticoagulants and thrombolytic drugs contraindicated? Select all that apply. *(697)*

1. _____    Venous thrombosis
2. _____    Active bleeding
3. _____    Recent surgery
4. _____    Patients on bed rest
5. _____    Uncontrolled hypertension

U. **Aneurysms.** Which are complications of aneurysms? Select all that apply. *(705)*

1. _____    Emboli
2. _____    Infection
3. _____    Rupture
4. _____    Thrombus forms, obstructing blood flow
5. _____    Pressure on surrounding structures
6. _____    Liver failure

**V.** Using Figure 36-2 (p. 686) below, label the structures of the artery, vein, and capillary using the following numbers. Structures may be used more than once. *(686)*

1. Tunica adventitia
2. Endothelial cells
3. Tunica media
4. External elastic membrane
5. Tunica intima
6. Internal elastic membrane
7. Valve

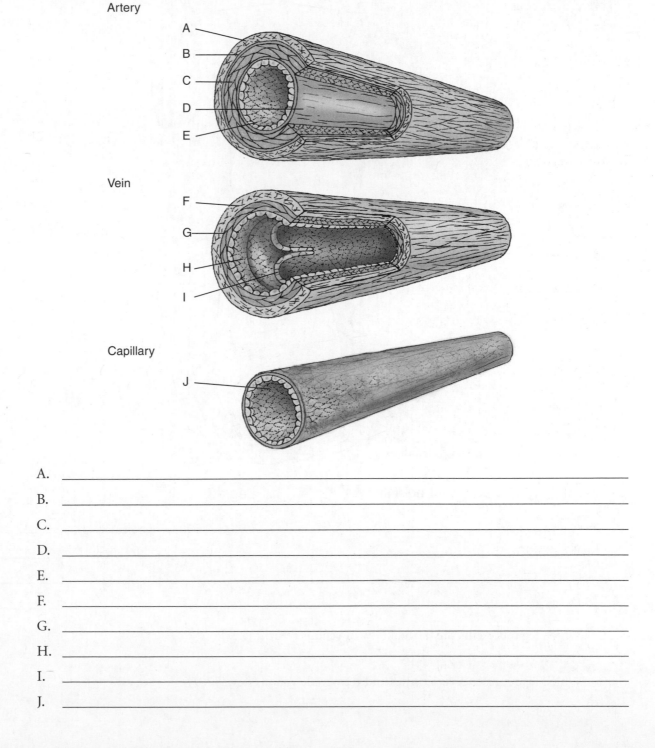

Artery

Vein

Capillary

A. _____

B. _____

C. _____

D. _____

E. _____

F. _____

G. _____

H. _____

I. _____

J. _____

## W.  Venous Return.

1.   Using Figure 36-8 (p. 707) below, label the veins involved in varicosities using the following numbers. *(707)*
     1.   Small saphenous veins
     2.   Great saphenous veins
     3.   External iliac veins
     4.   Femoral veins

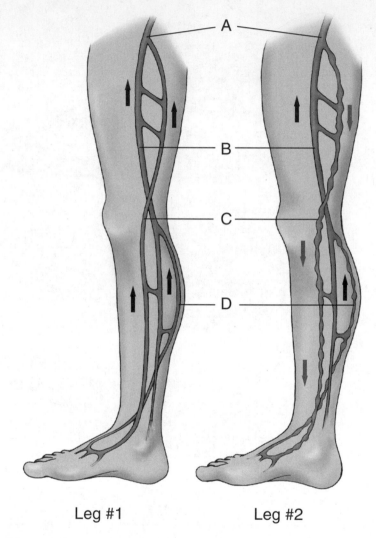

Leg #1              Leg #2

A.   _____

B.   _____

C.   _____

D.   _____

2.   Which leg represents the normal flow of venous return? *(707)*


3.   Which leg represents varicosities and retrograde venous flow? *(707)*

4. Which are factors contributing to varicosities? Select all that apply. *(706)*

    1. _____ Hereditary weakness
    2. _____ Aging
    3. _____ Pregnancy
    4. _____ Prolonged standing
    5. _____ Orthostatic hypotension

5. Match the description in the numbered column with the type of varicose veins in the lettered column. *(706)*

    1. _____ Characterized by deep     A.   Primary
                         vein obstruction.         B.   Secondary

    2. _____ Only superficial veins
                         are affected.

6. What are common sites for varicosities? Select all that apply. *(706)*

    1. _____ Esophageal veins
    2. _____ Renal veins
    3. _____ Coronary veins
    4. _____ Peripheral veins
    5. _____ Hemorrhoidal veins

**X. Venous Thrombi.** Which are primary diagnostic examinations used in the detection of venous thrombi? Select all that apply. *(706)*

    1. _____ Doppler ultrasonography
    2. _____ Duplex ultrasonography
    3. _____ Exercise treadmill test
    4. _____ Venography

## MULTIPLE-CHOICE QUESTIONS

**Y.** Choose the most appropriate answer.

1. Any interruption of the blood flow to the distal regions of the body, as occurs in peripheral vascular disease (PVD), results in: *(685)*
   1. kidney failure.
   2. cardiac shock.
   3. dyspnea.
   4. hypoxia.

2. The nervous system that acts on the smooth muscles of vessels, resulting in dilation and constriction of the artery walls, is the: *(687)*
   1. autonomic.
   2. somatic.
   3. central.
   4. cranial.

3. The primary result of aging on the peripheral vessels is: *(688)*
   1. vasoconstriction of arteries.
   2. vasodilation of veins.
   3. increased elasticity of vessel walls.
   4. stiffening of vessel walls.

4. Aging in the vascular system causes a slowing of the heart rate and a decrease in the stroke volume, resulting in decreased: *(688)*
   1. cardiac output.
   2. tachycardia.
   3. peripheral resistance.
   4. hypertension.

5. The transportation of oxygen is compromised in the aging patient by decreased: *(688)*
   1. hematocrit.
   2. WBC count.
   3. hemoglobin.
   4. cardiac enzymes.

6. PVD is a common complication of: *(685)*
   1. pneumonia.
   2. myocardial infarction.
   3. diabetes.
   4. influenza.

7. If PVD causes limb-threatening ischemia, amputation of a limb may be necessary because of the development of: *(689)*
   1. cyanosis.
   2. tissue necrosis.
   3. fractures.
   4. hypersensitivity.

8. Skin temperature is palpated in patients with PVD to determine the existence of: *(689)*
   1. infection.
   2. bleeding.
   3. cyanosis.
   4. ischemia.

9. In the evaluation of edema, when the thumb is depressed in the area for 5 seconds and the depression of the thumb remains in the edematous area, the edema is said to be: *(690)*
   1. 1+.
   2. 2+.
   3. 3+.
   4. pitting.

10. If pain or severe skin color changes occur during exercises with PVD patients, the nurse should: *(693)*
    1. encourage the exercises to be done gradually.
    2. stop the exercises immediately.
    3. ambulate the patient to promote venous return.
    4. administer muscle relaxants as ordered.

11. It is important for patients with PVD to stop smoking because smoking causes: *(693)*
    1. intermittent claudication.
    2. skin ulceration.
    3. vasoconstriction.
    4. vasodilation.

12. The primary function of intermittent pneumatic compression devices is to prevent: *(694)*
    1. infection.
    2. hemorrhage.
    3. deep vein thrombosis.
    4. cyanosis.

13. Which position should be avoided by patients with PVD? *(695)*
    1. Extended standing
    2. Elevation of lower extremities
    3. Lowering extremities below the level of the heart
    4. Elevation of extremities to a nondependent position

14. Which works as a vasodilator that promotes arterial flow to the peripheral tissues? *(695)*
    1. TED hose
    2. Intermittent pneumatic compression
    3. Heat
    4. Cold

15. Elevation of the extremity following surgery for patients with PVD aids in the prevention of: *(696)*
    1. hemorrhage.
    2. edema.
    3. hypotension.
    4. ulceration.

16. Disappearance of a peripheral pulse during the postoperative care of patients with PVD alerts the nurse to the development of a: *(696)*
    1. thrombotic occlusion.
    2. massive hemorrhage.
    3. severe infection.
    4. varicose vein.

17. The main adverse action of anticoagulants is: *(697)*
    1. bleeding.
    2. infection.
    3. hypertension.
    4. oliguria.

18. Thrombolytic therapy is employed to: *(698)*
    1. shorten the clotting time.
    2. increase clot formation.
    3. prevent the formation of new clots.
    4. dissolve an existing clot.

19. The use of vasodilators results in increased blood flow by relaxing the vascular smooth muscle and causing: *(697)*
    1. increased clotting time.
    2. decreased elasticity in vessels.
    3. decreased resistance in vessels.
    4. increased narrowing in vessels.

20. A grave risk with a diagnosis of deep vein thrombosis is the development of: *(708)*
    1. hemorrhage.
    2. pneumonia.
    3. pulmonary embolus.
    4. infection.

21. Three precipitating factors (called Virchow's triad) for a thrombus to form include hypercoagulability, damage to the vessel walls, and: *(708)*
    1. hemorrhage.
    2. stasis of the blood.
    3. decreased hematocrit.
    4. damaged blood cells.

22. The primary diagnostic examinations used in the detection of thrombus formation are plethysmography, Doppler ultrasound, and: *(708)*
    1. venography.
    2. an ECG.
    3. myelography.
    4. angioplasty.

23. Patients with thrombosis should not be massaged or rubbed because of the possible development of: *(709)*
    1. severe infection.
    2. hemorrhage.
    3. skin breakdown.
    4. pulmonary emboli.

24. The placement of antiembolism hose on patients with thrombosis is done to improve circulation and to prevent: *(709)*
    1. infection.
    2. stasis.
    3. hemorrhage.
    4. ulceration.

25. A life-threatening event that requires immediate attention is: *(699)*
    1. arterial embolism.
    2. thrombophlebitis.
    3. varicose vein disease.
    4. thrombosis.

26. The absence of a peripheral pulse below the occlusive area is a clinical manifestation of: *(701)*
    1. Raynaud's disease.
    2. aneurysms.
    3. peripheral arterial occlusive disease.
    4. thrombophlebitis.

27. During repair of an abdominal aneurysm, the aorta is clamped for a period of time. This poses a risk of: *(706)*
    1. dyspnea.
    2. renal failure.
    3. pneumonia.
    4. incontinence.

28. Varicose veins develop as a result of faulty: *(706)*
    1. elasticity.
    2. smooth muscle.
    3. thickness.
    4. valves.

29. Chronic venous insufficiency may develop from: *(710)*
    1. varicose veins.
    2. plaque formations.
    3. thrombophlebitis.
    4. aortic dissection.

30. Signs of chronic venous insufficiency include edema of lower legs and: *(710)*
    1. redness.
    2. infection.
    3. stasis dermatitis.
    4. cyanosis.

31. The medical management of lymphangitis necessitates the administration of: *(712)*
    1. antimicrobial agents.
    2. thrombolytic agents.
    3. anticoagulants.
    4. analgesics.

32. Elastic support hose are utilized for several months following an acute attack of lymphangitis to prevent the formation of: *(712)*
    1. infection.
    2. hemorrhage.
    3. lymphedema.
    4. dermatitis.

33. The primary age-related change in peripheral vessels is: *(688)*
    1. thrombosis.
    2. arteriosclerosis.
    3. varicose vein disease.
    4. chronic venous insufficiency.

34. Aging in the vascular system causes: *(688)*
    1. increased hemoglobin.
    2. increased stroke volume.
    3. increased heart rate.
    4. decreased cardiac output.

35. A patient complains of severe aching pain in his left foot after lying quietly in bed. This type of pain is a symptom of: *(688)*
    1. severe arterial occlusion.
    2. PVD.
    3. deep vein thrombosis.
    4. Raynaud's disease.

36. A priority in caring for patients with PVD is: *(688)*
    1. pain management.
    2. stress management.
    3. regular exercise.
    4. a low-sodium diet.

37. When intermittent claudication occurs, the patient should: *(688)*
    1. stop smoking.
    2. avoid constrictive clothing.
    3. use antiembolism hose.
    4. stop exercise.

38. Intermittent pneumatic compression is used for patients: *(694)*
    1. with paresthesia.
    2. with intermittent claudication.
    3. on bed rest following surgery.
    4. on moderate exercise programs.

39. Which medications intensify anticoagulant effects? *(697)*
    1. Antacids
    2. Barbiturates
    3. Oral contraceptives
    4. NSAIDs

40. Which herbal remedy decreases the effectiveness of warfarin? *(697)*
    1. Garlic
    2. Ginger root
    3. St. John's wort
    4. Ginkgo

41. Patients taking vasodilators for PVD must be monitored for: *(698)*
    1. hypotension.
    2. hemorrhage.
    3. increased vascular resistance.
    4. hypocalcemia.

42. Intermittent claudication is the classic sign of: *(688)*
    1. hypertension.
    2. arterial embolism.
    3. deep vein thrombosis.
    4. PVD.

43. Buerger's disease (thromboangiitis obliterans) is uncommon in people living in: *(703)*
    1. India.
    2. Korea.
    3. Japan.
    4. the United States.

44. Chronically cold hands and numbness are symptoms of: *(704)*
    1. Buerger's disease.
    2. Raynaud's disease.
    3. atherosclerosis.
    4. deep vein thrombosis.

45. An alternative therapy for vasospastic episodes of Raynaud's disease is: *(704)*
    1. guided imagery.
    2. meditation.
    3. biofeedback.
    4. yoga.

46. Occupations requiring prolonged standing and the aging process increase the risk for: *(706)*
    1. PVD.
    2. varicosities.
    3. aneurysms.
    4. aortic dissection.

47. Which food should be avoided in patients with PVD? *(712)*
    1. Grapefruit
    2. Ham
    3. Milk
    4. Pasta

48. What is the "related to" term in the ineffective tissue perfusion nursing diagnosis for a patient with Raynaud's disease? *(704)*
    1. Compromised circulation
    2. Vascular occlusion
    3. Graft thrombosis
    4. Vasoconstriction

## ALTERNATE FORMAT QUESTIONS

**Z.** 1. Which are characteristics of venous insufficiency in the legs? Select all that apply. *(710)*
    1. Capillary refill greater than 3 seconds
    2. Lower leg edema
    3. Pale skin color when elevated
    4. Varicose veins may be visible
    5. Dark reddish color in dependent position
    6. Bronze-brown pigmentation
    7. Cool skin
    8. Intermittent claudication or rest pain
    9. Dull ache, heaviness in calf or thigh
    10. Absent peripheral pulses

2. Which groups experience an increased incidence of Raynaud's disease? Select all that apply. *(704)*
    1. Men
    2. Women
    3. Peaople who live in a hot climate
    4. People who live in a cold climate

**AA. Nursing Care Plan.** Refer to Nursing Care Plan, The Patient with a Venous Stasis Ulcer, p. 711 in the textbook.

1. Which eight findings on the physical examination are abnormal? *(711)*
    1.                    5.

    2.                    6.

    3.                    7.

    4.                    8.

2. How does this patient describe his pain? *(711)*

3. What is a risk factor of PVD for this patient? *(711)*

4. What is the priority nursing diagnosis? *(711)*

5. What are steps this patient can take to lessen his pain? *(711)*

6. Which tasks can be assigned to unlicensed assistive personnel? Select all that apply. *(711)*
   1. Check vital signs.
   2. Instruct the patient in measures to improve circulation.
   3. Assess condition of ulcer, peripheral pulses, skin color and warmth, pain, and edema.
   4. Teach hygienic techniques of hand-washing and wound care.
   5. Teach signs and symptoms of infection that should be reported to physician.
   6. Teach pain relief measures.
   7. Explain the use of analgesics.
   8. Assist the patient with ambulation.
   9. Document the condition of the ulcer during each clinic visit.
   10. Weigh the patient.

# CHAPTER 37

# Hypertension

---

## OBJECTIVES

1. Define hypertension.

2. Explain the physiology of blood pressure regulation.

3. Discuss the risk factors, signs and symptoms, diagnosis, treatment, and complications of hypertension.

4. Identify the nursing considerations when administering selected antihypertensive drugs.

5. List the data to be obtained in the nursing assessment of a person with known or suspected hypertension.

6. Identify the nursing diagnoses, goals, and outcome criteria for the patient with hypertension.

7. Describe the nursing interventions for the patient with hypertension.

---

## LEARNING ACTIVITIES

**A. Key Terms.** Match the definition in the numbered column with the most appropriate term in the lettered column.

1. _____ Sudden drop in systolic blood pressure when changing from a lying or sitting position to a standing position *(722)*

2. _____ Stationary blood clot *(717)*

3. _____ Nosebleed *(717)*

4. _____ Persistent elevation of arterial blood pressure of 140/90 mm Hg or greater *(715)*

5. _____ Fainting *(726)*

6. _____ Enlargement *(717)*

7. _____ Abnormal amounts of lipids or lipoproteins in the blood *(717)*

A. Hypertension
B. Syncope
C. Thrombus
D. Dyslipidemia
E. Orthostatic hypotension
F. Epistaxis
G. Hypertrophy

**B.** **Risk Factors.** What are significant risk factors for primary (essential) hypertension? Select all that apply. *(717)*

1. _____      Varicose veins
2. _____      Dyslipidemia
3. _____      Tobacco use
4. _____      Obesity
5. _____      Thrombophlebitis

**C.** **Peripheral Vascular Resistance.** Complete the statements in the numbered column with the most appropriate term in the lettered column. Some terms may be used more than once, and some terms may not be used.

1. Epinephrine constricts blood vessels and increases blood pressure, causing the heart rate to _____. *(716)*

2. When body position is altered from supine to standing, the diastolic blood pressure normally _____ . *(724)*

3. In response to decreased ability of the aorta to distend, pulse pressure _____. *(717)*

4. In response to increased peripheral vascular resistance, the systolic pressure _____. *(717)*

5. Epinephrine constricts blood vessels and increases the force of cardiac contraction, causing blood pressure to _____. *(716)*

6. When there is a narrowing of the arteries and arterioles, peripheral vascular resistance _____. *(716)*

A. Increase(s)
B. Decrease(s)
C. Widen(s)
D. Narrow(s)

**D.** **Hypertension.**

1. Which factors contribute to hypertension? Select all that apply. *(716)*

    1. _____      Cardiac stimulation
    2. _____      Retention of fluid
    3. _____      Vasodilation

2. Which stimulants may contribute to hypertension? Select all that apply. *(717)*

1. _____ Caffeine

2. _____ Nicotine

3. _____ Alcohol

4. _____ Amphetamines

3. Which are symptoms of hypertensive crisis? Select all that apply. *(727)*

1. _____ Nausea

2. _____ Restlessness

3. _____ Drowsiness

4. _____ Blurred vision

**E. Lifestyle Modifications.** Match the description in the numbered column with the correct lifestyle modification in the lettered column. Some modifications may be used more than once, and some may not be used. *(719)*

1. _____ Reduces water in the body, decreasing the circulating blood volume

2. _____ Decreases blood glucose and cholesterol levels, increasing sense of well-being

3. _____ Eliminates vasoconstriction caused by nicotine

4. _____ Reduces stress and lowers blood pressure

5. _____ Improves cardiac efficiency by increasing cardiac output and decreasing peripheral vascular resistance

6. _____ Reduces blood pressure by reducing the workload of the heart

A. Weight reduction
B. Smoking cessation
C. Sodium reduction
D. Exercise
E. Relaxation therapy or biofeedback

F.  **Drug Therapy.** Match the actions of the drugs in the numbered column with the correct classification of drugs in the lettered column. Some classifications may be used more than once, and some may not be used.

1. _____    Block alpha receptor effects, lowering blood pressure by reducing peripheral resistance *(722)*

2. _____    Decrease fluid retention by decreasing the production of aldosterone *(722)*

3. _____    Reduce blood pressure by blocking the beta effects of catecholamines *(721)*

4. _____    Inhibit impulses from the vasomotor center in the brain, reducing peripheral resistance and lowering blood pressure *(722)*

5. _____    Block receptors for angiotensin II and reduce aldosterone secretion *(722)*

6. _____    Reduce blood volume through promotion of renal excretion of sodium and water *(721)*

7. _____    Block the movement of calcium into cardiac and vascular smooth muscle cells, reducing heart rate, decreasing force of cardiac contraction, and dilating peripheral blood vessels *(722)*

8. _____    Relax arteriolar smooth muscle *(722)*

9. _____    Prevent the conversion of angiotensin I to angiotensin II, a potent vasoconstrictor, decreasing peripheral resistance *(722)*

A.  Central-adrenergic blockers
B.  Calcium channel blockers
C.  Alpha-adrenergic receptor blockers
D.  ACE inhibitors
E.  Direct vasodilators
F.  Beta-adrenergic receptor blockers
G.  Diuretics
H.  Angiotensin II receptor antagonists

**G. Drug Therapy.** Match the side effect or caution in the numbered column with the correct classification of drugs in the lettered column. Some classifications may be used more than once.

1. _____ Palpitations, dizziness, headache, drowsiness *(720)*
2. _____ Hypoglycemia *(720)*
3. _____ Hypovolemia and hypokalemia *(721)*
4. _____ Flushing, dizziness, headache *(721)*
5. _____ Skin rash, cough *(721)*
6. _____ Use cautiously in patients with asthma, diabetes, and COPD *(720)*
7. _____ Fluid and electrolyte imbalances *(721)*
8. _____ Dry mouth, weakness *(720)*

A. Centrally acting drugs
B. Beta blockers
C. Calcium channel blockers
D. Alpha-adrenergic receptor blockers
E. Diuretics
F. ACE inhibitors

**H. Drug Therapy.** Match the names of the drugs in the numbered column with the correct classification of drugs in the lettered column.

1. _____ Prazosin (Minipress) *(720)*
2. _____ Hydrochlorothiazide (HCTZ) and furosemide (Lasix) *(721)*
3. _____ Losartan potassium (Cozaar) *(721)*
4. _____ Clonidine (Catapres) and methyldopa (Aldomet) *(720)*
5. _____ Propranolol (Inderal) *(720)*
6. _____ Hydralazine (Apresoline), diazoxide (Hyper-stat), and sodium nitroprusside (Nitropress) *(721)*
7. _____ Captopril (Capoten) and enalapril (Vasotec) *(721)*
8. _____ Verapamil (Calan) and diltiazem (Cardizem) *(721)*

A. Calcium channel blockers
B. Beta blockers
C. Direct vasodilators
D. Angiotensin II receptor antagonists
E. Diuretics
F. Alpha-adrenergic receptor blockers
G. Centrally acting drugs (alpha 2 agonists)
H. ACE inhibitors

I.  **Complications.**

1.  Using this figure, list four body structures (A–D) damaged by long-term blood pressure elevation. *(717-718)*

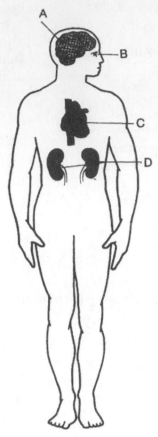

A.  _____

B.  _____

C.  _____

D.  _____

2.  As blood pressure rises, what are complications that occur? Select all that apply. *(717)*

    1.  _____    Heart failure
    2.  _____    Heart attack
    3.  _____    Blindness
    4.  _____    Kidney disease
    5.  _____    Hypoglycemia

3.  What are long-term effects of hypertension on the eyes? Select all that apply. *(718)*

    1.  _____    Retinal hemorrhages
    2.  _____    Pupil dilation
    3.  _____    Papilledema
    4.  _____    Narrowing of retinal arterioles

4. What are long-term effects of hypertension on the heart? Select all that apply. *(717)*
   1. _____ Angina
   2. _____ Myocardial infarction
   3. _____ Vasodilation
   4. _____ Coronary artery disease

5. What are long-term effects of hypertension on the brain? Select all that apply. *(717)*
   1. _____ Dehydration
   2. _____ Transient ischemic attacks
   3. _____ Strokes

6. At what age do complications of hypertension increase? *(715)*
   1. 20 years
   2. 30 years
   3. 40 years
   4. 50 years

7. What is the leading cause of death in people with hypertension? *(715)*
   1. Stroke
   2. Kidney failure
   3. Cardiac disease
   4. Pneumonia

8. How does aging affect blood pressure? Select all that apply. *(717)*
   1. _____ Increased elasticity of arteries
   2. _____ Decreased cardiac output
   3. _____ Increased peripheral vascular resistance
   4. _____ Decreased systolic blood pressure
   5. _____ Pulse pressure widens

## MULTIPLE-CHOICE QUESTIONS

J.  Choose the most appropriate answer.

1. The most common cardiovascular problem in the United States today is: *(715)*
   1. arteriosclerosis.
   2. coronary artery disease.
   3. myocardial infarction.
   4. hypertension.

2. The cause of primary (essential) hypertension is: *(716)*
   1. kidney disease.
   2. drugs.
   3. pregnancy.
   4. unknown.

3. Hypertension is usually detected in which age group? *(715)*
   1. 20–29
   2. 30–50
   3. 51–60
   4. over 60

4. A blood pressure of 135/87 is considered to be: *(716)*
   1. hypertension, stage 1.
   2. normal.
   3. prehypertension.
   4. hypertension, stage 2.

5. In which risk group is a hypertensive patient who smokes half a pack of cigarettes a day and who has no heart disease or heart damage, classified? *(715)*
   1. Risk A
   2. Risk B
   3. Risk C
   4. Risk D

6. Isolated systolic blood pressure elevations of 160 mm Hg in older adults are most often due to: *(716)*
   1. decreased cardiac output.
   2. atherosclerosis.
   3. increased peripheral vascular resistance.
   4. increased pulse pressure.

7. The diameter of blood vessels is regulated primarily by: *(716)*
   1. the heart muscle.
   2. adrenal gland hormones.
   3. the vasomotor center.
   4. thyroid gland hormones.

8. Patients with systolic pressures between 120 and 139 and with diastolic pressures between 80 and 89 are said to have: *(716)*
   1. normal hypertension
   2. Risk Group B
   3. prehypertension
   4. Stage I

9. An older patient taking furosemide (Lasix) for hypertension complains of muscle weakness, confusion, and irritability. Which patient teaching is correct for this patient? *(721)*
   1. Decrease sodium in the diet.
   2. Increase potassium in the diet.
   3. Increase fluid intake.
   4. Decrease vitamin K intake.

10. Beta blockers are contraindicated in patients with: *(721)*
    1. hypertension.
    2. edema.
    3. osteoporosis.
    4. asthma.

11. When people with diabetes are taking beta blockers for hypertension, the only sign of hypoglycemia may be: *(721)*
    1. diaphoresis.
    2. fatigue.
    3. hunger.
    4. excessive thirst.

12. Older patients taking beta blockers are at greater risk than younger people for: *(721)*
    1. bradycardia.
    2. hypoglycemia.
    3. bronchoconstriction.
    4. GI upset.

13. Which group of patients responds better to diuretics as treatment for hypertension? *(720)*
    1. Caucasians
    2. African-Americans
    3. Asians
    4. Hispanics

14. Older patients taking antihypertensives are more susceptible to orthostatic hypotension, increasing their risk for: *(727)*
    1. confusion.
    2. myocardial infarction.
    3. falls.
    4. congestive heart failure.

15. When body position is changed from supine to standing, the systolic pressure normally: *(724)*
    1. rises about 5 mm Hg.
    2. rises about 10 mm Hg.
    3. falls about 5 mm Hg.
    4. falls about 10 mm Hg.

16. If a patient's diastolic pressure is 120 mm Hg, the nurse should: *(724)*
    1. reassess it in 10 minutes.
    2. reassess it in 30 minutes.
    3. notify the physician.
    4. encourage the patient to stay on bed rest.

17. What is the danger of suddenly stopping antihypertensive drugs? *(726)*
    1. Orthostatic hypotension
    2. Bradycardia
    3. Hypokalemia
    4. Rebound hypertension

18. People with increased blood pressure should not take over-the-counter: *(726)*
    1. analgesics.
    2. cold remedies.
    3. antacids.
    4. laxatives.

19. A common side effect of many antihypertensives is: *(727)*
    1. GI distress.
    2. sexual dysfunction.
    3. respiratory depression.
    4. rebound hypertension.

20. Without appropriate treatment, the patient in hypertensive crisis may develop: *(727)*
    1. cerebrovascular accident.
    2. hyperglycemia.
    3. respiratory acidosis.
    4. adrenal insufficiency.

21. What percentage of people with hypertension do not know they have it? *(715)*
    1. 10%
    2. 20%
    3. 30%
    4. 40%

22. Although 59% of people with hypertension are being treated, in what percentage of people is hypertension controlled? *(715)*
    1. 20%
    2. 28%
    3. 34%
    4. 42%

23. What is the medical treatment goal for patients with diabetes or renal disease? *(719)*
    1. Lower than 110/70
    2. 120/80
    3. 130/80
    4. 140/90

24. Which drug is recommended for initial therapy for hypertension, according to JNC-7? *(720)*
    1. Thiazide-type diuretic
    2. ACE inhibitor
    3. Calcium channel blocker
    4. Beta adrenergic blocker

25. How does a blood pressure cuff which is too small affect the blood pressure reading? *(723-724)*
    1. False high reading
    2. False low reading
    3. Systolic reading too high
    4. Diastolic reading too low

26. Patients taking antihypertensive medications are encouraged to rise slowly from a lying or sitting position in order to prevent: *(726)*
    1. syncope.
    2. orthostatic hypotension.
    3. hypertensive crisis.
    4. confusion.

27. What may occur if antihypertensive drugs are stopped abruptly? *(726)*
    1. Hypotensive crisis
    2. Orthostatic hypotension
    3. Rebound hypertension
    4. Kidney failure

28. What is the percentage of people with hypertension who have primary or essential hypertension? *(716)*
    1. 10–15%
    2. 25–30%
    3. 45–50%
    4. 90–95%

## ALTERNATE FORMAT QUESTIONS

K. 1. Which food groups are emphasized in the DASH diet? Select all that apply. *(725)*
    1. Vegetables
    2. Fruits
    3. Nuts and seeds
    4. Whole milk

2. Which blood studies are usually ordered for people with hypertension? Select all that apply. *(718)*
   1. Hematocrit
   2. Glucose
   3. Potassium
   4. Calcium
   5. Creatine
   6. Prothrombin time
   7. Thyroid function
   8. Lipid profile

3. Which of the following are teaching points for patients with orthostatic hypotension? Select all that apply. *(726)*
   1. Eat a low-sodium diet.
   2. Avoid prolonged standing.
   3. Avoid cholesterol in diet.
   4. Avoid hot baths and showers.
   5. Rise slowly.

4. What are causes of secondary hypertension? Select all that apply. *(723)*
   1. Renal disease
   2. Sedentary lifestyle
   3. Tobacco use
   4. Narrowing of the aorta
   5. Increased intracranial pressure

**L.** Refer to Table 37-1, p. 716 in the textbook.

   1. What is the category for a person with blood pressure of 150/95? *(716)*

   2. What is the category for a person with blood pressure of 122/84? *(716)*

   3. What is the category for a person with blood pressure of 118/78? *(716)*

   4. What is the category for a person with blood pressure of 180/110? *(716)*

**M.** Refer to Table 37-2, p. 719 in the textbook.

   1. What is the average systolic blood pressure reduction range for a person who walks briskly 30 minutes per day, most days of the week? *(719)*

   2. What is the average systolic blood pressure reduction range for a person who adopts the DASH eating plan? *(719)*

   3. What is the average systolic blood pressure reduction range for a person who maintains body weight with a body mass index between 18.5–24.9 kg/m$^2$? *(719)*

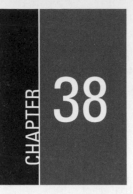

# 38 Digestive Tract Disorders

---

## OBJECTIVES

1. Identify the nursing responsibilities in the care of patients undergoing diagnostic tests and procedures for disorders of the digestive tract.

2. List the data to be included in the nursing assessment of the patient with a digestive disorder.

3. Describe the nursing care of patients with gastrointestinal intubation and decompression, tube feedings, total parenteral nutrition, digestive tract surgery, and drug therapy for digestive disorders.

4. Describe the pathophysiology, signs and symptoms, complications, and medical treatment of selected digestive disorders.

5. Assist in developing nursing care plans for patients receiving treatment for digestive disorders.

---

## LEARNING ACTIVITIES

**A. Mouth Disorders.** Match the definition in the numbered column with the most appropriate term in the lettered column.

1. _____ Difficulty swallowing *(756)*       A. Stomatitis
2. _____ Indigestion *(756)*                  B. Dysphagia
3. _____ Inflammation of the oral             C. Caries
             mucosa *(751)*                        D. Dyspepsia
4. _____ Tooth decay *(752)*

**341**

**B. Stomach Disorders.** Complete the statements in the numbered column with the most appropriate term in the lettered column. Some terms may be used more than once, and some terms may not be used.

1. The head of the bed is elevated during tube feedings to prevent _____. *(740)*
2. An inflammation of the lining of the stomach is called _____. *(763)*
3. The most serious complication of gastric endoscopy is _____. *(739)*
4. The best means of diagnosing gastritis is _____. *(764)*
5. Opiates (such as morphine) are not given to patients with diverticulosis to avoid the common side effect of _____. *(789)*
6. A complication that occurs following gastric surgery or when tube feedings of concentrated formula are given rapidly is _____. *(742)*
7. The most serious complication of gastric ulcers is _____. *(765, 766)*

A. Gastroscopy
B. Hemorrhage
C. Headache
D. Constipation
E. Perforation of the digestive tract
F. Dumping syndrome
G. Diarrhea
H. Aspiration
I. Drowsiness
J. Gastritis

**C. Esophageal Disorders.** Complete the statements in the numbered column with the most appropriate term in the lettered column. Some terms may be used more than once, and some terms may not be used.

1. Acidic gastric fluids can cause inflammation of the esophagus, called _____. *(763)*
2. The procedure used to assess bowel sounds is _____. *(734)*
3. Hiatal hernia is thought to be caused by weakness in the _____. *(761)*
4. The opening in the diaphragm through which the esophagus passes is the esophageal _____. *(760)*
5. Direct examination of the esophagus with an endoscope is called _____. *(761)*
6. The procedure used to detect the presence of air, fluid, or masses in tissues is known as _____. *(735)*
7. The protrusion of the lower esophagus and stomach upward through the diaphragm into the chest is _____. *(760)*
8. A surgical procedure that strengthens the lower esophageal sphincter by suturing the fundus of the stomach around the esophagus and anchoring it below the diaphragm is _____. *(761)*
9. Many patients with hiatal hernia report a feeling of burning and tightness rising from the lower sternum to the throat, which is called _____. *(761)*

A. Hiatus
B. Pyloric sphincter
C. Hiatal hernia
D. Esophagoscopy
E. Gastrectomy
F. Esophagitis
G. Heartburn
H. Palpation
I. Stomatitis
J. Auscultation
K. Fundoplication
L. Percussion
M. Lower esophageal sphincter

**D.   Intestinal Disorders.** Complete the statements in the numbered column with the most appropriate term in the lettered column. Some terms may be used more than once, and some terms may not be used.

1.   Two tests that allow the physician to confirm the presence of diverticula are colonoscopy and _____. *(789)*

2.   Ulcerative colitis and Crohn's disease are types of _____. *(786)*

3.   A loss of tissue from the lining of the digestive tract is _____. *(765)*

4.   Regional enteritis is also known as _____. *(786)*

5.   A break in the wall of the stomach or the duodenum that permits digestive fluids to leak into the peritoneal cavity is _____. *(786)*

6.   A common complication of peptic ulcers is _____. *(766)*

7.   Normally, the barrier that protects the digestive tract lining from digestive juices is _____. *(765)*

8.   The most common symptoms of inflammatory bowel disease are bloody diarrhea and _____. *(786)*

9.   A condition characterized by small saclike pouches in the intestinal wall is called _____. *(788)*

10.   A complication of diverticulitis in which an abnormal opening develops between the colon and the bladder is called _____. *(789)*

11.   Most diverticula are found in the _____. *(788)*

A.   Crohn's disease
B.   Hemorrhage
C.   Hiatal hernia
D.   Sigmoid colon
E.   Diverticulosis
F.   Barium enema
G.   Mucus
H.   Perforation
I.   Duodenum
J.   Fistula
K.   MRI
L.   Inflammatory bowel disease
M.   Abdominal pain
N.   Peptic ulcer

E.  **Bariatric Surgery.** Complete the statements in the numbered column with the most appropriate term in the lettered column. Some terms may be used more than once, and some terms may not be used.

1. _____  Procedure for decreasing size of stomach by creating a small upper pouch that receives food from the esophagus and connecting the pouch to the jejunum is called _____. *(775)*

2. _____  Complications of this bariatric procedure include dumping syndrome and iron and calcium deficiencies. *(775)*

3. _____  Complications of this bariatric procedure include metabolic and nutritional problems. *(775)*

4. _____  The newest restrictive bariatric procedure involving the laparoscopic placement of an adjustable band around the fundus of the stomach, creating a small pouch. *(775)*

5. _____  Restrictive bariatric surgery procedure that decreases the stomach capacity and bypasses much of the absorptive section of the GI tract. *(775)*

6. _____  Bariatric procedure in which the stomach is stapled to reduce its capacity, leaving a small opening for food to move from the small pouch into the lower stomach. *(775)*

7. _____  Best tolerated bariatric surgery procedure with low rate of complications. *(775)*

8. _____  The most common malabsorptive bariatric procedure that includes removal of the stomach and anastomosis of the duodenum to the distal ileum, shortening the digestive tract. *(775)*

A.  Gastrectomy
B.  Obesity
C.  Roux-en-Y gastric bypass (RNYGBP)
D.  Exercise
E.  Bulimia
F.  Anorexia
G.  Psychotherapy
H.  Liposuction
I.  Lipectomy
J.  Vertical banded gastroplasty (VBG)
K.  Lap-band system (LBS)
L.  Biliopancreatic division
M.  Extreme obesity
N.  Overweight

9. _____ Surgical excision of flabby folds of adipose tissue. *(775)*

10. _____ Removal of adipose tissue through a suction cannula. *(775)*

11. _____ Increased body weight caused by excessive body fat. *(774)*

12. _____ Term used when a person's body mass index is 40 kg/m² or more. *(774)*

## F. Surgical Treatment.

1. Which factors can cause persistent vomiting in patients with vertical banded gastroplasty? Select all that apply. *(775)*

   1. _____ Rupture of the staple line
   2. _____ Erosion of the band into the stomach tissue
   3. _____ Infection
   4. _____ Hemorrhage
   5. _____ Consuming solids too rapidly
   6. _____ Distention of walls of functional pouch

2. Which are interventions for the bariatric surgical patient related to imbalanced nutrition? Select all that apply. *(777)*

   1. _____ Imaging studies are done just after the patient is fed to assure that there are no leaks in the surgical sites.
   2. _____ The patient is advanced from water to full liquids, and then to clear liquids.
   3. _____ Once solid food is permitted, the typical diet is 800–1200 calories per day.
   4. _____ Small, frequent meals are recommended.
   5. _____ The meals are high in protein.
   6. _____ The meals are low in fat and high in carbohydrates.

3. Which are special needs of the obese surgical patient? Select all that apply. *(776)*

   1. _____ Risk of postoperative atelectasis and pneumonia
   2. _____ Risk of deep vein thrombosis and pulmonary emboli
   3. _____ Increased pressure ulcers
   4. _____ Increased risk for hemorrhage

**G. Intestinal Disorders.** Complete the statement in the numbered column with the most appropriate term in the lettered column. Some terms may be used more than once, and some terms may not be used.

1. A common symptom of malabsorption is the presence of excessive fat in the stool, which is called _____. *(777)*

2. A condition in which the large intestine loses the ability to contract effectively enough to propel the fecal mass toward the rectum is _____. *(780)*

3. The passage of loose, liquid stools with increased frequency is called _____. *(777)*

4. Increased pressure in the chest and abdominal cavities caused by straining to have a bowel movement is called _____. *(779)*

5. A term used to describe a condition in which one or more nutrients are not digested or absorbed is _____. *(777)*

6. Celiac sprue is treated by avoiding products that contain _____. *(777)*

7. A condition in which a person has hard, dry, infrequent stools that are passed with difficulty is _____. *(779)*

8. The retention of a large mass of stool in the rectum that the patient is unable to pass is called _____. *(780)*

9. The diet recommended for acute diarrhea is _____. *(778)*

10. Two examples of malabsorption are lactase deficiency and _____. *(777)*

11. Lactase deficiency is treated by eliminating _____. *(777)*

A. Valsalva's maneuver
B. Diarrhea
C. Fecal impaction
D. Gluten
E. High-fiber foods
F. Steatorrhea
G. Anorexia
H. Sprue
I. Constipation
J. Malabsorption
K. Paralytic ileus
L. Milk and milk products
M. Clear liquids
N. Megacolon

**H. Abdominal Hernia Disorders.** Complete the statements in the numbered column with the most appropriate term in the lettered column. Some terms may be used more than once, and some terms may not be used.

1. The repair of the muscle defect in abdominal hernia by suturing is called _____. *(785)*

2. For patients who cannot tolerate the stress of surgical hernia repair, a pad called a(n) _____ is placed over the hernia to provide support for the weak muscles. *(785)*

3. The bulging portion of the large intestine pushing through the abdominal wall is _____. *(784)*

4. Factors that cause hernias include heavy lifting and _____. *(784)*

5. Weak locations where hernias occur include the lower inguinal areas of the abdomen and the _____. *(784)*

6. Nausea, vomiting, pain, fever, and tachycardia may be signs and symptoms of a hernia complication called _____. *(784)*

7. Following inguinal hernia repair, a common complication is _____. *(785)*

8. An irreducible hernia, sometimes called _____, may impair blood flow to the trapped loop of intestine. *(784)*

A. Umbilicus
B. Hernia
C. Fecal incontinence
D. Scrotal swelling
E. Truss
F. Incarcerated
G. Coughing
H. Gangrene
I. Herniorrhaphy
J. Strangulation

**I. Drug Therapy.** Match the drugs in the numbered column with their actions in the lettered column.

1. _____ Anticholinergics *(746)*
2. _____ H$_2$-receptor antagonists *(746)*
3. _____ Antiemetics *(748)*
4. _____ Antacids *(746)*
5. _____ Mucosal barriers (cytoprotective) *(746)*
6. _____ Antidiarrheals *(748)*
7. _____ Antibacterials *(749)*
8. _____ Antifungals *(749)*
9. _____ Proton pump inhibitors *(746)*
10. _____ 5-HR receptor antagonists *(747)*
11. _____ Antibacterial agents *(748)*

A. Treat ulcerative colitis and *H. pylori*
B. Neutralize gastric acid
C. Cling to the surface of the ulcer and protect it so that healing can take place
D. Treat yeast infections in the mouth
E. Decrease hydrochloric acid production by competing at receptor sites
F. Prevent and treat nausea
G. Decrease intestinal motility so liquid portion of feces is reabsorbed
H. Reduce gastrointestinal motility and secretions; block acetylcholine
I. Treat diarrhea caused by pathogens
J. Prevent nausea and vomiting caused by chemotherapy
K. Inhibit gastric acid secretion and are used in peptic ulcer disease and GERD

**J.  Age-Related Changes.** Which of the following are normal age-related changes of the digestive tract? Select all that apply. *(732, 733)*

1. _____     Gums recede
2. _____     Taste buds increase
3. _____     Walls of the esophagus and stomach thin
4. _____     Increased stomach secretions
5. _____     Atrophy of muscle layer and mucosa in large intestine
6. _____     Constipation
7. _____     Tooth loss
8. _____     Esophageal sphincters are more rigid
9. _____     Anal sphincter strength decreases
10. _____    Vitamin A absorption decreases

**K.  Constipation.** Which factors may cause constipation in older adults? Select all that apply. *(779)*

1. _____     Low fluid intake
2. _____     Inactivity
3. _____     Hyperthyroidism
4. _____     Depression
5. _____     Medications

**L.  Capsule Endoscopy.** Which of the following statements are true about capsule endoscopy? Select all that apply. *(739)*

1. _____     Transmits video images of the entire digestive tract
2. _____     May detect obscure GI bleeding
3. _____     Detects inflammation caused by NSAIDs and radiotherapy
4. _____     Measures HCl and pepsin secreted in the stomach
5. _____     Detects parasitic infections
6. _____     Detects small bowel tumors
7. _____     Patients fast overnight before swallowing the capsule

**M.  Bowel Sounds.** Which are terms used to describe bowel sounds? Select all that apply. *(734)*

1. _____     Crackles
2. _____     Present or absent
3. _____     High-pitched
4. _____     Gurgling
5. _____     Increased or decreased

**N. Dumping Syndrome.** Match the description in the numbered column with the stages of symptoms of dumping syndrome in the lettered column. Answers may be used more than once. *(772)*

1. _____ Occurs 1–3 hours after eating.

2. _____ Patient experiences abdominal fullness and nausea within 10–20 minutes of eating.

3. _____ Patient feels flushed and faint.

4. _____ Patient has abdominal bloating and flatulence.

5. _____ Symptoms in this stage are probably caused by distention of the small intestine by the consumed food and fluids.

6. _____ Patient experiences symptoms such as cramps and diarrhea 20–60 minutes after eating.

7. _____ Patient may perspire and feel weak, anxious, shaky, or hungry.

8. _____ Symptoms in this stage probably caused a shift of a modest amount of fluid from the circulation into the intestines.

9. _____ Patient's heart rate races and patient breaks into a sweat as a result of pooling of blood in the abdominal organs.

10. _____ Symptoms in this stage are a result of hypoglycemia caused by an exaggerated rise in insulin secretion in response to the rapid delivery of carbohydrates into the intestine.

A. First stage
B. Intermediate stage
C. Third stage

**O. Dumping Syndrome.** Which aspects of care should the nurse teach the patient who experiences dumping syndrome? Select all that apply. *(772)*

1. _____ Follow a diet low in fat and protein.

2. _____ Drink fluids between meals, not with them.

3. _____ Lie down for about 30 minutes after meals.

4. _____ Follow a low carbohydrate diet.

**P.  Digestive Tract.** In the Figure 38-1 (p. 731) below, label the parts (A–W) of the digestive tract. *(731)*

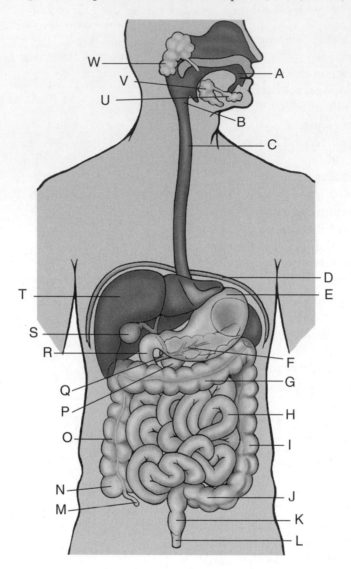

A. _____

B. _____

C. _____

D. _____

E. _____

F. _____

G. _____

H. _____

I. _____

J. _____

K. _____

L. _____

M. _____

N. _____

O. _____

P. _____

Q. _____

R. _____

S. _____

T. _____

U. _____

V. _____

W. _____

**Q. GI Tubes.**

1. Using the Figure 38-5 (p. 741) below, label the gastrointestinal tubes using the letters below. *(741)*

   1. Miller-Abbott tube _____

   2. Sengstaken-Blakemore tube _____

   3. Levin tube _____

   4. Weighted-flexible feeding tube _____

   5. Lavacuator tube (orogastric) _____

   6. Salem sump tube _____

   7. Cantor tube _____

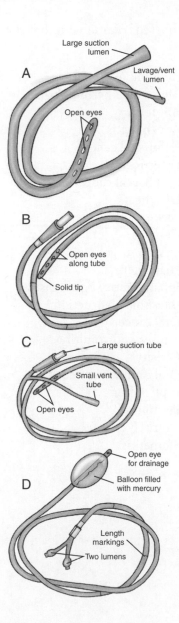

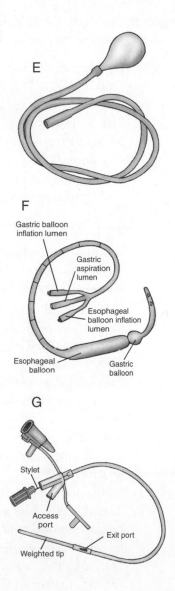

2. Which nasogastric tubes are used for gastric decompression (GI suction)? *(741)*

3. Which nasoenteric tubes are weighted and used for intestinal decompressions? *(741)*

4. Which esophageal-gastric balloon tube is used to control bleeding in the esophagus, usually in patients with severe complications of liver disease? *(741)*

**R. Nursing Diagnoses.** Match the nursing diagnosis in the numbered column with the related disorder in the lettered column. Answers may be used more than once.

1. _____ Deficient fluid volume *(760, 764, 778, 781, 783, 786)*

2. _____ Risk for injury related to hernia strangulation or distention *(762)*

3. _____ Risk for infection (peritonitis) related to rupture *(783)*

4. _____ Acute pain related to abdominal cramping and rectal irritation *(778)*

5. _____ Acute pain *(778, 786, 787)*

6. _____ Impaired oral mucous membranes related to tumor, edema, and secretions *(754)*

7. _____ Pain related to ulceration of the stomach or duodenum *(769)*

8. _____ Anxiety related to threat of serious illness and invasive treatment *(784)*

9. _____ Ineffective tissue perfusion related to effects of anesthesia, immobility *(790)*

10. _____ Impaired urinary elimination related to abdominal surgery, anesthesia *(785)*

11. _____ Sexual dysfunction related to perineal surgery *(790)*

12. _____ Impaired skin integrity related to pressure created by the truss *(785)*

A. Abdominal hernia
B. Abdominal hernia repair
C. Anorexia
D. Appendicitis
E. Colorectal cancer
F. Diverticulosis
G. Esophageal cancer
H. Diarrhea
I. Feeding problems
J. Gastritis
K. Gastric surgery
L. Hiatal hernia
M. Inflammatory bowel disease
N. Intestinal obstruction
O. Oral cancer
P. Nausea and vomiting
Q. Obesity
R. Oral cancer postoperative
S. Peptic ulcer
T. Peritonitis
U. Stomach cancer
V. Stomatitis

13. _____ Acute pain related to inflammation from diverticula *(789)*

14. _____ Feeding self-care deficit related to paralysis, weakness, poor coordination, confusion, visual impairment *(751)*

15. _____ Deficient fluid volume related to vomiting and bleeding *(764)*

16. _____ Imbalanced nutrition: less than body requirements related to inability to consume or retain food *(760)*

17. _____ Impaired oral mucous membranes related to trauma, infection, adverse drug effects *(752)*

18. _____ Acute pain related to scrotal swelling *(785)*

19. _____ Acute pain related to esophageal lesion, effect of radiation therapy *(757)*

20. _____ Risk for aspiration related to regurgitation of gastric contents *(762)*

21. _____ Imbalanced nutrition: more than body requirements related to excessive calorie intake for metabolic needs *(776)*

22. _____ Imbalanced nutrition: less than body requirements related to inadequate food intake *(750)*

23. _____ Pain related to tumor or surgical trauma, or both *(774)*

24. _____ Risk for injury related to wound dehiscence *(785)*

25. _____ Impaired skin integrity related to irritation of loose stool *(778)*

26. _____ Risk for injury related to gastric dilatation, obstruction, perforation *(771)*

27. _____ Deficient fluid volume related to vomiting, intestinal suction *(781)*

28. _____ Imbalanced nutrition: less than body requirement related to malabsorption *(786)*

29. _____ Acute pain related to tissue trauma in mouth *(754)*

30. _____ Imbalanced nutrition: less than body requirements related to dysphagia *(757)*

31. _____ Decreased cardiac output related to hypovolemia secondary to dumping syndrome *(771)*

32. _____ Diarrhea related to intestinal inflammation *(786)*

33. _____ Acute pain related to distention in abdomen *(781)*

34. _____ Risk for infection related to complications of obstruction *(781)*

## MULTIPLE-CHOICE QUESTIONS

**S.**  Choose the most appropriate answer.

1. The type of acid-base imbalance that results from prolonged vomiting is: *(759)*
   1. metabolic acidosis.
   2. metabolic alkalosis.
   3. respiratory acidosis.
   4. respiratory alkalosis.

2. Normal bowel sounds include: *(734)*
   1. minimal clicks and gurgles.
   2. clicks and gurgles 5–30 times/minute.
   3. steady, consistent gurgling sounds.
   4. no sounds for 1 full minute.

3. Which herb is effective in calming an upset
   stomach, reducing flatulence, and preventing motion sickness? *(760)*
   1. Ginkgo
   2. Ginseng
   3. Ginger root
   4. Garlic

4. After insertion of a gastric tube, feedings
   are not started until: *(740)*
   1. the patient requests food.
   2. adequate oxygen levels are achieved on
      blood gases.
   3. placement of tube is certain.
   4. oral fluids are tolerated.

5. Severe or prolonged vomiting puts the
   patient at risk for: *(760)*
   1. fluid volume deficit.
   2. altered tissue perfusion.
   3. hemorrhage.
   4. infection.

6. The vomiting patient who is also unconscious or who has impaired swallowing is at
   risk for aspiration and should be placed in
   which position? *(760)*
   1. Lying flat in bed
   2. With head of bed elevated at least 90
      degrees
   3. Side-lying
   4. With head of bed slightly elevated, for
      example, at 30 degrees

7. To prevent night-time reflux, the sleeping position for patients with hiatal hernia
   should be: *(762)*
   1. side-lying.
   2. with head of bed at 90-degree angle.
   3. flat.
   4. with head of bed elevated 6–12 inches.

8. Sudden, sharp pain starting in the mide-
   pigastric region and spreading across the
   entire abdomen in patients with peptic
   ulcer may indicate: *(771)*
   1. infection.
   2. perforation.
   3. dyspnea.
   4. kidney failure.

9. If the patient's abdomen becomes rigid and
   tender and he or she draws the knees up to
   the chest, this may indicate: *(771)*
   1. peritonitis.
   2. perforation.
   3. kidney failure.
   4. pyloric obstruction.

10. The most prominent symptom of pyloric
    obstruction is persistent: *(766)*
    1. eructation.
    2. heartburn.
    3. vomiting.
    4. hemorrhage.

11. A complication of stomach surgery that
    occurs because the absence or decreased
    size of the stomach prevents the normal
    pacing of chyme moving into the intestine
    is: *(772)*
    1. malabsorption.
    2. dumping syndrome.
    3. coffee-ground emesis.
    4. obstructed pyloric sphincter.

12. Severe constipation accompanied by trick-
    ling of liquid stool suggests: *(780)*
    1. pyloric obstruction.
    2. fecal impaction.
    3. intestinal hemorrhage.
    4. steatorrhea.

13. A major complication of appendicitis is: *(782)*
    1. diarrhea.
    2. constipation.
    3. fluid volume deficit.
    4. peritonitis.

14. The classic symptom of appendicitis is pain at: *(782)*
    1. McBurney's point.
    2. the xiphoid process.
    3. right hypochondriac region.
    4. inguinal node.

15. When appendicitis is suspected, the patient is allowed: *(782)*
    1. clear liquids.
    2. full liquids.
    3. nothing by mouth.
    4. soft foods.

16. In addition to deficient fluid volume, patients with peritonitis may go into shock because of: *(784)*
    1. edema.
    2. convulsions.
    3. septicemia.
    4. paralysis.

17. Pain is severe for several postoperative days following abdominoperineal resection. At first, the patient will probably be most comfortable in which position? *(791)*
    1. Supine
    2. Side-lying
    3. Prone
    4. Fowler's

18. Following abdominoperineal resection, a procedure that cleans, soothes, and increases circulation to the perineum is: *(791)*
    1. use of a TENS unit.
    2. Kegel exercises.
    3. the sitz bath.
    4. débridement.

19. What is the cause of most peptic ulcers? *(766)*
    1. *Helicobacter pylori*
    2. *E. coli*
    3. Stress
    4. Infection

20. A patient who should not use Ephedra sinica (Ma Huang) as an over-the-counter weight loss product is a person with: *(775)*
    1. a urinary tract infection.
    2. arthritis.
    3. dermatitis.
    4. hypertension.

21. Which natural substance can help control diarrhea? *(778)*
    1. Garlic
    2. Rice water
    3. Kava kava
    4. *Ephedra sinica*

22. Which type of laxative may not be effective for several days? *(779)*
    1. Bulk-producing laxative
    2. Intestinal stimulant
    3. Osmotic suppository
    4. Stool softener

23. Which type of diet is prescribed for moderate inflammatory bowel disease? *(787)*
    1. Low residue diet
    2. High-fiber diet
    3. Low-potassium diet
    4. Low-salt diet

24. The major nutritional goal of therapy for diarrhea is to replace: *(788)*
    1. potassium.
    2. sodium.
    3. calcium.
    4. fluids.

25. Which is a sign of intestinal rupture in a patient with intestinal obstruction? *(782)*
    1. Sudden vomiting of blood
    2. Sudden sharp pain
    3. Sudden increased temperature and chills
    4. Sudden diarrhea

26. The Roux-en-Y gastric bypass and the vertical-banded gastroplasty are restrictive procedures used to treat: *(775)*
    1. peptic ulcer.
    2. extreme obesity.
    3. stomach cancer.
    4. hiatal hernia.

27. Which bariatric procedure does not cause dumping syndrome or malabsorption, but does result in less weight loss than the other procedures? *(775)*
    1. Simple gastroplasty (stomach stapling)
    2. Roux-en-Y bypass
    3. Biliopancreatic diversion
    4. Vertical banded gastroplasty

**T. Nursing Care Plan.** Refer to Nursing Care Plan, The Patient with a Peptic Ulcer, p. 770 in the textbook.

1. What is the priority nursing diagnosis? *(770)*

2. What are this patient's risk factors for duodenal ulcers? *(770)*

3. What findings indicate the presence of duodenal ulcers? *(770)*

4. What diet is this patient on? *(770)*

5. What are signs and symptoms of bleeding you would be monitoring with this patient? Select all that apply. *(770)*
    1. Clay-colored stools
    2. Bradycardia
    3. Pallor
    4. Hypotension

6. If hemorrhage occurs in this patient, what will you do? *(770)*

7. What is the main symptom of perforation for which you would monitor? *(770)*

8. What is the main sign of pyloric obstruction for which you would monitor in this patient? *(770)*

9. What are the basic types of medications for peptic ulcer disease? Select all that apply. *(766)*
    1. Proton pump inhibitors
    2. H$_2$ antagonists
    3. Antacids
    4. Anticoagulants
    5. Mucosal barrier agents

10. What is triple therapy (two antibiotics and a proton pump inhibitor) used to treat? *(766)*

# Disorders of the Liver, Gallbladder, and Pancreas

---

## OBJECTIVES

1. Identify nursing assessment data related to the functions of the liver, gallbladder, and pancreas.

2. Identify the nurse's role in tests and procedures performed to diagnose disorders of the liver, gallbladder, and pancreas.

3. Describe the care of the patient who has an esophageal balloon tube in place.

4. Explain the pathology, signs and symptoms, diagnosis, complications, and medical treatment of selected disorders of the liver, gallbladder, and pancreas.

5. Assist in developing a nursing care plan care for the patient with liver, gallbladder, or pancreatic dysfunction.

---

## LEARNING ACTIVITIES

**A. Key Terms.** Match the definition in the numbered column with the most appropriate term in the lettered column.

1. _____ Chronic, progressive liver disease *(808)*

2. _____ Accumulation of excess fluid in the peritoneal cavity *(799)*

3. _____ Removal of ascitic fluid from the peritoneal cavity *(810)*

4. _____ Enlargement of the liver *(799)*

5. _____ Removal of the gallbladder *(819)*

6. _____ Presence of gallstones in the gallbladder *(818)*

7. _____ Obstruction in common bile duct *(819)*

8. _____ Excess fat in stools *(819)*

9. _____ Jaundice *(799)*

10. _____ Enlargement of breast tissue in males *(799)*

A. Paracentesis
B. Steatorrhea
C. Hepatomegaly
D. Icterus
E. Cirrhosis
F. Gynecomastia
G. Cholecystectomy
H. Choledocholithiasis
I. Cholelithiasis
J. Ascites

**B.  Anatomy and Physiology.** Complete the statements in the numbered column with the most appropriate term in the lettered column. Some terms may be used more than once, and some terms may not be used.

1.  Bile is produced in the _____. *(796)*

2.  Specialized reticuloendothelial cells in the liver that ingest old red blood cells and bacteria are called _____. *(796)*

3.  When fats pass into the duodenum, the gallbladder and the liver respond by delivering bile to the small intestine through the _____. *(796)*

4.  A product of the normal breakdown of old red blood cells in the liver is _____. *(796)*

5.  The vessel that delivers blood from the aorta to the liver is the _____. *(796)*

6.  The vessel that delivers blood from the intestines to the liver is the _____. *(796)*

7.  Bile produced in the liver passes into the gallbladder for storage through the _____. *(799)*

8.  Bile is stored in the _____. *(799)*

9.  When the sclera turns yellow in patients with liver disease, this condition is called scleral _____. *(799)*

A.  Bilirubin
B.  Portal vein
C.  Pancreas
D.  Kupffer cells
E.  Gallbladder
F.  Hepatic artery
G.  Pancreatic duct
H.  Common bile duct
I.  Icterus
J.  Liver
K.  Cystic duct
L.  Jaundice

**C.  Diagnostic Procedures.** Match the statements in the numbered column with the most appropriate term in the lettered column. Some terms may be used more than once, and some terms may not be used.

1.  _____    A procedure in which a radioactive substance is injected into a vein and visualized in a radiograph to reveal tumors and abscesses *(802)*

2.  _____    The use of sound waves to create an image of the liver, spleen, pancreas, gallbladder, and biliary system that is noninvasive and painless *(800)*

3.  _____    A procedure that involves removal of a small specimen of liver tissue for examination *(801)*

4.  _____    A primary complication of liver biopsy that occurs because of the liver's rich blood supply and potential for impaired coagulation *(801)*

5.  _____    A primary complication of liver biopsy that occurs if the lung is accidentally punctured during the biopsy *(804)*

A.  Liver biopsy
B.  Pneumothorax
C.  Ultrasonography
D.  Hemothorax
E.  Liver scan
F.  Hemorrhage
G.  PET scan

**D. Hepatitis.** Match the statements in the numbered column with the most appropriate term in the lettered column. Some terms may be used more than once, and some terms may not be used.

1. _____ The second phase of hepatitis, which lasts from 2–4 weeks, characterized by jaundice and clay-colored stools *(805)*

2. _____ Serum hepatitis transmitted in body fluids *(804)*

3. _____ Elevation in serum bilirubin when bile channels are compressed due to inflammation in the liver *(804)*

4. _____ The third phase of hepatitis, in which fatigue, malaise, and liver enlargement last for several months *(805)*

5. _____ Infectious hepatitis or epidemic hepatitis, transmitted by water, food, or contaminated medical equipment *(804)*

6. _____ The first phase of hepatitis, which lasts from 1–21 days, when the patient is most infectious *(805)*

7. _____ The most common type of hepatitis *(804)*

A. Hepatitis B
B. Preicteric phase
C. Angioedema
D. Jaundice
E. Icteric phase
F. Anorexia
G. Posticteric phase
H. Hepatitis A

**E. Cirrhosis.** Match the definition or description in the numbered column with the most appropriate term in the lettered column. Some terms may be used more than once, and some terms may not be used.

1. _____ A symptom common in cirrhosis that is characterized by tingling or numbness in the extremities thought to be caused by vitamin B deficiencies *(809)*

2. _____ Obstructive cirrhosis that develops as a result of obstruction to bile flow *(808)*

3. _____ Results from venous congestion and hypoxia *(808)*

4. _____ A chronic, progressive disease of the liver that is characterized by degeneration and destruction of liver cells *(808)*

5. _____ Liver enlarges, becomes "knobby," and shrinks later *(808)*

A. Alcoholic cirrhosis (Laennec's disease)
B. Peripheral neuropathy
C. Cirrhosis
D. Postnecrotic cirrhosis
E. Biliary cirrhosis
F. Dyspepsia
G. Cardiac cirrhosis

**F.  Cirrhosis Complications.** Match the effects of cirrhosis complications in the numbered column with the most appropriate complication of cirrhosis in the lettered column. Some terms may be used more than once, and some may not be used. *(809)*

1. _____  Results in leaking of lymph fluid and albumin-rich fluid from the diseased liver

2. _____  Renal failure following diuretic therapy, paracentesis, or GI hemorrhage

3. _____  Caused by excessive ammonia in the blood, resulting in cognitive disturbances

4. _____  May cause fatal hemorrhage

5. _____  Development of collateral vessels

A.  Hepatic encephalopathy
B.  Esophageal varices
C.  Portal hypertension
D.  Epistaxis
E.  Hepatorenal syndrome
F.  Peripheral neuropathy
G.  Ascites

**G.  Bile Duct Obstruction.** Which of the following are signs of bile duct obstruction that should be taught to patients? Select all that apply. *(822)*

1. _____  Blood in the stool

2. _____  Dark urine

3. _____  Jaundice

4. _____  Steatorrhea

**H.  Gallstones.** In Figure 39-10 (p. 818) below, label the anatomic parts (A–G). *(818)*

A.  _____

B.  _____

C.  _____

D.  _____

E.  _____

F.  _____

G.  _____

**I.   Cirrhosis.** Using Figure 39-5 (p. 800) below, list the five areas of clinical manifestations of cirrhosis. *(800)*

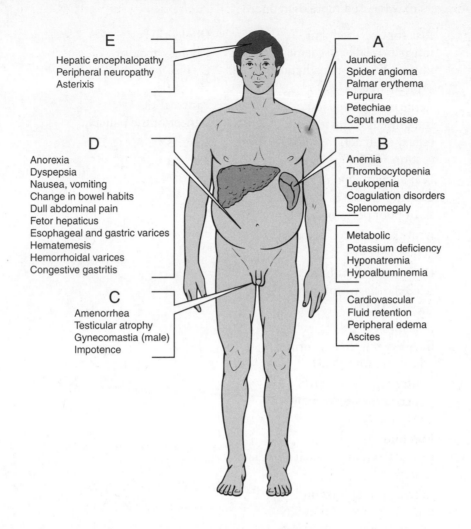

E
Hepatic encephalopathy
Peripheral neuropathy
Asterixis

A
Jaundice
Spider angioma
Palmar erythema
Purpura
Petechiae
Caput medusae

D
Anorexia
Dyspepsia
Nausea, vomiting
Change in bowel habits
Dull abdominal pain
Fetor hepaticus
Esophageal and gastric varices
Hematemesis
Hemorrhoidal varices
Congestive gastritis

B
Anemia
Thrombocytopenia
Leukopenia
Coagulation disorders
Splenomegaly

Metabolic
Potassium deficiency
Hyponatremia
Hypoalbuminemia

C
Amenorrhea
Testicular atrophy
Gynecomastia (male)
Impotence

Cardiovascular
Fluid retention
Peripheral edema
Ascites

A. _____

B. _____

C. _____

D. _____

E. _____

**J.   Nursing Diagnoses.** Match the nursing diagnosis in the numbered column with the disorder in the lettered column. Answers may be used more than once.

1. _____     Risk for impaired skin integrity related to edema, immobility, pruritus, hypoproteinemia *(814)*

2. _____     Acute pain related to inflammation, infection, biliary obstruction, autodigestion *(827)*

3. _____     Fear and anticipatory grieving related to diagnosis or poor prognosis *(832)*

4. _____     Acute pain related to biliary colic *(821)*

5. _____     Deficient fluid volume related to gastrointestinal suction *(822)*

6. _____     Risk for impaired skin integrity related to pruritus and scratching *(806)*

7. _____     Acute pain related to obstruction, extensive malignancy *(832)*

8. _____     Risk for injury (bleeding) related to vitamin K deficiency *(821)*

9. _____     Activity intolerance and impaired physical mobility related to fatigue, impaired metabolism, prescribed bed rest *(806)*

10. _____    Risk for infection related to tissue necrosis *(827)*

11. _____    Disturbed thought processes related to elevated blood ammonia *(814)*

12. _____    Disturbed body image related to jaundice *(806)*

13. _____    Ineffective breathing patterns related to ascites *(814)*

14. _____    Risk for injury related to impaired coagulation *(814)*

15. _____    Acute pain related to surgical incision, nasogastric tube *(822)*

A.   Cholelithiasis
B.   Cholecystectomy
C.   Cirrhosis
D.   Hepatitis
E.   Pancreatitis
F.   Cancer of the pancreas

## MULTIPLE-CHOICE QUESTIONS

**K.** Choose the most appropriate answer.

1. Patients with liver disease are at increased risk for drug: *(797)*
   1. incompatibilities.
   2. toxicities.
   3. idiosyncrasies.
   4. synthesis.

2. Clay-colored stools are characteristic of: *(819)*
   1. bile obstruction.
   2. pancreatitis.
   3. gastritis.
   4. Crohn's disease.

3. The prescribed diet for patients with hepatitis usually contains: *(806)*
   1. high carbohydrates and vitamins, low protein, low to moderate fat.
   2. low carbohydrates, moderate to high protein, high fat.
   3. high carbohydrates and vitamins, moderate to high protein, low to moderate fat.
   4. low carbohydrates, low protein, low to moderate fat.

4. Patients with hepatitis may have impaired skin integrity due to: *(807)*
   1. jaundice.
   2. pruritus or scratching.
   3. nausea and vomiting.
   4. fluid volume deficit.

5. The nurse should explain to patients with hepatitis that rest is necessary to allow the liver to heal by: *(806)*
   1. producing more white blood cells to fight infection.
   2. producing more platelets to assist in clotting.
   3. regenerating new cells to replace damaged cells.
   4. regenerating new blood vessels to replace damaged ones.

6. The nurse should be alert for signs of fluid retention in patients with hepatitis, which include increasing abdominal girth, rising blood pressure, and: *(807)*
   1. dry mucous membranes.
   2. tachycardia.
   3. edema.
   4. concentrated urine.

7. Which drugs may be ordered for pruritus, which occurs with hepatitis? *(807)*
   1. Antihistamines
   2. Antiemetics
   3. Antibiotics
   4. Analgesics

8. The patient with hepatitis may be self-conscious about his or her appearance because of: *(807)*
   1. cyanosis.
   2. redness.
   3. ulcerations.
   4. jaundice.

9. Health care workers who work with hospitalized patients should receive: *(808)*
   1. hepatitis B vaccinations.
   2. RhoGAM.
   3. influenza virus vaccine.
   4. immune globulin.

10. A frequent problem in cirrhosis for which small, semisolid meals are recommended is: *(814)*
    1. peripheral neuropathy.
    2. jaundice.
    3. anorexia.
    4. ascites.

11. The medical management of ascites aims to promote reabsorption and elimination of the fluid by means of salt restriction and: *(810)*
    1. antihistamines.
    2. analgesics.
    3. diuretics.
    4. antibiotics.

12. Potential complications of peritoneal-venous shunts used to allow ascitic fluid to drain from the abdomen and return to the bloodstream are tubing obstruction and: *(811)*
    1. jaundice.
    2. peripheral neuropathy.
    3. pruritus.
    4. peritonitis.

13. The best position for patients with ascites to help them breathe more easily is: *(815)*
    1. side-lying.
    2. prone.
    3. supine.
    4. with the head of the bed elevated.

14. The patient with cirrhosis is at great risk for injury or hemorrhage due to impaired: *(808)*
    1. coagulation.
    2. immunity.
    3. skin integrity.
    4. breathing patterns.

15. Since the esophagus and the trachea are adjacent to each other, upward movement of the esophageal balloon in the patient with cirrhosis may cause: *(815)*
    1. impaired circulation.
    2. airway obstruction.
    3. cardiac shock.
    4. perforated intestine.

16. Bile ducts respond to obstruction (such as gallstones) with spasms in an effort to move the stone; the intense spasmodic pain is called: *(818)*
    1. hepatic encephalopathy.
    2. renal colic.
    3. biliary colic.
    4. peripheral neuropathy.

17. A common symptom of cholecystitis is right upper quadrant pain that radiates to the: *(819)*
    1. sternum.
    2. shoulder.
    3. umbilicus.
    4. jaw.

18. When the cholecystectomy patient first returns from surgery, the drainage from the T tube may be bloody, but it should soon become: *(821)*
    1. dark amber.
    2. clay-colored.
    3. bright red.
    4. greenish brown.

19. What type of diet is recommended for patients with cholecystitis to decrease attacks of biliary colic? *(822)*
    1. Low protein
    2. Low fat
    3. Low carbohydrate
    4. Low salt

20. Patients with obstructed bile flow may have a deficiency of vitamin: *(822)*
    1. A.
    2. C.
    3. D.
    4. K.

21. A complication of endoscopic sphincterotomy is pancreatitis caused by accidental entry of the endoscope into the pancreatic duct. Early signs of pancreatitis are: *(820)*
    1. jaundice and confusion.
    2. nausea and vomiting.
    3. ascites and hypertension.
    4. pain and fever.

22. A gland that has both endocrine and exocrine functions is the: *(823)*
    1. pancreas.
    2. adrenal gland.
    3. thyroid gland.
    4. sebaceous gland.

23. Vitamin K is needed for the production of: *(822)*
    1. bile.
    2. calcium.
    3. prothrombin.
    4. thyroxine.

24. Specific blood studies used to assess pancreatic function include serum: *(824)*
    1. bilirubin.
    2. amylase.
    3. prothrombin.
    4. albumin.

25. The most prominent symptom of pancreatitis is: *(825)*
    1. jaundice.
    2. abdominal pain.
    3. hypertension.
    4. diarrhea.

26. To remove the stimulus for secretion of pancreatic fluid in acute pancreatitis, the patient is usually allowed: *(827)*
    1. nothing by mouth.
    2. a low-fat diet.
    3. a clear-liquid diet.
    4. a low-sodium diet.

27. Which drugs do patients with chronic pancreatitis need to take in order to digest food? *(827)*
    1. Analgesics
    2. Anticholinergics
    3. Antiemetics
    4. Pancreatic enzymes

28. Early signs of shock that may occur in patients with pancreatitis include: *(827)*
    1. restlessness.
    2. bradycardia.
    3. hypotension.
    4. easy bruising.

29. When patients with pancreatitis are on TPN in order to restrict oral intake and reduce pancreatic fluid secretion, the nurse must monitor for: *(830)*
    1. hyperkalemia.
    2. hypernatremia.
    3. hyperchloremia.
    4. hyperglycemia.

30. Which herb can harm the liver? *(798)*
    1. Garlic
    2. Ginkgo
    3. Comfrey
    4. Ginseng

31. The bile channels in the liver are compressed in patients with hepatitis, resulting in elevated: *(804)*
    1. serum creatinine.
    2. BUN.
    3. bilirubin.
    4. hemoglobin.

32. Which is a finding that supports the diagnosis of hepatitis? *(804)*
    1. Increased serum bilirubin
    2. Decreased prothrombin time
    3. Increased albumin
    4. Decreased urinary bilirubin

33. What is the prescribed diet for hepatitis? *(807)*
    1. Increased protein
    2. Increased fat
    3. Decreased carbohydrate
    4. Decreased calories

34. Which cultural group has the highest rate of death from cirrhosis of the liver? *(808)*
    1. Hispanics
    2. African-Americans
    3. Caucasians
    4. Asians

35. The medical treatment of hepatic encephalopathy is directed toward: *(809)*
    1. raising hemoglobin.
    2. reducing ammonia formation.
    3. decreasing urea.
    4. increasing prothrombin time.

36. In patients with hepatitis and in patients with cirrhosis, most of the calories should come from: *(807)*
    1. carbohydrates.
    2. protein.
    3. saturated fats.
    4. unsaturated fats.

37. Which is a common lab finding consistent with hepatitis? *(806)*
    1. Decreased levels of serum enzymes (AST, ALT, GT)
    2. Prolonged prothrombin time
    3. High albumin
    4. Low gamma globulin

38. Why is a liver biopsy sometimes done for a patient with hepatitis? *(806)*
    1. Confirm the diagnosis of hepatitis
    2. Determine if cancer is present
    3. Evaluate the harm caused by chronic HBV or HCV
    4. Examine the extent of inflammation

39. Which group of drugs is now being used in the treatment of patients with hepatitis (HBV and HBC)? *(806)*
    1. Antimicrobials
    2. Antivirals
    3. Anticoagulants
    4. Anticholinergics

## ALTERNATE FORMAT QUESTIONS

L. 1. Which are interventions for a patient who has just had a liver biopsy? Select all that apply. *(804)*
    1. Check pressure dressing every 15 minutes for the first hour, every 30 minutes for the next hour, and then hourly.
    2. Monitor the patient for signs of blood loss, which include bradycardia and hypertension.
    3. Keep the patient on the right side at least 2 hours.
    4. The patient may be kept flat up to 14 hours.

2. What are primary complications you would watch for in a patient with a liver biopsy? Select all that apply. *(804)*
    1. Hemorrhage
    2. Pneumothorax
    3. Hypertensive crisis
    4. Increased intracranial pressure

3. Which of the following results of blood tests and procedures are consistent with cirrhosis? Select all that apply. *(806)*
    1. Elevated serum and urine bilirubin
    2. Decreased serum enzymes
    3. Increased total serum protein
    4. Decreased cholesterol
    5. Prolonged prothrombin time

4. What neurologic symptoms are caused by a failing liver and excessive ammonia in the blood? Select all that apply. *(809)*
    1. Cognitive disturbances
    2. Declining level of consciousness
    3. Changes in neuromuscular function
    4. Numbness and tingling in extremities
    5. Edema in extremities

M. **Nursing Care Plan.** Refer to Nursing Care Plan, The Patient with Pancreatitis, p. 830 in the textbook.

1. What is the priority nursing diagnosis for this patient? *(830)*

2. What are the patient's risk factors? *(824, 830)*

3. What data was collected about this patient, indicating the presence of pancreatitis? *(830)*

4. What are causes of pancreatitis? Select all that apply. *(824)*
    1. Biliary tract disorders
    2. Alcoholism
    3. Peptic ulcer disease
    4. Hyperthyroidism
    5. Smoking

5. Which are common complications of pancreatitis? Select all that apply. *(826)*
    1. Pseudocyst
    2. Abscess
    3. Hypercalcemia
    4. Renal complications

6. What is a diet that is prescribed for patients with pancreatitis to avoid stimulating the pancreas and promote healing? Select all characteristics that apply. *(829)*
    1. Full liquid
    2. Bland
    3. High carbohydrate
    4. High fat

# Urologic Disorders

---

## OBJECTIVES

1.  List the data to be collected when assessing a patient who has a urologic disorder.

2.  Describe the diagnostic tests and procedures for patients with urologic disorders.

3.  Explain the nursing responsibilities for patients having tests and procedures to diagnose urologic disorders.

4.  Describe the nursing responsibilities for common therapeutic measures used to treat urologic disorders.

5.  Explain the pathophysiology, signs and symptoms, complications, and treatment of disorders of the kidney, ureters, bladder, and urethra.

6.  Assist in developing a nursing care plan for patients with urologic disorders.

---

## LEARNING ACTIVITIES

**A.  Physiology of Urinary System.** Complete the statement in the numbered column with the most appropriate term in the lettered column. Some terms may be used more than once, and some terms may not be used.

1.  Some nonelectrolyte substances that are not reabsorbed by the tubules include uric acid, urea, and _____. *(838, 839)*

2.  Reabsorption of water by the tubules occurs through the process of _____. *(838)*

3.  The end product of glomerular filtration and tubular reabsorption is _____. *(838)*

4.  Aldosterone is secreted by the adrenal glands in response to _____. *(839)*

5.  Aldosterone causes the reabsorption of water and _____. *(839)*

6.  Substances secreted by the tubules are called _____. *(839)*

7.  The amount of water reabsorbed in the kidneys is influenced by antidiuretic hormone and _____. *(839)*

8.  Urine is moved from the kidney to the bladder by means of _____. *(839)*

A.  Aldosterone
B.  Glucose
C.  Ions
D.  Peristalsis
E.  Concentrated urine
F.  Urethra
G.  Urine
H.  Creatinine
I.  Osmosis
J.  Sodium
K.  Dilute urine

**B.  Physiology.** Match the description or definition in the numbered column with the most appropriate term in the lettered column. Some terms may be used more than once, and some terms may not be used.

1.  _____  Causes reabsorption of water in the renal tubules, decreasing urine volume *(840)*

2.  _____  Is released in response to inadequate renal blood flow or low arterial pressure *(840)*

3.  _____  The hormone secreted in the kidneys that stimulates the bone marrow to produce red blood cells *(840)*

4.  _____  The hormone that is released from the pituitary gland when stimulated by hypertonic plasma *(840)*

5.  _____  Influences increased concentration of blood *(839)*

6.  _____  A common condition that leads to increased blood osmolality *(839)*

A.  Erythropoietin
B.  Angiotensin II
C.  Osmolality
D.  Calcium
E.  Renin
F.  Hypotonic
G.  Antidiuretic hormone
H.  Dehydration

**C. Diagnostic Procedures.** Complete the statements in the numbered column with the most appropriate term in the lettered column. Some terms may be used more than once, and some terms may not be used. *(842)*

1. With normally functioning kidneys, the serum creatinine level is _____.

2. _____ is a general indicator of the kidneys' ability to excrete urea; values are raised by high-protein diets, gastrointestinal bleeding, dehydration, and some drugs.

3. A better measurement of kidney functioning than the BUN because it is elevated only in kidney disorders is the _____.

4. With normally functioning kidneys, the urine creatinine level is _____.

5. The best test of overall kidney function is _____.

6. Two tests that are compared to each other and that should be opposite each other if kidneys are functioning normally are the creatinine clearance and the _____.

A. Blood urea nitrogen (BUN)
B. High
C. Serum electrolytes
D. Urine culture
E. Very low
F. Serum creatinine
G. Creatinine clearance

**D. Diagnostic Procedures.** Match the definition or description in the numbered column with the most appropriate term in the lettered column. Some terms may be used more than once, and some terms may not be used.

1. _____ A catheter is inserted into the bladder, and fluid is instilled until the patient reports the urge to void *(847)*

2. _____ Measures the rate of urine flow during voiding *(847)*

3. _____ Outlines the contour of the bladder and shows reflux of urine *(846)*

4. _____ The backward movement of urine from the bladder into the ureters *(847)*

5. _____ Dye is injected IV, radiographs of kidney, ureters, and bladder are taken; used to assess kidney function *(846)*

6. _____ A catheter is inserted into the bladder, dye is injected, and radiographs are taken *(846)*

7. _____ Used to evaluate bladder tone in the patient with incontinence or with a neurogenic bladder *(846)*

A. Reflux
B. Urodynamic study
C. Ultrasonography
D. Flat plate (KUB)
E. Cystometrogram
F. Cystogram
G. Intravenous pyelogram

E.  **Urologic Disorders.** Complete the statement in the numbered column with the most appropriate term in the lettered column. Some terms may be used more than once, and some terms may not be used.

1.  _____ is the condition in which calculi are formed in the kidneys. *(858)*

2.  Three diagnostic tests to confirm the presence and location of calculi in the urinary tract include ultrasound, IVP, and the _____. *(858)*

3.  _____ is inflammation of the renal pelvis. *(855)*

4.  A hereditary disorder in which grape-like cysts replace normal kidney tissue is _____. *(856)*

5.  _____ is the removal of a calculus. *(859)*

6.  The removal of a calculus from the renal pelvis is _____. *(859)*

7.  Inflammation of the urinary bladder is _____. *(853)*

8.  A urinalysis is done in patients with glomerulonephritis to detect red blood cell casts and _____. *(857)*

9.  The formation of calculi in the urinary tract is called _____. *(858)*

10. The formation of calculi in the kidneys is called _____. *(858)*

11. The intense, colicky pain of renal calculi may be relieved by narcotic analgesics and _____. *(860)*

12. Possible complications of lithotripsy include bruising and _____. *(859)*

13. Inflammation of the capillary loops in the glomeruli is _____. *(857)*

A.  Polycystic kidney disease
B.  Anticholinergics
C.  Pyelolithotomy
D.  Hemorrhage
E.  Polycystic kidney disease
F.  KUB
G.  MRI
H.  Proteinuria
I.  Glomerulonephritis
J.  Lithotomy
K.  Antispasmodics
L.  Urolithiasis
M.  Cystitis
N.  Platelets
O.  Nephrolithiasis
P.  Pyelonephritis

F.  **Urologic Surgery.** Match the definition or description in the numbered column with the most appropriate term in the lettered column. Some terms may be used more than once, and some terms may not be used. *(848)*

1.  _____    Removal of a kidney

2.  _____    A noninvasive procedure to break up calculi

3.  _____    Removal of the bladder

4.  _____    An incision made to open the bladder

5.  _____    A surgical procedure that reroutes the flow of urine

A.  Urinary diversion
B.  Lithotripsy
C.  Cystoscopy
D.  Cystectomy
E.  Nephrectomy
F.  Cystotomy

**G. Kidney Disorders.** Complete the statement in the numbered column with the most appropriate term in the lettered column. Some terms may be used more than once, and some terms may not be used.

1. _____ can be caused by the accumulation of calcium phosphate crystals and urea in the skin. *(872)*
2. Following the removal of a kidney, the condition in which peristalsis does not return within 3–4 days is called _____. *(864)*
3. When a calculus obstructs urine flow, the urine may back up into the kidney, causing _____. *(862)*
4. The placement of a tube in the kidney so that urine may drain through the tube into an external collection device is called _____. *(862)*
5. In patients with hydronephrosis, urine is usually strained and examined for _____. *(861)*
6. Distention of the kidney with urine is called _____. *(861)*

A. Hydronephrosis
B. Red blood cells
C. Nephrectomy
D. Cystectomy
E. Calculi
F. Paralytic ileus
G. Nephrostomy
H. Itching

**H. Chronic Kidney Disease.** Complete the statement in the numbered column with the most appropriate term in the lettered column. Some terms may be used more than once, and some terms may not be used.

1. _____, which is most often noted around the mouth, is a very late sign in chronic renal failure. *(872)*
2. Most patients with chronic renal failure retain water and _____. *(871)*
3. Emotional responses to chronic renal failure include depression, disturbed body image, and _____. *(871)*
4. Ovulation and _____ usually cease in females with chronic renal failure. *(871)*
5. The skeletal changes characteristic of chronic renal failure are known as _____. *(872)*
6. A diet high in carbohydrates and low in protein is prescribed to reduce the accumulation of _____. *(872)*
7. _____ is the condition in which calcium is lost from bones and replaced with fibrous tissue. *(872)*
8. Related to endocrine function, patients with chronic renal failure usually have _____. *(872)*
9. The effects of chronic renal failure on the male reproductive system typically include low sperm counts and _____. *(872)*

A. Anxiety
B. Impotence
C. Osteitis fibrosa
D. Hypothyroidism
E. Osteomalacia
F. Sodium
G. Cholesterol
H. Uremic frost
I. Urea
J. Menstruation
K. Renal osteodystrophy

I.   **Dialysis.** Complete the statement in the numbered column with the most appropriate term in the lettered column. Some terms may be used more than once, and some terms may not be used.

1. _____ is the passage of molecules through a semipermeable membrane into a special solution. *(873)*

2. A "_____" is a rippling sensation palpable on the venous side of the cannula or fistula. *(874)*

3. A leading cause of death in hemodialysis patients is _____. *(874)*

4. Vascular access for hemodialysis may be accomplished by temporary catheter, cannula, graft, or _____. *(874)*

5. A process by which blood is removed from the body and circulated through an artificial kidney is called _____. *(873)*

6. The major complication of peritoneal dialysis is _____. *(875)*

7. Vascular access sites must be assessed for _____. *(874)*

8. _____ allows a patient to have dialysis performed at night by a machine, giving the patient freedom during the day and reducing the risk of infection. *(875)*

9. A rushing, roaring, or "swoosh" noise heard through a stethoscope with each heartbeat is known as a _____. *(874)*

10. _____ allows the patient freedom from a machine and the independence to perform dialysis alone. *(875)*

A.   Thrill
B.   Peritonitis
C.   Cerebrovascular accident
D.   Nausca
E.   Dialysis
F.   Bruit
G.   Continuous ambulatory peritoneal dialysis
H.   Hemodialysis
I.   Murmur
J.   Fistula
K.   Patency
L.   Trocar
M.   Automated peritoneal dialysis

**J. Diagnostic Procedures.** Match the description or definition in the numbered column with the appropriate diagnostic test in the lettered column. Some tests may be used more than once, and some tests may not be used. *(842)*

1. _____ Examination of voided urine (or from catheter) specimen for pH, blood, glucose, and protein

2. _____ Clean-catch or midstream urine specimen is collected to determine which antibiotics will be effective against the specific organisms found in the culture

3. _____ Collection of urine for 12 or 24 hours, which is an estimate of the glomerular filtration rate

4. _____ A blood test that is a general indicator of the kidneys' ability to excrete urea

5. _____ A blood test that is indicative of the kidney's ability to excrete wastes

6. _____ A blood test that may show elevated sodium and potassium levels and decreased calcium levels, which indicate renal failure

A. Creatinine clearance
B. Osmolality
C. Serum creatinine
D. Urinalysis
E. Serum electrolytes
F. Blood urea nitrogen (BUN)
G. Urine sensitivity

**K. Urinary Tract Calculi.** Match the description of pain in the numbered column with the location of pain in the lettered column. Some locations may be used more than once, and some locations may not be used. *(858)*

1. _____ Dull flank pain

2. _____ Excruciating abdominal pain that radiates to the groin or perineum

A. Calculus in urethra
B. Calculus in renal pelvis
C. Calculus in ureter

**L. Acute Renal Failure.** Match the characteristics of acute renal failure in the numbered column with the stage in which it occurs in the lettered column. Some stages may be used more than once, and some stages may not be used. *(868)*

1. _____ Urine output exceeds 400 mL/day and may rise above 4 liters/day

2. _____ Serum electrolytes, BUN, and creatinine return to normal

3. _____ Urine specific gravity becomes fixed at 1.010

4. _____ Primary treatment goal is reversal of failing renal function to prevent further damage

5. _____ Urine output decreased to 400 mL/day or less

6. _____ Lasts 1–12 months

7. _____ Lasts up to 14 days

8. _____ Few waste products are excreted despite the production of large quantities of urine

9. _____ Lasts 1–3 days

A. Onset stage
B. Oliguric stage
C. Diuretic stage
D. Recovery stage

**M. Drug Therapy.** For the following drugs, indicate whether it is used to treat (A) oliguria or (B) hyperkalemia. *(850-852)*

1. _____ Hypertonic glucose and insulin

2. _____ Furosemide (Lasix)

3. _____ Sodium bicarbonate

4. _____ Calcium gluconate

5. _____ Ethacrynic acid (Edecrin)

6. _____ Sodium polystyrene sulfonate (Kayexalate)

**N. Age-Related Changes.** Describe the age-related changes in the kidneys that occur with respect to the areas listed below. *(840)*

1. Function of kidneys:_____

2. Adaptation of kidneys under stress:_____

3. Number of nephrons:_____

4. Renal blood vessels: _____

5. Renal blood flow: _____

6. Glomerular filtration rate: _____

7. Plasma renin and aldosterone levels: _____

8. Antidiuretic hormone's effect on tubules: _____

9. Kidney's ability to concentrate and dilute urine: _____

10. Creatinine clearance rate: _____

11. Incidence of nocturia: _____

**O. Age-Related Changes.** Describe the age-related changes of the bladder that occur in the areas listed below. *(840)*

1. Bladder muscles: _____

2. Connective tissue in the bladder: _____

3. Capacity of bladder: _____

4. Emptying function of bladder: _____

**P. Urine Characteristics.** Describe what the following color or appearance of urine may indicate in patients with urinary disorders. *(846)*

1. Straw-colored: _____

2. Bright red: _____

3. Tea-colored: _____

4. Cloudy or hazy appearance: _____

5. Colorless: _____

**Q.** List four symptoms of an allergic reaction to iodine dye used for intravenous pyelogram procedures. *(844)*

1. _____

2. _____

3. _____

4. _____

**R. Diagnostic Procedures/Angiography.** List four signs of blood loss for which the nurse observes when a patient with kidney disease returns from undergoing angiography. *(844)*

1. _____

2. _____

3. _____

4. _____

**S.   Renal Calculi.** List eight factors that influence the development of renal calculi. *(858)*

1. _____

2. _____

3. _____

4. _____

5. _____

6. _____

7. _____

8. _____

**T.   Urinary System.** In Figure 40-1 (p. 837) below, label the parts (A–I) of the urinary system. *(837)*

A. _____

B. _____

C. _____

D. _____

E. _____

F. _____

G. _____

H. _____

I. _____

**U.** **Kidney.** In Figure 40-3 (p. 837) below, label the parts (A–K) of the kidney. *(837)*

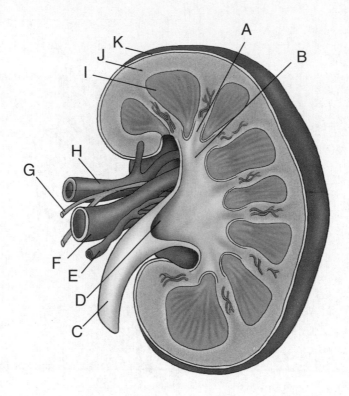

A. _____

B. _____

C. _____

D. _____

E. _____

F. _____

G. _____

H. _____

I. _____

J. _____

K. _____

**V. Nephron.** In Figure 40-4 (p. 838) below, label the parts (A–L) of the nephron. *(838)*

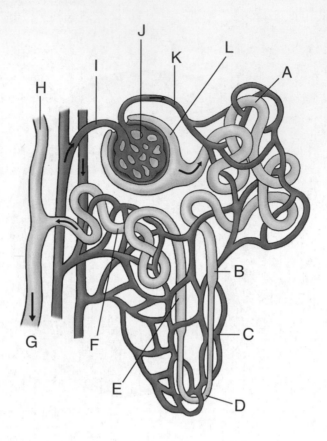

A. _____

B. _____

C. _____

D. _____

E. _____

F. _____

G. _____

H. _____

I. _____

J. _____

K. _____

L. _____

## MULTIPLE-CHOICE QUESTIONS

**W.** Choose the most appropriate answer.

1.  Glomerular filtrate and blood plasma are essentially the same, except that the filtrate does not have: *(838)*
    1.  water.
    2.  sodium.
    3.  potassium.
    4.  proteins.

2.  As the blood passes through the glomerulus, which element is too large to pass through the semipermeable membrane? *(838)*
    1.  Serum sodium
    2.  Serum potassium
    3.  Plasma protein
    4.  Glucose

3.  The normal pH of urine is: *(839)*
    1.  1.0–3.0.
    2.  4.5–8.0.
    3.  8.5–10.0.
    4.  10.5–3.0.

4.  The body normally excretes how many liters of urine per day? *(839)*
    1.  0.5 liter
    2.  1–2 liters
    3.  5 liters
    4.  7–10 liters

5.  Two substances that are present in blood but not normally present in urine are: *(839)*
    1.  sodium and chloride.
    2.  glucose and protein.
    3.  calcium and magnesium.
    4.  potassium and bicarbonate.

6.  Glomerular damage may be indicated by the presence of which of the following in the urine? *(839)*
    1.  Sodium
    2.  Chloride
    3.  Protein
    4.  Potassium

7.  The presence of how much urine usually causes the urge to urinate? *(839)*
    1.  100–150 mL
    2.  200–400 mL
    3.  500–600 mL
    4.  800–1000 mL

8.  Voiding is primarily controlled by: *(839)*
    1.  involuntary reflex.
    2.  voluntary muscles.
    3.  peristalsis.
    4.  tubular secretion.

9.  A hormone that helps maintain normal serum calcium and phosphate levels is: *(839)*
    1.  antidiuretic hormone.
    2.  epinephrine.
    3.  parathormone.
    4.  aldosterone.

10. Blood pressure is regulated through fluid volume maintenance and release of the hormone: *(840)*
    1.  aldosterone.
    2.  renin.
    3.  antidiuretic hormone.
    4.  parathormone.

11. A change in blood volume will result in a change in: *(840)*
    1.  body temperature.
    2.  heart rate.
    3.  blood pressure.
    4.  respiratory rate.

12. Decreased oxygen in renal blood triggers the secretion of: *(840)*
    1.  aldosterone.
    2.  antidiuretic hormone.
    3.  epinephrine.
    4.  erythropoietin.

13. Patients in renal failure have a deficiency of erythropoietin, which causes them to have: *(840)*
    1.  pneumonia.
    2.  anemia.
    3.  seizures.
    4.  hypertension.

14. A common age-related problem in males related to the urinary system is: *(840)*
    1. urethral obstruction.
    2. incontinence.
    3. relaxed pelvic musculature.
    4. lack of testosterone.

15. If crystals on the skin are observed during the examination of patients with urinary disorders, this is recorded as: *(841)*
    1. ashen skin.
    2. edema.
    3. uremic frost.
    4. scaly skin.

16. Tissue turgor is evaluated in patients with urinary disorders to detect: *(841)*
    1. uremic frost.
    2. Kussmaul respirations.
    3. infection.
    4. dehydration.

17. The eyes of patients with urinary disorders are examined for periorbital edema, the presence of which suggests: *(841)*
    1. dehydration.
    2. fluid retention.
    3. uremic frost.
    4. Kussmaul respirations.

18. If patients with urinary disorders have dyspnea, this may be a sign of: *(842)*
    1. dehydration.
    2. uremic frost.
    3. potassium imbalance.
    4. fluid overload.

19. If patients with urinary disorders have an odor of urine on their breath, this may indicate: *(842)*
    1. urinary tract infection.
    2. kidney failure.
    3. cardiac failure.
    4. diabetes mellitus.

20. Patients with urinary disorders who have potassium imbalances may have: *(842)*
    1. uremic frost.
    2. heart irregularities.
    3. hypertension.
    4. rapid respirations.

21. Swishing sounds caused by the turbulence of blood are called: *(842)*
    1. bruits.
    2. uremic frost.
    3. crackles.
    4. rhonchi.

22. An indication of renal artery stenosis (narrowing) is: *(842)*
    1. urinary tract infection.
    2. crackles.
    3. bruits.
    4. uremic frost.

23. The edema found in renal failure is described as: *(842)*
    1. dependent.
    2. peripheral.
    3. pitting.
    4. generalized.

24. In patients with renal failure, the skin over edematous areas is likely to be described as: *(842)*
    1. warm and moist.
    2. dry and flushed.
    3. pink and intact.
    4. pale and thick.

25. Inspection of the genitalia during the examination of patients with urinary disorders must always be done utilizing: *(842)*
    1. auscultation.
    2. palpation.
    3. standard precautions.
    4. aseptic technique.

26. Normal urine is: *(842)*
    1. bright red.
    2. straw-colored.
    3. tea-colored.
    4. smoke-colored.

27. Urine with a cloudy appearance may be indicative of: *(842)*
    1. bacterial infection.
    2. excessive fluid intake.
    3. dehydration.
    4. diabetes mellitus.

28. Normally, urine is sterile and slightly: *(842)*
    1. alkaline.
    2. acidic.
    3. pyuric.
    4. hematuric.

29. A diagnostic test for the identification of microorganisms present in urine is: *(842)*
    1. blood urea nitrogen.
    2. urinalysis.
    3. urine culture.
    4. creatinine clearance.

30. The best test of overall kidney function, which is an estimate of glomerular filtration rate, is: *(842)*
    1. blood urea nitrogen.
    2. urinalysis.
    3. urine culture.
    4. creatinine clearance.

31. Which blood test needs to be within normal limits before a renal biopsy is performed? *(845)*
    1. Electrolytes
    2. Blood urea nitrogen
    3. Serum creatinine
    4. Clotting studies

32. After a renal biopsy, what is the most important side effect to watch for? *(847)*
    1. Infection
    2. Dyspnea
    3. Bleeding
    4. Fatigue

33. Following cystoscopy, at first the urine will be: *(845)*
    1. colorless.
    2. pink-tinged.
    3. tea-colored.
    4. orange.

34. Following cystoscopy, urine should lighten to its usual color within: *(845)*
    1. 4–6 hours.
    2. 8–10 hours.
    3. 24–48 hours.
    4. 60–72 hours.

35. Following cystoscopy, belladonna and opium suppositories may be ordered to reduce: *(847)*
    1. bladder spasm.
    2. hematuria.
    3. infection.
    4. back pain.

36. Bladder perforation is rare following cystoscopy, but it may be indicated by severe: *(847)*
    1. hematuria.
    2. abdominal pain.
    3. tachycardia.
    4. hypotension.

37. The major concern with catheterization is the potential for: *(847)*
    1. hemorrhage.
    2. shock.
    3. kidney failure.
    4. infection.

38. To measure residual volume, the patient must be catheterized immediately after voiding; which of the following is an abnormal finding? *(848)*
    1. 5 mL
    2. 10 mL
    3. 25 mL
    4. 75 mL

39. Following urologic surgery, which of the following outputs should be reported to the physician? *(849)*
    1. Less than 30 mL/hour
    2. Less than 50 mL/hour
    3. Less than 70 mL/hour
    4. Less than 100 mL/hour

40. The most common nosocomial infections are: *(849)*
    1. skin infections.
    2. wound infections.
    3. urinary tract infections.
    4. blood infections.

41. Most urinary tract infections are caused by: *(849)*
    1. viruses.
    2. bacteria.
    3. yeasts.
    4. fungi.

42. Dysuria, frequency, urgency, and bladder spasms are common symptoms of: *(849)*
    1. pyelonephritis.
    2. kidney failure.
    3. vaginitis.
    4. urethritis.

43. The passage of renal calculi is facilitated by: *(859)*
    1. bed rest.
    2. opiates.
    3. restricted fluids.
    4. ambulation.

44. The pain of urethritis may be reduced by: *(853)*
    1. antiemetics.
    2. back massage.
    3. sitz baths.
    4. bubble baths.

45. A common symptom of pyelonephritis is: *(855)*
    1. polyuria.
    2. hypotension.
    3. bradycardia.
    4. flank pain.

46. When forcing fluids on patients with pyelonephritis, the nurse needs to be careful to prevent: *(856)*
    1. infection.
    2. hemorrhage.
    3. kidney failure.
    4. circulatory overload.

47. An older patient with pyelonephritis who experiences a suddenly increased fluid volume may develop: *(856)*
    1. hypotension.
    2. congestive heart failure.
    3. seizures.
    4. thrombophlebitis.

48. The most common type of glomerulonephritis follows a respiratory tract infection caused by: *(857)*
    1. *Staphylococcus.*
    2. a virus.
    3. a fungus.
    4. *Streptococcus.*

49. In addition to antibiotics, acute glomerulonephritis is treated medically with: *(857)*
    1. diuretics and antihypertensives.
    2. antihistamines and antiemetics.
    3. anticholinergics and analgesics.
    4. narcotics and anticonvulsants.

50. In the acute phase of glomerulonephritis, bed rest is ordered to prevent or treat heart failure and severe hypertension that result from: *(857)*
    1. fluid volume deficit.
    2. fluid overload.
    3. altered renal tissue perfusion.
    4. respiratory distress.

51. A common nursing diagnosis for patients with acute glomerulonephritis is: *(857)*
    1. fluid volume deficit.
    2. excess fluid volume.
    3. altered renal tissue perfusion.
    4. high risk for injury.

52. The incidence of uric acid stones is high among: *(858)*
    1. Jewish males.
    2. Caucasian females.
    3. African-American females.
    4. Hispanic males.

53. When a person is dehydrated, the kidneys conserve water, causing urine to be: *(846)*
    1. dilute.
    2. cloudy.
    3. alkaline.
    4. concentrated.

54. A diet that can contribute to calculus formation is one that is high in purines and: *(859)*
    1. sodium.
    2. potassium.
    3. calcium.
    4. fat.

55. In order to prevent renal calculi, the nurse should teach patients to: *(862)*
    1. follow a high-calcium diet.
    2. follow a high-purine diet.
    3. have a high fluid intake.
    4. limit physical activity.

56. A major nursing concern for patients with renal calculi is: *(860)*
    1. frequent ambulation.
    2. emotional support.
    3. range-of-motion exercises.
    4. pain relief.

57. The treatment of choice for renal cancer is: *(863)*
    1. lithotripsy.
    2. radical nephrectomy.
    3. cystectomy.
    4. nephrostomy.

58. The location of the flank incision following nephrectomy causes pain with expansion of the: *(864)*
    1. abdomen.
    2. pelvis.
    3. cerebrum.
    4. thorax.

59. When patients after nephrectomy protect the chest by not breathing deeply, this leads to the development of: *(864)*
    1. hemorrhage.
    2. infection.
    3. atelectasis.
    4. shock.

60. The most common malignancy of the urinary tract is: *(865)*
    1. cancer of the kidney.
    2. cervical cancer.
    3. bladder cancer.
    4. liver cancer.

61. The most frequent symptom of bladder cancer is intermittent: *(865)*
    1. glycosuria.
    2. proteinuria.
    3. pyuria.
    4. hematuria.

62. When the bladder is removed completely, urinary diversion is sometimes provided, which allows urine to be excreted through the: *(865)*
    1. urethra.
    2. ileal conduit.
    3. ureter.
    4. cystoscopy.

63. Preoperative care for an ileal or sigmoid conduit includes thorough preparation of the intestinal tract, which includes administration of an antibiotic that is not absorbed from the intestinal tract, called: *(866)*
    1. Keflex.
    2. penicillin.
    3. neomycin.
    4. tetracycline.

64. An effective means of assessing changes in fluid status of patients in acute renal failure is: *(870)*
    1. monitoring edema.
    2. recording intake and output.
    3. weighing daily.
    4. taking vital signs.

65. When 90–95% of kidney function is lost, the patient is considered to be in: *(871)*
    1. acute renal failure.
    2. chronic renal failure.
    3. renal shock.
    4. renal oliguria.

66. The most life-threatening effect of renal failure is: *(871)*
    1. hypernatremia.
    2. hyponatremia.
    3. hyperkalemia.
    4. hypokalemia.

67. When a kidney is obtained from a living related donor, the 1-year survival rate for transplantation is about: *(878)*
    1. 30–33%.
    2. 65–70%.
    3. 75–80%.
    4. 95–97%.

68. To control the body's response to foreign tissue, the transplant recipient is given: *(880)*
    1. analgesics.
    2. immunosuppressants.
    3. anticholinergics.
    4. antihistamines.

69. Specific nursing diagnoses related to possibility of organ rejection after renal transplantation may include: *(881)*
    1. Risk for injury.
    2. Altered role performance.
    3. Anxiety.
    4. Diarrhea.

70. Signs of dehydration in the patient who has had a renal transplant may include thready pulse, poor tissue turgor, and: *(880)*
    1. low blood pressure.
    2. high blood pressure.
    3. high fever.
    4. abnormally low body temperature.

71. Complications of lithotripsy include: *(859)*
    1. bruising.
    2. congestive heart failure.
    3. dyspnea.
    4. thrombus.

72. Risk factors for bladder cancer include: *(865)*
    1. obesity.
    2. cigarette smoking.
    3. a high-purine diet.
    4. a sedentary lifestyle.

73. Which procedure is contraindicated in patients with known renal insufficiency or diabetes mellitus? *(846)*
    1. Intravenous pyelogram (IVP)
    2. Flat plate
    3. Renal scan
    4. Ultrasonography

## OBJECTIVES

1. Define connective tissue.

2. Describe the function of connective tissue.

3. Describe the characteristics and prevalence of connective tissue diseases.

4. Describe the diagnostic tests and procedures used for assessing connective tissue diseases.

5. Discuss the drugs used to treat connective tissue diseases.

6. Describe the pathophysiology and treatment of basis for osteoarthritis (degenerative joint disease), rheumatoid arthritis, osteoporosis, gout, progressive systemic sclerosis, polymyositis, bursitis, carpal tun-nel syndrome, ankylosing spondylitis, polymyalgia rheumatica, Reiter's syndrome, Behçet's syndrome, and Sjögren's syndrome.

7. Identify the data to be collected in the nursing assessment of a patient with a connective tissue disorder.

8. Assist in developing a nursing care plan for a patient whose life has been affected by a connective tissue disease.

## LEARNING ACTIVITIES

**A.  Key Terms.** Match the definition in the numbered column with the most appropriate term in the lettered column.

| | | | |
|---|---|---|---|
| 1. | _I_ | Instrument used to measure joint range of motion *(885)* | A.  Hyperuricemia |
| 2. | _F_ | Within the joint *(894)* | B.  Ankylosis |
| 3. | _A_ | Elevated level of uric acid in the blood *(905)* | C.  Fibromyalgia |
| 4. | _J_ | Muscle pain *(911)* | D.  Tophus |
| 5. | _D_ | Deposit of sodium urate crystals under the skin *(906)* | E.  Vasculitis |
| 6. | _G_ | Protrusions of the distal interphalangeal finger joints; associated with osteoarthritis *(894)* | F.  Intra-articular |
| 7. | _L_ | Enlarged proximal interphalangeal joints of the fingers *(894)* | G.  Heberden's nodes |
| 8. | _C_ | Chronic musculoskeletal pain disorder *(901)* | H.  Crepitus |
| 9. | _K_ | Granulation of tissue surrounding cores of fibrous debris *(900)* | I.  Goniometer |
| 10. | _M_ | Plastic repair of a joint *(894)* | J.  Myalgia |
| 11. | _E_ | Inflammation of blood vessels *(901)* | K.  Rheumatoid nodule |
| 12. | _H_ | Crackling sound or sensation *(895)* | L.  Bouchard's nodes |
| 13. | _B_ | Joint immobility *(900)* | M.  Arthroplasty |

**B. Diagnostic Tests.** Match the purpose or description in the numbered column with the appropriate diagnostic test in the lettered column. Some tests may be used more than once, and some tests may not be used. *(887)*

1. __C__    Results of this test are elevated in any inflammatory process, especially RA

2. __E__    Detection of blood dyscrasias; differentiation of anemias, leukemia; decreased values in RA and SLE

3. __D__    Increased values with infection, tissue necrosis, and inflammation; sometimes decreased values in SLE

4. __B__    Determines the presence of antibodies; present in about 80% of persons with RA

5. __H__    Assesses renal function; elevated values in SLE, scleroderma, and polyarteritis

6. __A__    Positive reading in active inflammation, often positive for RA and SLE

7. __E__    Measures presence of antibodies that react with a variety of nuclear antibodies; positive in SLE, RA, scleroderma, Raynaud's disease, Sjögren's syndrome

A. C-reactive protein
B. Rheumatoid factor (RF)
C. Erythrocyte sedimentation rate (ESR)
D. White blood cell count (WBC)
E. Antinuclear antibodies (ANA)
F. Red blood cell count (RBC)
G. Platelet count
H. Creatinine

C. **Radiologic Tests.** Match the purpose or description in the numbered column with the appropriate radiologic test in the lettered column. Some tests may be used more than once, and some may not be used.

1. _____E_____ Intravenous radioactive material that is taken up by bone is injected for visualization of entire skeletal system; procedure detects malignancies, osteoporosis, osteomyelitis, and some fractures *(888)*

2. _____C_____ Determines density, texture, and alignment of bones; assesses soft tissue involvement *(888)*

3. _____G_____ Scans the soft tissues and bones by use of both radiographs and computers; determines presence of tumors or some spinal fractures *(888)*

4. _____H_____ Examines soft tissue joint structures; performed most commonly on shoulder or knee when a traumatic injury is suspected and determines presence of bone chips, torn ligaments, or other loose bodies *(887)*

5. _____D_____ Contrast medium injected directly into vertebral disk being examined *(888)*

6. _____A_____ Soft tissue visualization produced by sound waves *(888)*

7. _____B_____ A noninvasive procedure that makes use of magnetic energy sources to view soft tissue *(888)*

A. Ultrasound
B. Magnetic resonance imaging (MRI)
C. Radiography
D. Diskography
E. Nuclear scintigraphy (bone scan)
F. PET
G. Computed tomography (CT) scan
H. Arthrography

**D. Drug Therapy.** Match the description in the numbered column with the drug classification in the lettered column. Some answers may be used more than once.

1. _C_    Examples are Indocin and Clinoril. *(890)*

2. _E_    Examples are methotrexate (Folex) and sulfasalazine (Azulfidine). *(890)*

3. _G_    Examples are allopurinol and probenecid. *(891-892)*

4. _F_    Examples are etanercept (Enbrel) and infliximab (Remicade). *(891)*

5. _H_    Examples are Fosamax, calcitonon (Miacalcin), and raloxifene (Evista). *(892)*

6. _D_    Examples are hydrocortisone and prednisone. *(890)*

7. _B_    Example is celecoxib (Celebrex). *(890)*

8. _A_    Examples are aspirin, naproxen, and ibuprofen. *(890)*

9. _A_    Main side effect is GI bleeding. *(890)*

10. _C_    Indicated for severe ankylosing spondylitis and painful shoulders. *(890)*

11. _F_    A monoclonal antibody that neutralizes activity of tumor necrosis factor, decreasing inflammation. Used to treat RA. *(892)*

12. _G_    Drugs that inhibit synthesis of uric acid or increase urinary excretion of uric acid. *(891)*

13. _D_    Anti-inflammatory drugs that suppress normal immune response. *(890)*

A. First-generation nonsteroidal anti-inflammatory drugs (NSAIDs)
B. Second-generation nonsteroidal anti-inflammatory drugs: COX-2 inhibitors
C. Indole analogues
D. Glucocorticoids
E. Disease-modifying antirheumatic drugs (DMARDs)
F. Biologic response modifiers, antiarthritic
G. Antigout agents
H. Bone resorption inhibitors

**E.** **Osteoarthritis.** Complete the statement in the numbered column with the most appropriate term in the lettered column. Some terms may be used more than once, and some terms may not be used.

1. A device that is used after joint replacement surgery to move the joints through a set range of motions at a set rate of movements per minute is the ___C___. *(893)*

2. The most common form of arthritis, which is also called degenerative joint disease, is ___D___. *(893)*

3. The surgical treatment of choice for OA is ___A___. *(894)*

4. Joint activities are compromised because the basic structure of the cartilage is altered in ___D___. *(893)*

5. The primary indication for total joint replacement in patients with OA is ___F___. *(894)*

6. A condition that generally affects joints under pressure (such as the spine and knees) is ___D___. *(893)*

A. Total joint replacement
B. Physical therapy
C. Continuous passive movement machine
D. Osteoarthritis (OA)
E. Ankylosing spondylitis
F. Intractable pain

**F.** **Rheumatoid Arthritis.** Complete the statement in the numbered column with the most appropriate term in the lettered column. Some terms may be used more than once, and some terms may not be used.

1. The synovium thickens and fluid accumulates in the joint spaces of patients with ___A___. *(900)*

2. A loss of joint mobility occurring in RA is called ___G___. *(900)*

3. Morning stiffness lasting more than 1 hour is a common symptom of ___A___. *(900)*

4. If blood vessels are affected by RA, they become inflamed, a condition called ___E___. *(901)*

5. Subcutaneous nodules over bony prominences, which are often present in RA, are called ___C___. *(900-901)*

6. Inflammation of sacs at joints treated by lidocaine injections for temporary relief is ___D___. *(900)*

7. Compression of the median nerve in the wrist, causing pain and tenderness, is ___H___. *(911)*

8. A chronic, progressive inflammatory disease is ___A___. *(900)*

A. Rheumatoid arthritis (RA)
B. Osteoarthritis
C. Rheumatoid nodules
D. Bursitis
E. Vasculitis
F. Polymyositis
G. Ankylosis
H. Carpal tunnel syndrome

**G.** **Connective Tissue Disorders.** Complete the statements in the numbered column with the most appropriate term in the lettered column. Some terms may be used more than once, and some terms may not be used.

1. A disease characterized by dry mouth, dry eyes, and dry vagina is called ___F___. *(911)*
2. A condition in which there is loss of bone mass, making the patient susceptible to fractures, is ___G___. *(904)*
3. Common sites of fractures due to osteoporosis are the wrist, vertebrae, and ___D___. *(904)*
4. A technique for measuring bone mass is ___A___. *(904)*
5. A systemic disease characterized by the deposition of urate crystals in the joints and other body tissues is ___H___. *(905)*
6. An excessive rate of uric acid production or decreased uric acid excretion by the kidneys results in ___H___. *(905)*
7. The joint commonly affected by gout is that of the ___I___. *(906)*
8. A diet low in ___C___ is recommended for patients with gout. *(907)*

A. Absorptiometry
B. Hyperuricemia
C. Purines
D. Hip
E. Systemic lupus erythematosus
F. Sjögren's syndrome
G. Osteoporosis
H. Gout
I. Great toe

**H.** **Connective Tissue Disorders.** Complete the statement in the numbered column with the most appropriate term in the lettered column. Some terms may be used more than once, and some terms may not be used.

1. Decreased elasticity, stenosis, and occlusion of vessels are manifestations of ___C___. *(908)*
2. An inflammatory disease that primarily affects the vertebral column, causing spinal deformities, is ___F___. *(911)*
3. The management of Raynaud's phenomenon is aimed at elimination of anything that causes _____. *(908)*
4. Scleroderma may be brought into remission with high doses of immunosuppressants or ___D___. *(908)*
5. A condition characterized by inflammation and damage to blood vessels that is present in nearly all connective tissue diseases is ___C___. *(901)*
6. A condition characterized by degeneration of articular cartilage is _____. *(912)*
7. The primary symptom of polymyositis is ___A___. *(910)*
8. A chronic multisystem disease that draws its name from the characteristic hardening of the skin is ___E___. *(907)*

A. Muscle weakness
B. Osteoarthritis
C. Vasculitis
D. Steroids
E. Progressive systemic sclerosis (scleroderma)
F. Ankylosing spondylitis
G. Vasospasm
H. Dermatomyositis
I. Polymyositis

**I.** **Complications.** When mobility is severely impaired following hip replacement surgery, which of the following are complications for which the patient is at risk? Select all that apply. *(898)*

1. __✗_____ Contractures
2. __✗_____ Pulmonary and circulatory complications
3. __✗_____ Urinary retention
4. _____ Constipation
5. _____ Hemorrhage
6. __✗_____ Skin breakdown

**J.** **Synovial Joint.** In Figure 41-1 (p. 893) below, label the major structures (A–H) of the normal synovial joint. *(893)*

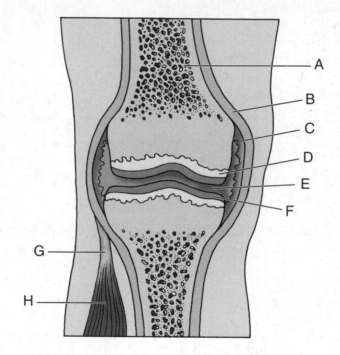

A. _____

B. _____

C. _____

D. _____

E. _____

F. _____

G. _____

H. _____

**K. Nursing Diagnoses.** Match the nursing diagnosis in the numbered column with the patient's disorder in the lettered column. Answers may be used more than once and some answers may not be used.

1. ___A___    Acute pain related to joint inflammation *(907)*
2. ___A___    Chronic pain related to swelling and tenderness *(903)*
3. ___B___    Risk for trauma related to loss of bone strength *(905)*
4. ___E___    Risk for injury related to improper alignment *(897)*
5. ___F___    Chronic pain with motion related to loss of smooth joint surfaces *(895)*
6. ___C___    Impaired urinary elimination related to urate kidney stones *(907)*

A. Rheumatoid arthritis (RA)
B. Osteoporosis
C. Gout
D. Scleroderma
E. Total joint replacement, postoperative
F. Osteoarthritis

## MULTIPLE-CHOICE QUESTIONS

**L.** Choose the most appropriate answer.

1. Important changes in the connective tissue of the body that occur with aging include loss of bone strength and bone: *(884)*
   1. nutrients.
   2. mass.
   3. vitamins.
   4. minerals.

2. Age-related joint changes are related primarily to changes in: *(884)*
   1. blood volume.
   2. bone strength.
   3. bone mass.
   4. cartilage.

3. During the physical examination of people with connective tissue disorders, what is assessed by asking the patient to move each extremity through the normal range of motion? *(885)*
   1. Joint pain and range of motion
   2. Fever and tachycardia
   3. Weight loss and nutritional deficiencies
   4. Tachypnea and bone function

4. When assessing patients for joint pain and range of motion, the nurse watches for signs of pain and listens for the crackling sound called: *(885)*
   1. bursitis.
   2. grinding.
   3. crepitus.
   4. scraping.

5. Besides a complete blood count, the routine blood studies for evaluation of musculoskeletal disorders should include the: *(885)*
   1. prothrombin time.
   2. BUN.
   3. electrolyte count.
   4. erythrocyte sedimentation rate.

6. Anti-inflammatory drugs used for musculoskeletal disorders include NSAIDs and: *(886)*
   1. hydrocortisone.
   2. morphine.
   3. furosemide.
   4. digoxin.

7. Following joint replacement surgery, a continuous passive motion (CPM) machine may be used to prevent formation of scar tissue and promote: *(893)*
   1. phagocytosis.
   2. clotting.
   3. flexibility.
   4. circulation.

8. Often the pain in osteoarthritis (OA) can be controlled with: *(894)*
   1. beta blockers.
   2. salicylates.
   3. anticholinergics.
   4. narcotics.

9. Symptoms of salicylate toxicity in older adults may be atypical; instead of the common symptoms of gastrointestinal complaints or ototoxicity, the older person may exhibit: *(894)*
   1. drowsiness.
   2. confusion.
   3. malaise.
   4. hypotension.

10. A nursing diagnosis that patients with OA may have related to pain and limited range of motion is: *(895)*
    1. Ineffective coping.
    2. Altered self-esteem.
    3. Impaired tissue perfusion.
    4. Impaired physical mobility.

11. Bathroom grab bars, a seat in the shower, and a raised toilet seat may promote independence and safety for the patient with poor: *(897)*
    1. shoulder mobility.
    2. ankle mobility.
    3. upper arm mobility.
    4. hip mobility.

12. A nursing diagnosis following total joint replacement that is related to improper alignment, dislocated prosthesis, and/or weakness is: *(897)*
    1. Altered peripheral tissue perfusion.
    2. Risk for injury.
    3. Risk for infection.
    4. Knowledge deficit.

13. Uncontrolled pain may make the patient reluctant to participate in rehabilitation measures following total joint replacement surgery; an intervention to improve patient participation is: *(898)*
    1. assess nerve and circulatory status before exercises.
    2. check vital signs at least every 4 hours.
    3. assist patient in and out of bed.
    4. administer analgesics 30 minutes to 1 hour before exercises.

14. Prosthetic joints can become dislocated if they are not maintained in proper alignment; after hip replacement, the affected leg must be kept in a position of: *(898)*
    1. abduction.
    2. adduction.
    3. slight elevation.
    4. supination.

15. Body areas distal to the operative joint are monitored for circulatory adequacy by assessing warmth, color, and: *(899)*
    1. peripheral pulses.
    2. ulceration.
    3. skin necrosis.
    4. wound drainage.

16. Pillows and pads should not be placed under the legs of patients with joint replacements in order to reduce the risk of: *(899)*
    1. ulceration.
    2. gangrene.
    3. deep vein thrombosis.
    4. infection.

17. A positive Homans' signs in patients who have had joint replacement surgery may be indicative of: *(899)*
    1. wound infection.
    2. deep vein thrombosis.
    3. septicemia.
    4. cardiac shock.

18. After joint replacement, the patient has ineffective tissue perfusion and is at risk for: *(899)*
    1. headache.
    2. hemorrhage.
    3. seizure.
    4. pneumonia.

19. If a patient shows signs of cerebral blood vessel occlusion, headache, confusion, or loss of consciousness, the patient may have: *(899)*
    1. deep vein thrombosis.
    2. hemorrhage.
    3. fat embolus.
    4. neuropathy.

20. Pressure caused by edema or constrictive dressings following joint replacement surgery can cause nerve damage, which may be manifested as: *(900)*
    1. paresthesia.
    2. infection.
    3. positive Homans' sign.
    4. hemorrhage.

21. If the nurse suspects that a dressing is too tight and is causing nerve damage, the nurse monitors sensations: *(900)*
    1. at the wound site.
    2. proximal to the joint.
    3. distal to the joint.
    4. within the joint.

22. A nursing intervention related to the patient's high risk for infection is that the nurse will: *(900)*
    1. place the call light in easy reach.
    2. instruct patient to keep legs slightly abducted.
    3. use strict sterile technique for dressing changes.
    4. assess nerve and circulatory status.

23. Drugs that are administered to patients with joint replacements who are at risk for infection are: *(900)*
    1. antihistamines.
    2. antimicrobials.
    3. antiemetics.
    4. anticoagulants.

24. A measure to control morning pain and stiffness in patients with RA is to: *(903)*
    1. take a warm shower.
    2. increase intake of fluids.
    3. eat foods low in purines.
    4. use aseptic technique.

25. A factor that slows bone loss and improves strength, balance, and reaction time (reducing the risk of falls and fractures) is: *(905)*
    1. vitamin C.
    2. increased fluid intake.
    3. regular exercise.
    4. protein.

26. Patients with gout may have altered urinary elimination related to: *(906)*
    1. dehydration.
    2. restricted fluid intake.
    3. kidney stones.
    4. edema.

27. To prevent the complication of kidney stones in patients with gout, patients are advised to: *(907)*
    1. protect affected joints from trauma.
    2. keep walking pathways lighted and free from obstacles.
    3. obtain assistance with activities of daily living.
    4. drink at least eight glasses of fluid daily.

28. Polymyalgia rheumatica, Reiter's syndrome, Behçet's syndrome, and Sjögren's syndrome all involve: *(910)*
    1. urinary tract disorders.
    2. connective tissue disorders.
    3. central nervous system disorders.
    4. cardiac disorders.

29. When a patient has pain from rheumatoid arthritis, which group is most likely to face pain stoically? *(903)*
    1. Dominican Republican
    2. Germans
    3. Caucasian Americans
    4. Italians

30. When a patient is taking NSAIDs for rheumatoid arthritis, the nurse monitors the patient for: *(890)*
    1. fatigue.
    2. edema.
    3. bruising.
    4. infection.

31. An important teaching point for patients taking antigout medications is to: *(907)*
    1. increase potassium intake.
    2. avoid foods high in vitamin K.
    3. rise slowly from a sitting position.
    4. increase fluids.

32. Which food should be avoided in patients with acute gout? *(908)*
    1. Sardines
    2. Aged cheese
    3. Bananas
    4. Orange juice

33. Which anti-inflammatory drugs work much like older NSAIDs but are less likely to cause stomach ulcers and bleeding? *(890)*
    1. COX-2 inhibitors
    2. Disease-modifying antirheumatic drugs (DMARDs)
    3. Biologic response modifiers (BRMs)
    4. Glucocorticoids

34. Fatigue, morning stiffness lasting more than 1 hour, and muscle aches are symptoms of: *(900)*
    1. rheumatoid arthritis.
    2. Sjögren's syndrome.
    3. ankylosing spondylitis.
    4. bursitis.

M. **Nursing Care Plan.** Refer to Nursing Care Plan, The Patient with a Total Hip Replacement, p. 896 in the textbook.

1. What are the four priority problems for which this patient is at risk? *(896)*
    1.

    2.

    3.

    4.

2. What are this patient's risk factors for total hip replacement surgery? *(896)*
    1.

    2.

3. What are interventions related to prevention of injury related to dislocation for this patient? *(896)*

4. What tasks for this patient could be assigned to unlicensed assistive personnel? *(896)*
    1.

    2.

    3.

    4.

    5.

# 42 Fractures

---

## OBJECTIVES

1. Identify the types of fractures.

2. Describe the five stages of the healing process.

3. Discuss the major complications of fractures, their signs and symptoms, and their management.

4. Compare the types of medical treatment for fractures, particularly reduction and fixation.

5. Describe common therapeutic measures for fractures, including casts, traction, crutches, walkers, and canes.

6. Discuss the nursing care of a patient with a fracture.

7. Describe specific types of fractures, including hip fractures, Colles' fractures, and pelvic fractures.

---

**397**

**NING ACTIVITIES**

**Key Terms.** Match the definition in the numbered column with the most appropriate term in the lettered column.

1. _____K_____  Condition in which fat globules are released from the marrow of the broken bone into the bloodstream, migrate to the lungs, and cause pulmonary hypertension *(916)*

2. _____D_____  Fracture in which the broken bone does not break through the skin *(914)*

3. _____N_____  Fracture in which the fragments of the broken bone break through the skin *(914)*

4. _____A_____  Serious complication of a fracture caused by internal or external pressure to the affected area, resulting in decreased blood flow, pain, and tissue damage *(917)*

5. _____H_____  Failure of a fracture to heal *(917)*

6. _____L_____  Fracture in which the break extends across the entire bone, dividing it into two separate pieces *(914)*

7. _____C_____  Procedure done during the open reduction surgical procedure to attach the fragments of the broken bone together when reduction alone is not feasible *(919)*

8. _____O_____  Process of bringing the ends of the broken bone into proper alignment *(919)*

9. _____F_____  Fracture in which the bone breaks only partially across, leaving some portion of the bone intact *(914)*

10. _____J_____  Nonsurgical realignment of the bones to their previous anatomic position using traction, angulation, rotation, or a combination of these *(919)*

A. Compartment syndrome
B. Open reduction
C. Fixation
D. Closed or simple fracture
E. Delayed union
F. Incomplete fracture
G. Fracture
H. Nonunion
I. Bone remodeling
J. Closed reduction or manipulation
K. Fat embolism
L. Complete fracture
M. Stress fracture
N. Open or compound fracture
O. Reduction
P. Comminuted fracture
Q. Greenstick fracture
R. Malunion

11. __B__ Surgical procedure in which an incision is made at the fracture site, usually on patients with open (compound) or comminuted fractures, to cleanse the area of fragments and debris *(919)*

12. __M__ Fracture caused by either sudden force or prolonged stress *(914)*

13. __I__ Process in which immature bone cells are gradually replaced by mature bone cells *(916)*

14. __E__ Healing of fracture does not occur in the normally expected time *(917)*

15. __G__ Break or disruption in the continuity of a bone *(914)*

16. __R__ Improper alignment of a fracture resulting in deformity *(917)*

17. __P__ Fracture in which the bone is broken or crushed into small pieces *(919)*

18. __Q__ Fracture in which the bone is broken on one side but only bent on the other; most common in children *(914)*

**B.  Casts.** Complete the statements in the numbered column with the most appropriate term in the lettered column. Some terms may be used more than once, and some terms may not be used.

1. __H__ A cast used for breaks in the forearm, elbow, or humerus *(922)*

2. __G__ A cast used for fracture of the distal femur, knee, or lower leg *(921)*

3. __A__ A cast that encircles the trunk; used for stable spine injuries of thoracic or lumbar spine *(921)*

4. __F__ A cast that encases the trunk plus two extremities; used for fractures of the femur, acetabulum, or pelvis *(921)*

5. __E__ Used for fractures of the foot, ankle, or distal tibia or fibula *(921)*

6. __G__ Used for injury to the knee or knee dislocation *(921)*

7. __I__ Used for injury to knee, allowing knee to bend *(921)*

8. _____ Used for postoperative immobilization following open reduction and internal fixation *(921, 922)*

9. __B__ Used for fracture of the hand or wrist *(922)*

A.  Body jacket cast
B.  Short arm cast
C.  Leg cylinder cast
D.  Spica cast
E.  Short leg cast
F.  Bilateral long leg hip spica cast
G.  Long leg cast
H.  Long arm cast
I.  Cast brace

**C. Traction.** Complete the statements in the numbered column with the most appropriate term in the lettered column. Some terms may be used more than once, and some terms may not be used. *(922)*

1. A pulling force on a fractured extremity to provide alignment of the broken bone fragments is called ___E___.

2. Traction applied directly to a bone is called ___H___.

3. Traction applied directly to the skin is called ___B___.

4. A type of traction used for immobilization of fractures of the cervical vertebrae is called ___G___.

5. A type of traction used for hip and knee contractures, muscle spasms, and alignment of hip fractures is called ___C___.

6. Crutchfield's traction and halo vest are examples of ___H___.

7. A type of traction in which tongs are inserted into either side of the skull is called _____.

A. Plastic traction
B. Skin traction
C. Buck's traction
D. Contracture traction
E. Traction
F. Vest traction
G. Crutchfield's traction
H. Skeletal traction

**D. Fracture Healing.**

1. Place the stages of fracture healing in the correct order. Refer to Figure 42-2, p. 916 in the textbook. *(916)*

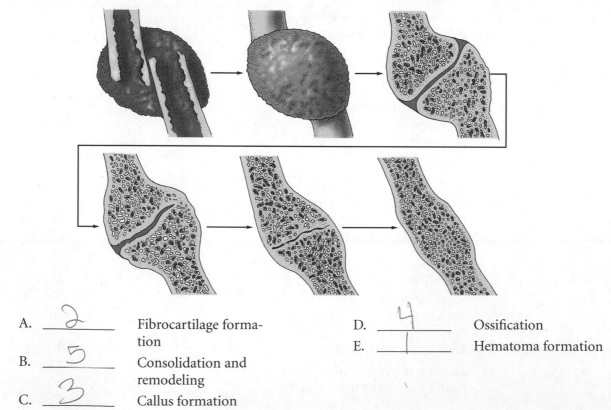

A. ___2___  Fibrocartilage formation

B. ___5___  Consolidation and remodeling

C. ___3___  Callus formation

D. ___4___  Ossification

E. ___1___  Hematoma formation

2. **Fracture Healing.** Match the definition or description in the numbered column with the most appropriate stage of healing in the lettered column. Some stages may be used more than once, and some may not be used. *(915)*

1. _____A_____ Granulation tissue forms a collar around each end of the broken bone, gradually becoming firm

2. _____C_____ Within 2–3 weeks after the break, a permanent bone callus forms; ends of the broken bone begin to "knit"

3. _____F_____ Formation of a clot between the two broken ends of the bones; occurs in 48–72 hours

4. _____E_____ The distance between bone fragments closes, and immature bone cells are replaced by mature bone cells

5. _____C_____ Formation of a temporary splint by the end of the first week; granulation tissue turns into formation of cartilage, osteoblasts, calcium, and phosphorus

6. _____F_____ Bleeding occurs with edema immediately after the fracture

A. Fibrocartilage formation
B. Consolidation and remodeling
C. Callus formation
D. Cellular proliferation
E. Ossification
F. Hematoma formation

**E.  Signs and Symptoms of Fracture.** Match the cause of the signs and symptoms of fracture in the numbered column with the most appropriate sign or symptom in the lettered column. Some signs and symptoms may be used more than once, and some may not be used. *(918)*

1. _____  Strong muscle pull may cause bone fragments to override

2. _____  Edema may appear rapidly from localization of serous fluid at the fracture site and extravasation of blood into adjacent tissues

3. _____  Caused by subcutaneous bleeding

4. _____  Involuntary muscle contraction near the fracture

5. ___K___  Occurs over fracture site due to underlying injuries

6. ___C___  Severe at the time of injury; following injury, this symptom may result from muscle spasm or damage to adjacent structures

7. ___F___  Results from nerve damage

8. ___B___  Grating sensations or sounds felt or heard if the injured part is moved; results from broken bone ends rubbing together

9. ___D___  Results from blood loss or other injuries

A.  Muscle spasm
B.  Crepitus
C.  Pain
D.  Hypovolemic shock
E.  Swelling
F.  Impaired sensation (numbness)
G.  Abnormal mobility
H.  Bruising (ecchymosis)
I.  Fever
J.  Deformity
K.  Tenderness

**F.  Positions for Patients with Fractures.** Match the proper positioning in the numbered column with the fracture in the lettered column. *(928)*

1. _____  Before medical treatment, keep patient supine and immobilize patient's neck; after treatment, turn with head well-supported

2. _____  Avoid high sitting positions; log roll

3. _____  When fracture is stable or after fixation, turn to side opposite fracture

4. _____  Elevate head of bed to comfort; turn to side opposite fracture

5. _____  Elevate distal portion of extremity higher than heart

A.  Pelvis fracture
B.  Forearm or foreleg fracture
C.  Cervical spine fracture
D.  Lumbar spine fracture
E.  Shoulder or humerus fracture

**G. Types of Fractures.**

1. In Figure 42-1 (p. 915) below, label each type of fracture (A–L) with numbers from the following list. *(915)*

   1. Greenstick
   2. Oblique
   3. Transverse
   4. Displaced
   5. Longitudinal
   6. Stress

   7. Comminuted (fragmented)
   8. Interarticular
   9. Spiral
   10. Avulsion
   11. Impacted
   12. Pathologic

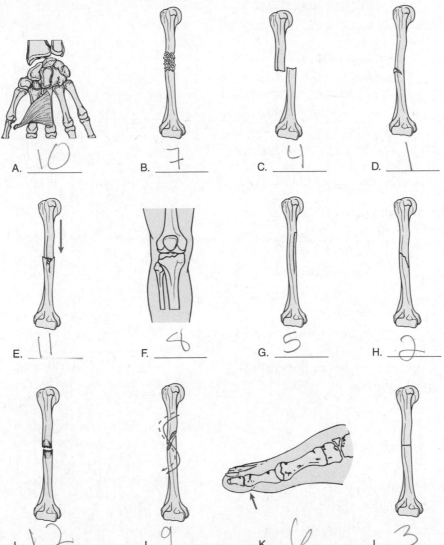

A. 10   B. 7   C. 4   D. 1

E. 11   F. 8   G. 5   H. 2

I. 12   J. 9   K. 6   L. 3

2. Which type of fracture is caused by a tumor in the bone? *(914)*

3. Which type of fracture occurs most frequently in children? *(914)*

4. Which type of fracture is often related to a sports injury, such as track? *(914)*

## H. Hip Fractures.

1. Using Figure 42-10 (p. 929) below, label the anatomic regions in A and the type of fractures in B–E. *(929)*

   A. _____

      1. _____

      2. _____

      3. _____

      4. _____

      5. _____

   B. _____

   C. _____

   D. _____

   E. _____

A. Anatomic Regions

B

C

D

E

2. Where do most hip fractures occur? Select all that apply. *(928)*

   1. _____ Femoral head
   2. _____ Femoral neck
   3. _____ Intertrochanteric region
   4. _____ Subtrochanteric region

3. What percentage of women by the age of 90 have sustained a hip fracture? *(928)*

   1. 10%
   2. 20%
   3. 30%
   4. 40%

4. What are signs and symptoms of a hip fracture? Select all that apply. *(928)*

   1. _____ History of a fall
   2. _____ Severe pain and tenderness in the region of the fracture site
   3. _____ Bleeding at the fracture site
   4. _____ Internal rotation of the hip on the affected side

5. What is the standard treatment for hip fractures? Select all that apply. *(929)*
    1. _____ Traction
    2. _____ External fixation
    3. _____ Femoral head replacement
    4. _____ Total hip replacement

**I. Skin Traction.**

1. In Figure 42-7 (p. 923) below, label each type of traction (A–E) using the following list. *(923)*
    1. _____ Head halter traction
    2. _____ Pelvic traction
    3. _____ Russell's traction
    4. _____ Buck's traction
    5. _____ Balanced suspension traction

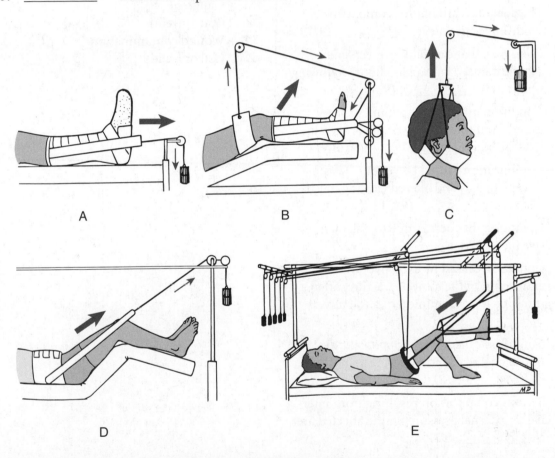

2. What are the purposes of traction? Select all that apply. *(922)*
    1. _____ Prevent or correct deformity
    2. _____ Decrease muscle spasm
    3. _____ Promote rest
    4. _____ Clean the area of fragments and debris
    5. _____ Use of rods, pins and metal plates to align bone fragments and keep them in place for healing
    6. _____ Maintain the position of the diseased or injured part

**J.**   **Complications of Fractures.** Match the description in the numbered column with the complication term in the lettered column. Some terms may be used more than once, and some terms may not be used.

1.  Primary symptom of compartment syndrome is ___K___. *(917)*

2.  First sign of a fat embolism is ___L___. *(917)*

3.  Likely to develop in deep, grossly contaminated fracture wound ___AM___. *(916)*

4.  Infection of the bone is ___N___. *(916)*

5.  Infections associated with fractures result from indwelling hardware used to repair the broken bone or from ___O___. *(916)*

6.  The goal of treatment for compartment syndrome is to relieve ___J___. *(917)*

7.  Condition that can cause irreversible muscle damage within 4–6 hours following fractures is ___P___. *(917)*

8.  Condition in which fat globules are released from the marrow of the broken bone into the blood is ___B___. *(916)*

9.  Complication caused by venous stasis, vessel damage, and altered clotting mechanisms is ___C___. *(917)*

10. Condition that occurs due to risk of excessive blood loss is ___E___. *(917)*

11. Condition caused by excessive stress and strain on the joint or fracture, often resulting from nonunion of a fracture, is ___G___. *(918)*

12. Condition called *reflex sympathetic dystrophy* characterized by severe pain is ___I___. *(918)*

13. Serious complication resulting from internal or external pressure on the affected area is ___D___. *(917)*

14. Condition caused by interference with blood supply after a bone injury is ___H___. *(918)*

A.  Infection
B.  Fat embolism
C.  Deep vein thrombosis
D.  Compartment syndrome
E.  Shock
F.  Stiffness and contractures
G.  Post-trauma arthritis
H.  Avascular necrosis
I.  Complex regional pain syndrome
J.  Pressure
K.  Pain
L.  Respiratory distress
M.  Gangrene
N.  Osteomyelitis
O.  Wound contamination
P.  Osteomyelitis

## MULTIPLE CHOICE QUESTIONS

**K.** Choose the most appropriate answer.

1. In adults, the bones most commonly fractured are: *(914)*
   1. femurs.
   2. ribs.
   3. pelvic bones.
   4. wrists.

2. In young and middle-aged adults, the most common fractures are those of the: *(914)*
   1. femur.
   2. rib.
   3. wrist.
   4. pelvis.

3. The most common fractures in older adults are fractures of the wrist and: *(914)*
   1. femur.
   2. rib.
   3. hip.
   4. shoulder.

4. Which is a characteristic of fat embolism following a fracture? *(917)*
   1. Bradycardia
   2. Decreased respirations
   3. Oliguria
   4. Petechiae

5. The most common diagnostic test used to reveal bone disruption, deformity, or malignancy following a fracture is: *(918)*
   1. myelography.
   2. standard radiography.
   3. ultrasonography.
   4. bone scan.

6. The use of rods, pins, nails, screws, or metal plates to align bone fragments is called: *(919)*
   1. external fixation.
   2. closed reduction.
   3. internal fixation.
   4. mechanical reduction.

7. Which is used for external fixation of extensive fractures and fractures of the extremities? *(919)*
   1. Casts
   2. Rods
   3. Pins
   4. Metal plates

8. A condition in which a patient in a body cast may have feelings of claustrophobia is called: *(922)*
   1. compartmental syndrome.
   2. cardiac shock.
   3. cast syndrome.
   4. fat embolus.

9. After a fracture of the lower extremity, crutches are used to assist with ambulation and to increase: *(923)*
   1. pain relief.
   2. deep breathing.
   3. mobility.
   4. circulation.

10. Crutch use requires good: *(923-924)*
    1. lower extremity function.
    2. cardiac function.
    3. lung expansion.
    4. upper body strength.

11. When walking with crutches, patients should put their weight on the: *(923-924)*
    1. top of the crutches.
    2. hand grips.
    3. lower extremities.
    4. shoulders.

12. The type of gait pattern used with bilateral lower extremity prostheses is called: *(924)*
    1. four-point.
    2. swing-to.
    3. swing-through.
    4. two-point.

13. When a patient is climbing stairs using crutches, which body part goes up the step first while the body is supported by the crutches? *(923-924)*
    1. Unaffected leg
    2. Affected leg
    3. Upper extremities
    4. Spine

14. Which gait is used with a walker? *(924)*
    1. Two-point
    2. Four-point
    3. Modified swing-to
    4. Modified swing-through

15. Canes should be held close to the body on the: *(924)*
    1. left side.
    2. right side.
    3. affected side.
    4. unaffected side.

16. When the nurse is assessing the patient with a fracture, the affected extremity is compared with the: *(925)*
    1. proximal body parts.
    2. distal body parts.
    3. unaffected extremity.
    4. normal skeleton.

17. In order to assess circulation and sensation in the affected and unaffected extremity, the nurse should perform neurovascular checks in the areas: *(925)*
    1. distal to the wound.
    2. proximal to the wound.
    3. surrounding the wound.
    4. inside the wound.

18. A good indication of circulation to the extremity in patients with a fracture is: *(925)*
    1. size of the wound.
    2. edema.
    3. skin color.
    4. infection.

19. If pallor is observed in the extremity of patients with fractures, this may be an indication of: *(925)*
    1. infection.
    2. poor circulation.
    3. hemorrhage.
    4. skin breakdown.

20. The primary method of pain relief for patients with fractures is: *(926)*
    1. application of cold to the affected part.
    2. application of heat to the affected part.
    3. wrapping the affected part with a blanket.
    4. immobilization of the affected part.

21. An appropriate intervention for patients with fractures who have impaired physical mobility is: *(926)*
    1. strict aseptic technique.
    2. monitor for fever.
    3. isolation precautions.
    4. gait training.

22. An appropriate intervention for patients with fractures who have ineffective tissue perfusion is: *(927)*
    1. strict aseptic technique.
    2. gait training.
    3. elevation of the affected part above the heart.
    4. rest periods to preserve strength.

23. Patients with fractures are at risk for impaired skin integrity; treatment measures such as casts or traction to immobilize parts may result in: *(928)*
    1. pressure sores.
    2. petechiae.
    3. palmar erythema.
    4. paralysis.

24. For older patients with hip fractures, the treatment of choice is: *(929)*
    1. immobilization.
    2. antibiotic therapy.
    3. surgical repair.
    4. traction.

25. Colles' fracture is a break in the distal: *(930)*
    1. humerus.
    2. tibia.
    3. radius.
    4. fibula.

26. Colles' fractures frequently occur in older adults when they use their hands to: *(930)*
    1. sew or knit.
    2. break a fall.
    3. write letters.
    4. reach for objects above their heads.

27. Interventions for Colles' fractures are aimed at relieving pain and preventing edema; for the first few days, the extremity should be: *(930)*
    1. below the heart.
    2. exercised.
    3. elevated.
    4. flat.

28. Patients with Colles' fractures are encouraged to move their fingers and thumb to promote circulation and reduce: *(930)*
    1. temperature.
    2. swelling.
    3. infection.
    4. dyspnea.

29. Patients with Colles' fractures are encouraged to move their shoulder to prevent: *(930)*
    1. infection.
    2. circulation.
    3. cyanosis.
    4. stiffness.

30. The most common cause of pelvic fractures in young adults is: *(930)*
    1. head injury.
    2. motor vehicle accidents.
    3. falls.
    4. myocardial infarction.

31. The main cause of pelvic fractures in older adults is: *(930)*
    1. motor vehicle accidents.
    2. head injury.
    3. falls.
    4. heart attacks.

32. The nurse needs to observe the patient with a pelvic fracture closely for signs of: *(930)*
    1. internal trauma.
    2. bone infection.
    3. kidney failure.
    4. dyspnea.

33. Which is restricted in patients with pelvic fractures until healing is complete? *(930)*
    1. Use of a trapeze while in bed
    2. Range-of-motion exercises
    3. Coughing and deep-breathing exercises
    4. Weight-bearing

34. Following total hip replacement, which patient teaching is incorrect? *(930)*
    1. Do not extend the affected hip more than 90 degrees.
    2. Use an elevated toilet seat.
    3. Sit in supportive chairs.
    4. Avoid crossing the legs.

L.  **Nursing Care Plan.** Refer to Nursing Care Plan, The Patient with a Fracture, on p. 927 of the textbook.

    1.  What is the priority nursing diagnosis? *(927)*

    2.  What are risk factors for this patient to have a fracture? *(927)*

    3.  What tasks can be assigned to unlicensed assistive personnel? *(927)*

# 43 Amputations

---

## OBJECTIVES

1. Identify the clinical indications for amputations.

2. Describe the different types of amputations.

3. Discuss the medical and surgical management of the amputation patient.

4. Identify appropriate nursing interventions during the preoperative and postoperative phases of care.

5. Assist in developing a nursing process to plan care for the amputation patient.

---

## LEARNING ACTIVITIES

**A. Key Terms.** Match the definition in the numbered column with the most appropriate term in the lettered column.

1. C, D, E    Type of amputation in which a limb or portion of a limb is severed from the body and the wound is left open; a type of open amputation *(936)*

2. C, D, E    Amputation that is done over the course of several surgeries; usually done to control the spread of infection or necrosis *(936)*

3. H    Amputation in which a limb or part of a limb is removed and the wound is surgically closed *(935)*

4. B    Individual who has undergone an amputation *(933)*

5. J    Necrosis, or death of tissue, usually due to a deficient or absent blood supply; may result from inflammatory processes, injury, arteriosclerosis, frostbite, or diabetes mellitus *(933)*

6. I    Deformity or absence of a limb or limbs occurring during fetal development in the uterus *(934)*

7. A    The sensation that a limb still exists following amputation of the limb *(942)*

8. CDE    Amputation in which the wound is left open; usually done in cases of infection or necrosis *(935)*

9. K.    Partial limb remaining after amputation *(935)*

10. J    Removal of a limb, part of a limb, or an organ; may be done by surgical means or may be the result of an accident *(933)*

11. G    Surgical reattachment of an organ to its original site; reimplantation *(933)*

A. Phantom limb
B. Amputee
C. Guillotine amputation
D. Staged amputation
E. Gangrene
F. Open amputation
G. Replantation
H. Closed amputation
I. Congenital amputation
J. Amputation
K. Residual limb

B. **Indications for Amputation.** Which of the following are diseases leading to impaired circulation that may result in the need for an amputation? Select all that apply. *(933)*

1. _____ Osteoporosis
2. ___X___ Peripheral vascular disease
3. ___X___ Diabetes mellitus
4. ___X___ Arteriosclerosis

C. **Open Amputation.** Which of the following are reasons for doing an open amputation instead of a closed amputation? Select all that apply. *(935)*

1. _____ Create a weight-bearing residual limb
2. ___X___ Done when an actual or potential infection exists
3. ___X___ Done in the case of gangrene or trauma
4. ___X___ Done for non–weight-bearing residual limb amputations

D. **Complications of Amputations.** Which complications are associated with amputations? Select all that apply. *(937)*

1. _____ Urinary retention
2. ___X___ Hemorrhage and hematoma
3. ___X___ Wound dehiscence
4. ___X___ Gangrene
5. _____ Hyperglycemia
6. ___X___ Contracture
7. ___X___ Infection
8. _____ Constipation
9. _____ Pulmonary complications
10. ___X___ Necrosis
11. ___X___ Phantom limb sensation
12. ___X___ Phantom limb pain

E. **Patient Teaching.** Which statements are true regarding patient instruction for residual limb and prosthesis care? Select all that apply. *(944)*

1. ___X___ Wash residual limb with soap and water every night. Rinse and dry skin thoroughly.
2. _____ Do not expose the residual limb to air.
3. ___X___ Keep prosthetic socket and residual limb sock clean. Use a clean sock every day.
4. _____ Lotions, ointments, and powders may be applied once a day.
5. ___X___ If redness or irritation develops on the residual limb, discontinue use of prosthesis and have area checked.
6. ___X___ The residual limb may shrink in size for up to 2 years after surgery. Annual visits to the prosthetist are recommended.

F. **Replantation.** What are signs that indicate the medical emergency of inadequate arterial circulation following replantation? Select all that apply. *(946)*

1. ___X___ No peripheral pulse
2. _____ Warm skin
3. ___X___ Pallor
4. ___X___ Slow capillary refill

**G. Types of Amputations.** Complete the statement in the numbered column with the most appropriate term in the lettered column. Some terms may be used more than once, and some terms may not be used.

1.  The removal of the lower leg at the middle of the shin is called a ___E___. *(933)*
2.  Removal of part or all of a limb during a serious accident is called ___C___. *(933)*
3.  Conditions that lead to the need for an amputation include trauma, disease, and ___A___. *(934)*
4.  An amputation through the joint is called ___D___. *(933)*

A.  Tumors
B.  Open amputation
C.  Traumatic amputation
D.  Disarticulation
E.  Below-knee amputation

**H. Diagnostic Tests.** Match the indication in the numbered column with the name of the appropriate diagnostic test relating to amputation in the lettered column.

1.  _____ Record heat present to measure amount of blood flow to certain part of body *(935)*
2.  _____ After imaging reveals suspicious lesions *(935)*
3.  _____ Infection *(934)*
4.  _____ Nature of tumor *(935)*
5.  _____ Volume of blood flow to extremity *(934)*
6.  _____ Pulses in extremities *(935)*
7.  _____ Compromised circulation *(934)*

A.  Bone biopsy
B.  Pulse volume recording (plethysmography)
C.  Doppler ultrasound
D.  WBC
E.  Transcutaneous $P_{O_2}$
F.  Vascular studies (angiography)
G.  Thermography

**I. Nursing Diagnoses.** Match the postoperative nursing diagnosis for patients with amputations in the numbered column with the "related to" statement in the lettered column. *(941)*

1.  _____ Ineffective coping
2.  _____ Acute pain
3.  _____ Self-care deficit
4.  _____ Disturbed sensory perception
5.  _____ Risk for infection
6.  _____ Decreased cardiac output
7.  _____ Impaired skin integrity
8.  _____ Disturbed body image
9.  _____ Anxiety or fear
10. _____ Activity intolerance
11. _____ Impaired physical mobility
12. _____ Risk for injury

A.  Blood loss
B.  Surgical incision, scar formation on a severed nerve
C.  Surgical wound
D.  Loss of a body part
E.  Surgical disruption of skin integrity
F.  Inability to carry out ADLs
G.  Perceived threat of disability
H.  Inadequate support system
I.  Incision
J.  Phantom limb
K.  Loss of limb, weakness, debilitation
L.  Loss of limb
M.  Prolonged bed rest, weakness

**J. Nursing Interventions.** Match the postoperative nursing diagnosis in the numbered column with the appropriate nursing intervention in the lettered column.

1. _____ Risk for injury *(942)*
2. _____ Decreased cardiac output *(941)*
3. _____ Disturbed body image *(944)*
4. _____ Impaired skin integrity *(942)*
5. _____ Impaired physical mobility *(943)*
6. _____ Risk for infection *(942)*
7. _____ Pain *(941)*
8. _____ Disturbed sensory perception *(942)*

A. Active and passive range-of-motion exercises; use of overbed trapeze, if indicated; prosthesis fitting
B. Check temperature; watch for foul or unpleasant odor from stump; check lab work (WBC)
C. Encourage patient to do exercises as ordered; keep environment free from clutter
D. Whirlpool, massage, or TENS stimulation if ordered
E. Check vital signs; observe for excessive bleeding
F. Use of imagery, acupuncture, analgesics
G. Wrap bandage smoothly; inspect residual limb for irritation and edema; elevate residual limb
H. Encourage patient to talk about changes and effects of amputation

**K. Nursing Care.** Match the nursing goal in the numbered column relating to the postoperative patient following amputation with the appropriate outcome criterion in the lettered column. *(941)*

1. _____ Positive body image
2. _____ Absence of infection
3. _____ Absence of new skin lesions
4. _____ Pain relief
5. _____ Healed wound
6. _____ Normal cardiac output
7. _____ Resumed self-care
8. _____ Absence of injury
9. _____ Patient states understanding of phantom limb sensation
10. _____ Improved activity tolerance results

A. Patient accepts limb loss, demonstrates proper care of residual limb
B. Patient states relief from phantom limb sensation
C. Pulse and blood pressure are consistent with patient norms
D. Body temperature returns to normal; drainage decreases
E. Patient states pain relief; has relaxed expression
F. Skin intact; no redness due to pressure
G. Patient demonstrates residual limb care within limits
H. Incision margins intact
I. No falls result from weakness or problems with balance
J. Patient carries out daily activities without excessive fatigue

**L. Nursing Interventions/Older Adult.** Match the characteristics of the older adult amputee in the numbered column with the nursing interventions in the lettered column. *(944)*

1. _____ May have one or more chronic health problems

2. _____ Sometimes easily distracted

3. _____ May have decreased appetite and poor nutritional status

4. _____ May feel foolish in describing phantom sensations

A. Emphasize high-calorie and high-protein diet
B. Remind patient that phantom sensations are not unusual or bizarre
C. Skip unnecessary details when teaching; make sure that patients with glasses or hearing aids have them in place
D. Provide a prosthesis with extra padding and support to patients with diabetes; recognize that poor vision and decreased sensation may keep older people from recognizing complications

**M. Nursing Care/Postoperative Replantation.** Match the nursing goal in the numbered column with the appropriate outcome criterion in the lettered column for postoperative replantation patients. *(946)*

1. _____ Improved body image

2. _____ Adequate circulation in the replanted limb

3. _____ Pain relief

A. Patient touches and looks at affected part
B. Patient states less pain; has relaxed expression
C. Warmth, normal skin color, and arterial pulses are present in the replanted limb

**N. Complementary Therapies.** Which are complementary therapies that are used with analgesics to control pain in patients after surgical amputation? Select all that apply. *(941)*

1. _____ Imagery

2. _____ Relaxation

3. _____ Aerobic exercises

4. _____ Meditation

5. _____ Acupuncture

## MULTIPLE-CHOICE QUESTIONS

**O.** Choose the most appropriate answer.

1. Replantation surgery is most likely to be performed on the: *(944)*
   1. shoulder.
   2. hand.
   3. forearm.
   4. upper arm.

2. The purpose of giving heparin to a postoperative replantation patient is to reduce the risk of: *(946)*
   1. thrombosis.
   2. edema.
   3. infection.
   4. hypersensitivity.

3. A complication of amputation due to inadequate hemostasis is: *(941)*
   1. necrosis.
   2. hemorrhage.
   3. gangrene.
   4. contracture.

4. A complication of amputation manifested by redness, warmth, swelling, and exudate formation at the residual limb site due to invasion of tissues by pathogens is called: *(942)*
   1. contracture.
   2. infection.
   3. edema.
   4. necrosis.

5. Which may be prevented by frequent position changes and range-of-motion exercises? *(943)*
   1. Infection
   2. Hemorrhage
   3. Necrosis
   4. Contractures

6. Which is an opening of the suture line (caused by early removal of sutures or falling) that requires reclosure? *(937)*
   1. Gangrene
   2. Necrosis
   3. Wound dehiscence
   4. Contracture

7. Which person will request that an amputated body part be present for burial? *(941)*
   1. Roman Catholic
   2. Mormon
   3. Orthodox Jew
   4. Muslim

8. Which diagnosis is a priority in the postoperative period for a patient after surgical amputation? *(941)*
   1. Disturbed body image
   2. Impaired skin integrity
   3. Pain
   4. Disturbed sensory perception

9. Which treatment for venous congestion of a replanted limb utilizes the saliva of parasites that extracts excess blood? *(946)*
   1. Anticoagulants
   2. Vasodilators
   3. Leeches
   4. Local anesthetics

10. What complication can occur if pillows are placed continuously under a below-knee amputation? *(943)*
    1. Infection
    2. Necrosis
    3. Phantom limb sensation
    4. Hip contractures

P. **Nursing Care Plan.** Refer to the Nursing Care Plan, The Patient with an Upper Extremity Amputation, on p. 939 in your textbook.

1. What is the priority nursing diagnosis for this patient? *(939)*

2. What are risk factors that led to this patient's need for an upper extremity amputation? *(939)*

3. What tasks can be assigned to unlicensed assistive personnel? *(939)*

# Pituitary and Adrenal Disorders

---

## OBJECTIVES

1. Identify nursing assessment data relevant to the function of the adrenal and pituitary glands.

2. Describe the tests and procedures used to diagnose disorders of the adrenal and pituitary glands, including relevant nursing considerations.

3. Describe the pathophysiology and medical treatment of adrenocortical insufficiency, excess adrenocortical hormones, hypopituitarism, diabetes insipidus, and pituitary tumors.

4. Assist in developing nursing care plans for patients with selected disorders of the adrenal and pituitary glands.

---

## LEARNING ACTIVITIES

**A. Key Terms.** Match the definition in the numbered column with the most appropriate term in the lettered column.

1. _____ Ductless gland that produces an internal secretion discharged into the lymph or bloodstream and circulated to all parts of the body; hormones, the active substances of these glands, cause an effect on certain organs or tissues *(948)*

2. _____ Disease resulting from a deficiency of adrenocorticotropic hormone (ACTH) caused by destruction or dysfunction of the adrenal glands; characterized by increased pigmentation of the skin and mucous membranes, weakness, fatigue, hypotension, nausea, weight loss, and hypoglycemia *(966)*

3. _____ Disease caused by inadequate secretion of antidiuretic hormone (ADH) by the posterior pituitary gland; symptoms include excessive urination, thirst, and dehydration *(961)*

4. _____ Disease of middle-aged adults resulting from overproduction of growth hormone (GH) by the anterior pituitary gland; characterized by enlargement of the facial bones, nose, lips, and jaw; also associated with decreased libido, moodiness, fatigue, muscle pains, sweating, and headache *(952)*

5. _____ Type of hormone secreted by the adrenal cortex and involved in the regulation of fluid and electrolyte levels in the body *(965)*

A.  Acromegaly
B.  Addison's disease
C.  Adrenaline
D.  Androgens
E.  Catecholamines
F.  Cushing's disease
G.  Cushing's syndrome
H.  Diabetes insipidus
I.  Endocrine gland
J.  Estrogens
K.  Gigantism
L.  Glucocorticoids
M.  Hypophysectomy
N.  Mineralocorticoids
O.  Syndrome of inappropriate antidiuretic hormone (SIADH)

6. _____ Disorder caused by excess antidiuretic hormone production; symptoms include decreased urination, edema, and fluid overload *(963)*

7. _____ Disorder resulting from excessive glucocorticoids in the body as a result of tumor or hypersecretion of the pituitary; may also be caused by prolonged administration of large doses of exogenous steroids; symptoms include fat deposits in the neck and abdomen, fatigue, weakness, edema, excess hair growth, glucose intolerances, skin discoloration, and mood swings *(973)*

8. _____ Class of adrenocortical hormones that affects protein and carbohydrate metabolism and helps protect the body against stress *(965)*

9. _____ Chemical (dopamine, epinephrine, norepinephrine) released at sympathetic nerve endings in response to stress *(965)*

10. _____ Hormones produced by the ovaries, adrenal glands, and fetoplacental unit in females that are responsible for the development and maturation of females *(966)*

11. _____ Disease caused by excessive growth hormone in children and young adolescents, resulting in excessive proportional growth *(952)*

12. _____ Disease caused by the hypersecretion of glucocorticoids as a result of excessive release of adrenocorticotropic hormone by the pituitary gland *(973)*

13. _____ Hormones produced by the adrenal cortex, and testes that stimulate the development of male characteristics *(966)*

14. _____ Surgical removal of all or part of the pituitary gland *(957)*

15. _____ Epinephrine; a powerful vasoactive substance produced by the medulla or adrenal gland in times of stress or danger, allowing the body to react by fighting or fleeing *(965)*

B.  **Pituitary Gland Disorders.** Complete the statements in the numbered column with the most appropriate term in the lettered column. Some terms may be used more than once, and some terms may not be used.

1.  The first symptom of a problem in hyper-
    pituitarism is often _____. *(954)*

2.  Radiographic films of the skull of people
    with hyperpituitarism may show a large
    sella turcica and increased _____.
    *(954)*

3.  For patients with a diagnosis of pitu-
    itary tumors, the treatment of choice is
    _____. *(954)*

4.  A disease that occurs in early childhood or
    puberty in which the diaphysis of the long
    bones grows to great lengths stimulated by
    excess GH is _____. *(952)*

5.  A disease that appears when adults are in
    their 30s and 40s in which bones increase
    in thickness and width after epiphyseal
    closure is _____. *(952)*

A.  Gigantism
B.  Hypothalamus
C.  Cushing's syndrome
D.  Hypophysectomy
E.  Bone density
F.  Parathyroid gland
G.  Acromegaly
H.  Visual deficit

C.  **SIADH.** Complete the statements in the numbered column with the most appropriate term in the lettered column. Some terms may be used more than once, and some terms may not be used.

1.  A syndrome characterized by a water
    imbalance related to an increase in ADH
    secretion is called _____. *(963)*

2.  Kidneys retain fluid due to the elevation of
    _____. *(963)*

3.  Plasma volume expands when ADH is
    elevated in SIADH, causing an increased
    _____. *(963)*

4.  When the ADH level is elevated, the pa-
    tient experiences water intoxication and
    the body's sodium is diluted, resulting in
    _____. *(963)*

5.  Weight gain without edema is one of the
    main symptoms of _____. *(963)*

6.  The treatment of SIADH promotes the
    elimination of _____. *(963)*

7.  In patients with SIADH, fluids are re-
    stricted and patients are given _____.
    *(964)*

8.  Patients with SIADH have fluid vol-
    ume excess related to excess secretion of
    _____. *(963)*

A.  Blood pressure
B.  Potassium
C.  Excess water
D.  SIADH
E.  Hyponatremia
F.  Heart rate
G.  ADH
H.  Diabetes insipidus
I.  Sodium chloride

**D. Addison's Disease.** Complete the statements in the numbered column with the most appropriate term in the lettered column. Some terms may be used more than once, and some terms may not be used.

1. Addison's disease results in the loss of aldosterone and _____. *(967)*

2. A test that is necessary for a definitive diagnosis of hypoadrenalism, such as Addison's disease, is _____. *(968)*

3. The mainstay of treatment of patients with Addison's disease is replacement therapy with mineralocorticoids and _____. *(969)*

4. Potassium excretion is decreased when cortisol is not secreted, resulting in _____. *(967)*

5. Secondary adrenal insufficiency is a result of dysfunction of the hypothalamus or the _____. *(967)*

6. Decreased levels of aldosterone alter the clearance of potassium, water, and _____. *(967)*

7. When sodium and water excretion rates accelerate, problems such as hyponatremia and _____ can result. *(967)*

8. Acute adrenal crisis is also called _____. *(968)*

9. Impaired secretion of cortisol results in decreased liver and muscle glycogen and decreased _____. *(967)*

10. Secondary adrenal insufficiency leads to decreased production of cortisol and _____. *(967)*

11. Primary adrenal insufficiency is also called _____. *(966)*

12. Decreased supplies of available glucose, which occurs as a result of impaired secretion of cortisol, is called _____. *(967)*

13. Patients with either primary or secondary adrenal insufficiency are at risk for episodes of _____. *(968)*

14. A condition that occurs because hyperkalemia promotes hydrogen ion retention is _____. *(967)*

A. Hypovolemia
B. Pituitary gland
C. Addison's disease
D. Gluconeogenesis
E. Norepinephrine
F. Glucocorticoids
G. Tachycardia
H. ACTH stimulation test
I. SIADH
J. Hypoglycemia
K. Hyperkalemia
L. Metabolic acidosis
M. Sodium
N. Androgen
O. Cortisol
P. Addisonian crisis
Q. Androgens

**E.   Cushing's Syndrome.** Complete the statements in the numbered column with the most appropriate term in the lettered column. Some terms may be used more than once, and some terms may not be used.

1.   Prolonged administration of high doses of corticosteroids may cause Cushing's syndrome; this is an example of a(n) _____ cause. *(973)*

2.   An initial screening for Cushing's syndrome is the overnight _____ test. *(973)*

3.   In the immediate postoperative period of adrenalectomy patients, _____ may be needed to maintain blood pressure. *(976)*

4.   The most common cause of Cushing's syndrome is long-term exogenous _____ use. *(973)*

5.   Corticotropin-secreting pituitary tumors may cause Cushing's syndrome; this is an example of a(n) _____ cause. *(973)*

6.   Patients with a pheochromocytoma exhibit episodes of hypertension, hypermetabolism, and _____. *(976)*

7.   Excessive production of ACTH resulting from a pituitary tumor is called _____. *(973)*

8.   Hypersecretion of the adrenal cortex may result in the production of excess amounts of _____. *(965)*

9.   The prevention of infections in adrenalectomy patients is maintained through observance of _____. *(976)*

10.  A tumor of the adrenal medulla that causes secretion of excessive catecholamines is a(n) _____. *(976)*

11.  The condition that results from excessive cortisol is called _____. *(973)*

12.  Patients who take drugs that suppress adrenal function are at risk of acute _____. *(974)*

A.   Cushing's disease
B.   SIADH
C.   Exogenous
D.   Pheochromocytoma
E.   Steroid
F.   Cushing's syndrome
G.   Hyperglycemia
H.   Corticosteroids
I.   Diabetes insipidus
J.   Dexamethasone
K.   Endogenous
L.   Adrenal crisis
M.   Vasopressors
N.   Asepsis

F. **Pituitary and Adrenal Hormones.** Match the definition or description in the numbered column with the most appropriate term in the lettered column. Some terms may be used more than once, and some may not be used.

1. _____ Stimulates the growth and development of bone, muscles, or organs (*949*)

2. _____ Controls ovulation or egg release in the female and testosterone production in the male (*950*)

3. _____ Controls the release of glucocorticoids and adrenal androgens (*949*)

4. _____ Stimulates the development of eggs in the ovary of the female and the production of sperm in the testes of the male (*950*)

5. _____ Another name for the somatotrophic hormone (*949*)

6. _____ Stimulates breast milk production in the female (*950*)

7. _____ Promotes pigmentation (*950*)

8. _____ Another name for the lactogenic hormone (*950*)

9. _____ Causes the reabsorption of water from the renal tubules of the kidney (*950*)

10. _____ Causes contractions of the uterus in labor and the release of breast milk (*950*)

11. _____ Another name for vasopressin (*950*)

12. _____ Controls the secretory activities of the thyroid gland (*949*)

A. Luteinizing hormone
B. Thyroid-stimulating hormone
C. Oxytocin
D. Melanocyte-stimulating hormone
E. Growth hormone
F. Norepinephrine
G. Antidiuretic hormone
H. Adrenocorticotropic hormone
I. Prolactin
J. Follicle-stimulating hormone

**G. Diabetes Insipidus.** Complete the statements in the numbered column with the most appropriate term in the lettered column. Some terms may be used more than once, and some terms may not be used. (*961*)

1. Increased plasma osmolarity stimulates the osmoreceptors, which in turn relay information to the cerebral cortex, causing the person to experience _____.

2. Massive dehydration leads to severe _____ imbalances.

3. With ADH deficiency, massive dehydration occurs, which leads to decreased intravascular volume, circulatory collapse, and _____.

4. Electrolyte imbalances contribute to circulatory collapse by causing arrhythmias and impaired contractility of the _____.

5. Massive diuresis results in increased plasma _____.

A. Thirst
B. Skeletal muscles
C. Heart
D. Electrolyte
E. Osmolarity
F. Hypotension

**H. Lab Results in Addison's Disease.** Indicate whether the following laboratory study results would be expected to (A) increase or (B) decrease in patients with Addison's disease. (*968*)

1. _____ Serum cortisol level

2. _____ Fasting glucose

3. _____ Sodium

4. _____ Potassium

5. _____ Blood urea nitrogen

**I. Cushing's Syndrome: Nursing Diagnoses.** Match the nursing diagnoses for patients with Cushing's syndrome in the numbered column with the most appropriate "related to" statements in the lettered column. (*975*)

1. _____ Risk for infection

2. _____ Disturbed thought processes

3. _____ Risk for impaired skin integrity

4. _____ Risk for injury (fracture)

5. _____ Disturbed body image

A. Changes in skin and connective tissue and edema
B. Changes in physical appearance and function
C. Fluid and electrolyte imbalance
D. Osteoporosis
E. High serum cortisol levels

J.  **Cushing's Syndrome: Nursing Interventions.** Match the interventions in the numbered column with the nursing diagnoses for patients with Cushing's syndrome in the lettered column. Some nursing diagnoses may be used more than once, and some may not be used.

1.  _____ Avoid exposure to infections (*975*)

2.  _____ Report minor signs, such as low-grade fever, sore throat, or aches to the physician (*975*)

3.  _____ Seek a psychiatric referral if mood swings continue to be a problem (*975*)

4.  _____ Assist patient to change positions at least every 2 hours (*975*)

5.  _____ Protect patient from falls or trauma (*975*)

6.  _____ Discuss bruises, abnormal fat distribution, and hirsutism with the patient if they cause embarrassment (*975*)

7.  _____ Teach patient about the importance of continuing drug therapy under medical supervision (*976*)

A.  Risk for injury
B.  Risk for impaired skin integrity
C.  Sexual dysfunction
D.  Disturbed body image
E.  Risk for infection
F.  Ineffective management of therapeutic regimen
G.  Disturbed thought processes

K.  **Age-Related Changes.** Which of the following are age-related changes in the healthy older person regarding pituitary function? Select all that apply. (*951*)

1.  _____ Pituitary function is not adequate.

2.  _____ ADH secretion may be increased.

3.  _____ Ability to concentrate urine may be decreased.

4.  _____ Risk for dehydration decreases.

L.  **Hypophysectomy.**

1.  Monitoring the postoperative hypophysectomy patient for signs and symptoms of infection is important; which are signs and symptoms that may be indications of meningitis? Select all that apply. (*958*)

    1.  _____ Decreased white blood cell (WBC) count

    2.  _____ Sudden rise in temperature

    3.  _____ Headache

    4.  _____ Neck rigidity

2.  Which medications are given as hormone replacement therapy following a complete hypophysectomy? Select all that apply. (*958*)

    1.  _____ Pituitary hormone suppressants

    2.  _____ Dopamine receptor antagonists

    3.  _____ Glucocorticoids

    4.  _____ Thyroid medications

3. The postoperative hypophysectomy patient is instructed to avoid any activities that can cause Valsalva's maneuver. Which activities may create enough intracranial pressure to disrupt the surgical site and cause CSF leakage? Select all that apply. (*959*)

   1. _____ Passive range-of-motion exercises
   2. _____ Coughing
   3. _____ Straining
   4. _____ Vomiting

**M. Acute Adrenal Crisis.**

1. Which are manifestations of acute adrenal crisis (addisonian crisis)? Select all that apply. (*968*)

   1. _____ Bradycardia
   2. _____ Dehydration
   3. _____ Confusion
   4. _____ Hyponatremia
   5. _____ Hypoglycemia
   6. _____ Hyperkalemia
   7. _____ Hypertension

2. Which types of stressors can initiate acute adrenal crisis (addisonian crisis)? Select all that apply. (*968*)

   1. _____ Infection
   2. _____ Illness
   3. _____ Steroid therapy use
   4. _____ Trauma

**N. Drug Therapy.** Match the descriptions of drugs used for adrenal disorders in the numbered column with the drug classification in the lettered column. Answers may be used more than once. (*970*)

| | | |
|---|---|---|
| 1. _____ | Used to suppress adrenocortical function | A. Glucocorticoids |
| 2. _____ | Stimulate reabsorption of sodium and excretion of potassium and hydrogen ions | B. Mineralocorticoids<br>C. Adrenocortical cytotoxic agents<br>D. Antifungal agents |
| 3. _____ | Stimulate the formation of glucose and promote the storage of glucose as glycogen | |
| 4. _____ | Used to treat adrenal insufficiency | |
| 5. _____ | Example of this category is Florinef | |
| 6. _____ | Example of this category is hydrocortisone (Cortef) | |

O. **Diagnostic Tests.** Match the description in the numbered column with the name of the procedure in the lettered column. (*953*)

1. _____   Used to detect diabetes mellitus and hyperpituitarism.

2. _____   Serum levels are measured to detect elevations or deficiencies of pituitary hormones.

3. _____   Given to stimulate release of ADH to detect diabetes insipidus (DI)

4. _____   Measures cortisol, which increases with adrenal hyperplasia and Cushing's syndrome

5. _____   Detects changes in specific gravity and osmolality after vasopressin is given; used to detect diabetes insipidus (DI)

6. _____   Radiographs taken to study cerebral blood flow and blood vessels

7. _____   Uses radiographs to create images of internal structures and detect tumors

A. Cerebral computed tomography scan
B. Cerebral angiogram
C. Glucose tolerance test
D. Dexamethasone suppression tests
E. Pituitary hormone serum levels
F. Hypertonic saline test
G. Fluid deprivation test

P. **Diagnostic Test Results/Addison's Disease.** Which are diagnostic test results used to determine the presence of Addison's disease? Select all that apply. (*968, 969*)

1. _____   Decreased fasting glucose

2. _____   Decreased BUN

3. _____   Hyponatremia

4. _____   ECG changes of increased peaked T waves

**Q. Nursing Diagnoses.** Match the nursing diagnosis in the numbered column with the disorder in the lettered column.

1. _____   Excess fluid volume related to excess ADH secretion *(964)*

2. _____   Risk for infection related to high serum cortisol levels *(975)*

3. _____   Ineffective tissue perfusion related to electrolyte imbalances *(971)*

4. _____   Disturbed body image related to changes in physical appearance *(957)*

5. _____   Deficient fluid volume related to excessive urine output *(962)*

6. _____   Sexual dysfunction related to hormone deficiency *(960)*

A.   SIADH
B.   Hypopituitarism
C.   Hyperpituitarism
D.   Cushing's syndrome
E.   Addison's disease
F.   Diabetes insipidus

**R. Endocrine System.** Using Figure 44-1 (p. 949) below, label the organs of the endocrine system (A–G). (*949*)

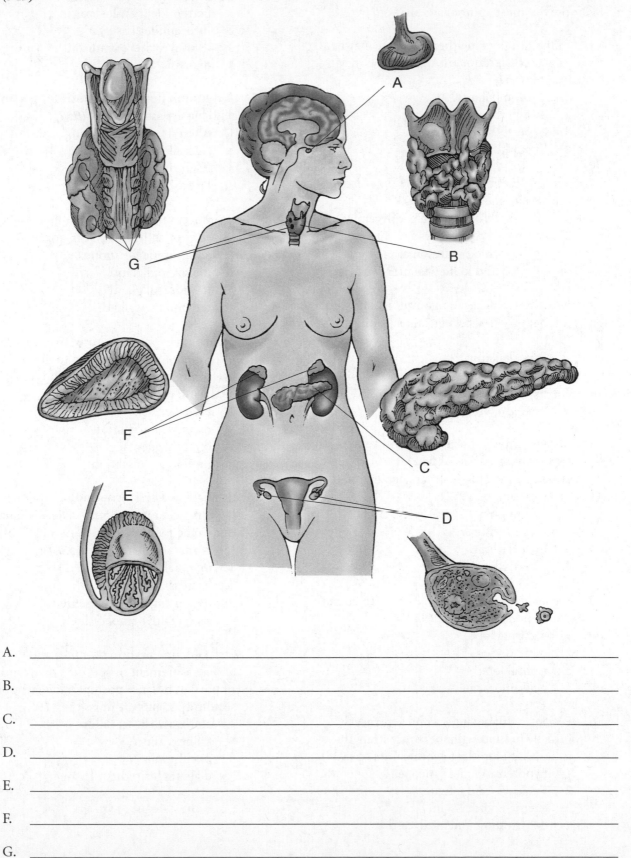

A. _____

B. _____

C. _____

D. _____

E. _____

F. _____

G. _____

## MULTIPLE-CHOICE QUESTIONS

**S.** Choose the most appropriate answer.

1. In the healthy older person, there may be increased secretion of ADH, which may lead to: *(951)*
   1. fluid imbalance.
   2. dyspnea.
   3. hypertension.
   4. hypopituitarism.

2. The production of excess GH may lead to the development of: *(952)*
   1. atherosclerosis and hyperglycemia.
   2. edema and congestive heart failure.
   3. dyspnea and pneumonia.
   4. oliguria and kidney failure.

3. Growth hormone antagonizes insulin and interferes with its effects, thus leading to: *(952)*
   1. hyperkalemia.
   2. hypokalemia.
   3. hyperglycemia.
   4. hypoglycemia.

4. Because growth hormone mobilizes stored fat for energy, levels of free fatty acids are elevated in the bloodstream, leading to the development of: *(952)*
   1. pneumonia.
   2. kidney failure.
   3. hypotension.
   4. atherosclerosis.

5. Visual problems occur in hyperpituitarism due to pressure on the: *(954)*
   1. occipital lobe.
   2. optic nerves.
   3. frontal lobe.
   4. oculomotor nerves.

6. Patients with gigantism and acromegaly initially present with increased strength, progressing rapidly to complaints of: *(954)*
   1. hypotension and syncope.
   2. weakness and fatigue.
   3. edema and dry skin.
   4. dehydration and bradycardia.

7. One drug commonly prescribed for patients with acromegaly is: *(954)*
   1. octreotide (Sandostatin).
   2. furosemide (Lasix).
   3. levothyroxine (Synthroid).
   4. digoxin.

8. A common nursing diagnosis for patients with hyperpituitarism is: *(957)*
   1. Altered tissue perfusion.
   2. Altered skin integrity.
   3. High risk for infection.
   4. Disturbed body image.

9. Bromocriptine (Parlodel) inhibits the release of prolactin and GH from: *(957)*
   1. antidiuretic hormone.
   2. the thyroid gland.
   3. the adrenal gland.
   4. the pituitary gland.

10. Following hypophysectomy, the nurse asks the patient to place the chin to the chest to assess for nuchal rigidity, which is associated with: *(958)*
    1. bone density.
    2. meningeal irritation.
    3. cerebral edema.
    4. impaired circulation.

11. Changes in assessment findings following hypophysectomy that may reflect edema due to the manipulation of tissues or bleeding intracranially include: *(958)*
    1. unequal pupil size.
    2. decreasing alertness.
    3. decreasing blood pressure.
    4. rising body temperature.

12. Strict documentation of intake and output and measurement of specific gravity are important because postoperative hypophysectomy patients are at risk for: *(958)*
    1. congestive heart failure.
    2. kidney failure.
    3. pneumonia.
    4. diabetes insipidus.

13. Because CSF leaks sometimes occur in postoperative hypophysectomy patients, the nurse should check: *(958)*
    1. intake and output.
    2. pupil reactivity.
    3. nasal packing.
    4. vital signs.

14. A bedside test can be done with a chemical strip to detect whether drainage in a postoperative hypophysectomy patient is CSF, since CSF has a high content of: *(958)*
    1. glucose.
    2. protein.
    3. white blood cells.
    4. red blood cells.

15. Decreased pigmentation of the skin results in: *(960)*
    1. edema.
    2. pallor.
    3. pruritus.
    4. erythema.

16. The patient who has a complete hypophysectomy requires hormone replacement: *(958)*
    1. preoperatively.
    2. during the postoperative recovery period.
    3. for 6 months to 1 year.
    4. for a lifetime.

17. In patients with hypopituitarism, insufficient thyroid hormone is available for normal metabolism and: *(960)*
    1. visual acuity.
    2. muscle tone.
    3. heat production.
    4. bone growth.

18. If there is a lack of melanocyte-stimulating hormone, the skin exhibits decreased: *(960)*
    1. sensory perception.
    2. immunity.
    3. pigmentation.
    4. thermoregulation.

19. Deficiency of thyroid-stimulating hormones necessitates thyroid replacement with a drug such as: *(960)*
    1. octreotide acetate (Sandostatin).
    2. bromocriptine (Parlodel).
    3. levothyroxine (Synthroid).
    4. vasopressin (Pitressin Synthetic).

20. To produce or maintain libido, secondary sexual characteristics, and well-being, males with hypopituitarism should receive: *(960)*
    1. testosterone.
    2. estrogen.
    3. levothyroxine (Synthroid).
    4. bromocriptine (Parlodel).

21. Drug-related diabetes insipidus is often caused by: *(961)*
    1. bromocriptine (Parlodel).
    2. lithium carbonate (Eskalith).
    3. levothyroxine (Synthroid).
    4. digitalis.

22. A 24-hour urine output of greater than 4 liters of fluid suggests a diagnosis of: *(962)*
    1. hypertension.
    2. kidney infection.
    3. congestive heart failure.
    4. diabetes insipidus.

23. In order to maintain adequate blood volume in patients with diabetes insipidus, two measures that are required include intravenous fluid volume replacement and: *(962)*
    1. diuretics.
    2. vasopressors.
    3. anticholinergics.
    4. antihistamines.

24. The level of consciousness deteriorates and the patient may have seizures or lapse into a coma when water intoxication affects the: *(963)*
    1. respiratory system.
    2. urinary system.
    3. cardiovascular system.
    4. central nervous system.

25. A nursing diagnosis for patients with SI-ADH is Risk for injury related to confusion associated with: *(964)*
    1. acute adrenal insufficiency.
    2. impaired physiologic response to stress.
    3. water intoxication.
    4. decreased ADH secretion.

26. To prevent progressive cerebral edema in patients with SIADH, patients are placed in which position in bed? *(964)*
    1. Semi-Fowler's
    2. Flat
    3. Fowler's
    4. Side-lying

27. In postmenopausal women, the primary source of endogenous estrogen is the: *(965)*
    1. hypothalamus.
    2. thyroid gland.
    3. adrenal cortex.
    4. ovarian follicle.

28. A common skin finding in patients with adrenal dysfunction is: *(966)*
    1. protruding bones.
    2. erythema.
    3. bronze pigmentation.
    4. pruritus.

29. An age-related change that affects the adrenal glands is that adrenal function: *(966)*
    1. decreases in epinephrine.
    2. remains adequate.
    3. becomes hyperactive.
    4. increases in metabolism.

30. The response to sodium restriction and to position changes is less efficient in older adults because of declines in the secretion of plasma renin and: *(966)*
    1. thyroxine.
    2. aldosterone.
    3. estrogen.
    4. androgens.

31. Signs and symptoms of hyperkalemia that should be reported to the physician by patients with Addison's disease include: *(971)*
    1. dyspnea and coughing.
    2. oliguria and flank pain.
    3. constipation and fatty stools.
    4. weakness and paresthesia.

32. Which substance may be used liberally in the diet of patients with Addison's disease? *(971)*
    1. Carbohydrates
    2. Salt
    3. Saturated fats
    4. Caffeine

33. What is a common sign of diabetes insipidus? *(961)*
    1. Massive diuresis
    2. Edema
    3. Hyperglycemia
    5. Oliguria

34. What is a priority nursing diagnosis specific to the patient who has had an adrenalectomy? *(976)*
    1. Ineffective tissue perfusion related to fluid volume deficit
    2. Risk for injury related to acute adrenal insufficiency
    3. Fatigue related to fluid and electrolyte imbalance
    4. Risk for injury related to infection

T. **Nursing Care Plan.** Refer to Nursing Care Plan, The Patient with Addison's Disease, on p. 972 in the textbook.

1. What is the priority nursing diagnosis for this patient? *(972)*

2. What is the most common cause of primary Addison's disease? *(972)*

3. What are the manifestations of adrenal insufficiency exhibited by this patient? Select
   all that apply. *(972)*
   1. Hypoglycemia
   2. Nausea, vomiting and diarrhea
   3. Weight loss
   4. Weakness
   5. Darkening of the skin on his face and
      arms
   6. Irritability
   7. Dehydration
   8. Hypokalemia
   9. Hypotension

4. What type is diet is this patient on? *(972)*

5. Which tasks can be assigned to unlicensed
   assistive personnel for this patient? *(972)*

# 45 Thyroid and Parathyroid Disorders

---

## OBJECTIVES

1. Identify nursing assessment data related to the functions of the thyroid and parathyroid glands.

2. Describe tests and procedures used to diagnose disorders of the thyroid and parathyroid glands and identify nursing responsibilities relevant for each.

3. Describe the pathophysiology, signs and symptoms, complications, and treatment of hyperthyroidism, hypothyroidism, hyperparathyroidism, and hypoparathyroidism.

4. Assist in the development of nursing care plans for patients with disorders of the thyroid or parathyroid glands, including assessment, nursing diagnoses, goals, interventions, and outcome criteria.

---

## LEARNING ACTIVITIES

**A. Key Terms.** Match the definition in the numbered column with the most appropriate term in the lettered column.

1. _____ Facial edema that develops with severe, long-term hypothyroidism; sometimes used as a synonym for hypothyroidism *(988)*
2. _____ Enlargement of the thyroid gland, causing the neck to appear swollen *(993)*
3. _____ Steady muscle contraction caused by hypocalcemia *(987)*
4. _____ Small mass of tissue that can be palpated *(979)*
5. _____ Spasmodic closure of the larynx *(987)*
6. _____ Permanent mental and physical retardation caused by congenital deficiency of thyroid hormones *(988)*
7. _____ Excessive metabolic stimulation caused by elevated thyroid hormone level *(982)*
8. _____ Inflammation of the parotid (salivary) gland *(983)*
9. _____ Inflammation of the thyroid gland *(983)*
10. _____ Substance that suppresses thyroid function *(988)*
11. _____ Protrusion of the eyeballs associated with hyperthyroidism *(980)*

A. Goiter
B. Goitrogen
C. Exophthalmos
D. Myxedema
E. Nodule
F. Cretinism
G. Parotiditis
H. Tetany
I. Laryngospasm
J. Thyroiditis
K. Thyrotoxicosis

**B. Hyperthyroidism/Hypothyroidism.** For each of the following signs or symptoms, indicate whether it is characteristic of (A) hyperthyroidism or (B) hypothyroidism. *(982, 989, 990)*

1. _____ Heat intolerance
2. _____ Apathy
3. _____ Increased appetite
4. _____ Tachycardia
5. _____ Cold intolerance
6. _____ Weight loss
7. _____ Anorexia
8. _____ Bradycardia
9. _____ Nervousness and restlessness
10. _____ Weight gain
11. _____ Coarse, dry skin and hair
12. _____ Systolic hypertension

C. **Thyroidectomy.**

1. Which two things should be placed at the bedside before the patient who is having a thyroidectomy returns from surgery? *(987)*

   1. _____ Thromboembolic stockings
   2. _____ Suction equipment
   3. _____ Emergency tracheotomy tray

2. What are two reasons that respiratory distress can result following thyroidectomy? Select all that apply. *(987)*

   1. _____ Compression of the trachea
   2. _____ Aspiration leading to atelectasis
   3. _____ Spasms of the larynx due to nerve damage or hypocalcemia

3. Following thyroidectomy surgery, where should the nurse check for bleeding? Select all that apply. *(988)*

   1. _____ Inspect the dressing on the front of the neck.
   2. . _____ Check behind the neck.
   3. _____ Check in the midclavicular area.

D. **Thyroid Enlargement.** If thyroid enlargement is mild and thyroid hormone production is normal, what treatment is required? *(993)*

E. **Radioactive Iodine.** Explain why thyroidectomy surgery may be followed with radioactive iodine treatment. *(983)*

F. **Thyroid and Parathyroid Hormones.** Complete the statements below with either (A) increase(s) or (B) decrease(s). *(982)*

1. When thyroid hormones are elevated, the pulse rate _____.
2. Excess thyroxine _____ the body's metabolic rate.
3. High levels of PTH _____ retention of calcium.
4. When thyroid hormones are elevated, blood pressure _____.
5. High levels of PTH _____ loss of phosphates by the kidneys.

**G. Hyperthyroidism.** Complete the statement in the numbered column with the most appropriate term in the lettered column. Some terms may be used more than once, and some terms may not be used.

1. The most common forms of hyperthyroidism are Graves' disease and _____. *(982)*
2. If untreated, hyperthyroidism may lead to _____. *(982)*
3. Symptoms of thyrotoxicosis include tachycardia, heart failure, and _____. *(982)*
4. Drugs that block the synthesis, release, or activity of thyroid hormones are _____. *(983)*
5. The two classes of drugs commonly used as antithyroid drugs are thioamides and _____. *(983)*
6. When a patient is taking drugs that interfere with thyroxine secretion, the nurse should monitor for edema, weight gain, and _____. *(983)*
7. Examples of thioamides are methimazole (Tapazole) and _____. *(983)*
8. One main disadvantage of the thioamides is that they can cause _____. *(983)*

A. Antithyroids
B. Cold intolerance
C. Agranulocytosis
D. Heat intolerance
E. Hyperthermia
F. Iodides
G. Propylthiouracil (PTU)
H. Multinodular goiter
I. Hypothermia
J. Thyrotoxicosis (thyroid storm)

**H. Complications.** Complete the statements in the numbered column with the most appropriate term in the lettered column. Some terms may be used more than once, and some terms may not be used.

1. A condition in which deposits of fat and fluid behind the eyeballs make them bulge forward is called _____. *(986)*
2. A complication in patients undergoing thyroidectomies that can be prevented by preoperative treatment with antithyroid drugs is _____. *(982)*
3. Signs and symptoms of poor oxygenation due to airway obstruction that may occur after thyroidectomy include restlessness, increased pulse, and _____. *(987)*
4. Signs of laryngeal nerve damage include inability to speak and _____. *(987)*
5. A complication of thyroidectomies includes injury to the parathyroid glands, which results in _____. *(987)*
6. The most serious side effect of hypocalcemia is _____. *(987)*
7. Signs of severe hyperthyroidism include fever, confusion, and _____. *(988)*
8. Symptoms of infection that should be reported after thyroidectomy include fever, wound swelling, and _____. *(988)*
9. The result of inadequate secretion of thyroid hormones is called _____. *(988)*

A. Hyperthyroidism
B. Dyspnea
C. Laryngospasm
D. Bradycardia
E. Tetany
F. Hypothyroidism
G. Calcium salts
H. Foul discharge
I. Hoarseness
J. Exophthalmos
K. Tachycardia
L. Thyroid crisis
M. Tetany

I. **Hyperparathyroidism.** Complete the statement in the numbered column with the most appropriate term in the lettered column. Some terms may be used more than once, and some terms may not be used.

1. Parathyroid hormone (parathormone, PTH) plays a critical role in regulating _____. *(995)*

2. The most notable effect of hyperparathyroidism is _____. *(995)*

3. People who undergo kidney transplantation after being on dialysis for a long time may experience _____. *(995)*

4. When the serum calcium level falls, _____ is secreted. *(993)*

5. Generally, calcium retention by the kidney is balanced by the loss of _____. *(993)*

6. A spasm of the facial muscle when the face is tapped over the facial nerve is _____. *(994)*

7. A carpopedal spasm that occurs when a blood pressure cuff is inflated beyond a patient's systolic blood pressure and is left in place for several minutes is _____. *(994)*

8. _____ is an element that is an important component of strong bones and that plays a vital role in the functions of nerve and tissue cells. *(993)*

9. The secretion of excess PTH is called _____. *(995)*

A. Trousseau's sign
B. Phosphates
C. Hypoparathyroidism
D. Chvostek's sign
E. Calcium
F. PTH
G. Hyperparathyroidism
H. TSH
I. Hypercalcemia
J. Sodium

J. **Diagnostic Tests.** Match the description in the numbered column with the diagnostic procedure in the lettered column. Answers may be used more than once. *(981)*

1. _____ After radioactive iodine is given and the amount of iodine taken up is measured, a high uptake indicates hyperthyroidism.

2. _____ Provides high-quality images of thyroid and any nodules.

3. _____ An elevated $T_3$ serum level indicates Graves' disease.

4. _____ After iodine isotope is given, a scanner detects pattern of uptake by the thyroid gland.

5. _____ Elevated $T_4$ serum levels indicated hyperthyroidism.

6. _____ Assesses response of the pituitary to TRH; differentiates types of hypothyroidism.

7. _____ Test that can differentiate benign and malignant nodules and detect other abnormalities.

8. _____ Material from thyroid nodules is aspirated and is guided by ultrasonography.

A. Serum $T_3$ and $T_4$ measurements
B. Serum thyroid-stimulating hormone (TSH) levels
C. Radioactive iodine uptake test
D. Thyroid scan
E. Thyroid ultrasonography
F. Fine needle aspiration biopsy
G. TRH stimulation test

K. **Drug Therapy.** Match the description in the numbered column with the drug classification in the lettered column.

1. _____ Used to treat hyperthyroidism by interfering with synthesis of thyroid hormones (*984*)

2. _____ Concentrates in thyroid tissue for diagnostic scans (*984*)

3. _____ Used to treat hypothyroidism and thyroiditis (*984*)

4. _____ Reduces the size and vascularity of thyroid gland in hyperthyroidism (*984*)

5. _____ Promotes calcium absorption from digestive tract (*997*)

6. _____ Corrects calcium deficiency due to hypoparathyroidism (*997*)

7. _____ Inhibits bone resorption and reduces serum calcium (*997*)

8. _____ Increases the metabolic rate (*984*)

A. Thyroid hormone replacement drugs
B. Antithyroid drugs
C. Iodides
D. Radioactive iodine
E. Calcium salts
F. Vitamin D
G. Biphosphonates

L. **Hypoparathyroidism.** Which are manifestations of hyperparathyroidism? Select all that apply. (*995*)

1. _____ Cramps
2. _____ Poor muscle tone
3. _____ Bone pain
4. _____ Demineralization
5. _____ Twitching
6. _____ Fractures

**M. Nursing Diagnoses.** Match the nursing diagnoses in the numbered column with the disorder in the lettered column.

1. _____ Hyperthermia related to increased metabolic energy production *(985)*

2. _____ Ineffective airway clearance related to laryngeal spasm *(986)*

3. _____ Risk for impaired skin integrity related to dryness and edema *(990)*

4. _____ Risk for injury related to hypocalcemia *(998)*

5. _____ Risk for injury related to weakness and decreased bone mass *(996)*

6. _____ Decreased cardiac output related to blood loss *(986)*

7. _____ Risk for injury related to exophthalmos *(985)*

8. _____ Hypothermia related to cold intolerance *(990)*

9. _____ Impaired urinary elimination related to urinary calculi *(996)*

10. _____ Decreased cardiac output related to dysrhythmias and heart failure secondary to hypocalcemia *(998)*

11. _____ Decreased cardiac output related to excessive thyroid hormone stimulation *(985)*

A. Hyperthyroidism
B. Hypothyroidism
C. Thyroidectomy
D. Hyperparathyroidism
E. Hypoparathyroidism

**N. Neck, Thyroid, and Parathyroid glands.** Referring to Figure 45-7 (p. 994) below, fill in the spaces with the correct letters. *(994)*

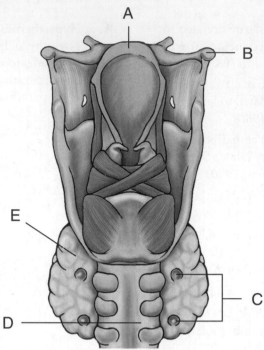

1. _____ Parathyroid glands

2. _____ Epiglottis

3. _____ Thyroid gland (posterior surface)

4. _____ Hyoid bone

5. _____ Trachea

## MULTIPLE-CHOICE QUESTIONS

**O.** Choose the most appropriate answer.

1. Which is secreted when serum calcium levels are high to limit the shift of calcium from the bones into the blood? *(996)*
   1. Calcitonin
   2. Thyroxine
   3. Thymine
   4. Phosphorus

2. Hyperthyroid patients often experience sleep disturbances and: *(982)*
   1. sedation.
   2. bradycardia.
   3. restlessness.
   4. hypotension.

3. Poor tolerance of heat and excessive perspiration are symptoms of: *(982)*
   1. hyperparathyroidism.
   2. hypoparathyroidism.
   3. hyperthyroidism.
   4. hypothyroidism.

4. If untreated, hyperthyroidism may lead to: *(982)*
   1. thyrotoxicosis (thyroid storm).
   2. hypotension.
   3. bradycardia.
   4. decreased metabolism.

5. Signs of iodine toxicity include: *(983)*
   1. bradycardia and hypotension.
   2. urinary retention and oliguria.
   3. esophageal ulcers and pyloric sphincter spasms.
   4. swelling and irritation of mucous membranes and increased salivation.

6. Elevated thyroid hormones result in: *(982)*
   1. decreased pulse and blood pressure.
   2. increased pulse and blood pressure.
   3. decreased temperature and infection.
   4. increased temperature and infection.

7. An important nursing diagnosis for the patient with exophthalmos is: *(986)*
   1. Risk for infection.
   2. Knowledge deficit (of disease process).
   3. Decreased cardiac output.
   4. Disturbed body image.

8. A complication of thyroidectomies includes injury to the parathyroid glands, which results in: *(987)*
   1. bradycardia.
   2. cyanosis.
   3. tetany.
   4. headache.

9. Results of two tests that are indicative of hypocalcemia are: *(987)*
   1. positive Chvostek's and Trousseau's signs.
   2. increased blood urea nitrogen and potassium levels.
   3. increased WBC and decreased RBC levels.
   4. increased phosphorus and decreased iodine levels.

10. An early symptom of tetany is: *(987)*
    1. flank pain with hematuria.
    2. difficulty breathing.
    3. a tingling sensation around the mouth, fingers, and toes.
    4. muscle cramps in leg and arm muscles.

11. Graves' disease (toxic diffuse goiter) is characterized by: *(988)*
    1. increased secretion of thyroid hormones.
    2. a decreased metabolic rate.
    3. intolerance to cold.
    4. constipation.

12. Which drug stains the teeth and should be sipped through a straw? *(983)*
    1. Iron
    2. Saturated solution of potassium iodide (SSKI)
    3. Levothyroxine (Synthroid)
    4. Propylthiouracil

13. In patients with toxic diffuse goiter, there is a risk for injury related to: *(985)*
    1. increased metabolic energy production.
    2. exophthalmos.
    3. increased thyroid hormone stimulation.
    4. intolerance to heat.

14. Lack of iodine is associated with: *(993)*
    1. goiter.
    2. hypoparathyroidism.
    3. tetany.
    4. thyrotoxicosis.

15. Thyroxine (T4), triiodothyronine (T3), and calcitonin are hormones produced by the: *(979)*
    1. adrenal gland.
    2. thymus gland.
    3. thyroid gland.
    4. parathyroid gland.

16. Which drug is used to treat hypothyroidism? *(989)*
    1. SSKI
    2. Synthroid
    3. methimazole (Tapazole)
    4. Lugol's solution

P. **Nursing Care Plan.** Refer to Nursing Care Plan, The Patient with Hypothyroidism, p. 992 in the textbook.

1. What is the priority nursing diagnosis for this patient? *(992)*

2. What are data collected for this patient that indicate the presence of hypothyroidism? *(992)*

3. What tasks can be assigned to unlicensed assistive personnel? *(992)*

# Diabetes Mellitus and Hypoglycemia

---

## OBJECTIVES

1.  Describe the role of insulin in the body.

2.  Explain the pathophysiology of diabetes mellitus and hypoglycemia.

3.  Describe the signs and symptoms of diabetes mellitus and hypoglycemia.

4.  Explain tests and procedures used to diagnose diabetes mellitus and hypoglycemia.

5.  Discuss treatment of diabetes mellitus and hypoglycemia.

6.  Explain the difference between type 1 and type 2 diabetes mellitus.

7.  Differentiate between acute hypoglycemia and diabetic ketoacidosis.

8.  Describe the treatment of a patient experiencing acute hypoglycemia or diabetic ketoacidosis.

9.  Describe the complications of diabetes mellitus.

10. Identify nursing interventions for a patient diagnosed with diabetes mellitus or hypoglycemia.

11. Identify nursing interventions for a patient diagnosed with ketoacidosis.

---

## LEARNING ACTIVITIES

A.  **Key Terms.** Complete the statement in the numbered column with the most appropriate term in the lettered column. Some terms may be used more than once, and some terms may not be used.

1.  An inadequate amount of insulin to meet daily requirements characterizes _____. *(1002)*

2.  Insulin is released in the body in response to the ingestion of _____. *(1002)*

3.  The absence of endogenous insulin characterizes _____. *(1002)*

4.  When insulin is absent, the blood becomes thick with glucose, causing the patient to experience _____. *(1002)*

5.  Tissue breakdown and burning of lean body mass send hunger signals to the hypothalamus; consequently, the patient experiences _____. *(1002)*

6.  The hormone that stimulates the active transport of glucose into the cells of muscle and adipose tissue is _____. *(1002)*

7.  A precursor to diabetes mellitus is thought to be _____. *(1003)*

A.  Weight loss
B.  Insulin
C.  Type 1 diabetes mellitus
D.  Type 2 diabetes mellitus
E.  Glycogen
F.  Polydipsia
G.  Carbohydrates
H.  Polyphagia
I.  Metabolic syndrome (insulin resistance syndrome)

**B. Complications.** Match the description in the numbered column with the complication in the lettered column. Answers may be used more than once.

1. _____ Life-threatening emergency caused by a relative or absolute deficiency of insulin *(1006)*

2. _____ Complication in which signs and symptoms are classified as adrenergic and neuroglucopenic *(1006)*

3. _____ Complication caused by rough shoe linings, burns, or chemical irritation *(1005)*

4. _____ Symptoms range from tingling, numbness, and burning to complete loss of sensation caused by sensory and autonomic nerve impairment *(1005)*

5. _____ Glycosuria, along with hypertension, gradually destroy the capillaries that supply the renal glomeruli *(1004)*

6. _____ Characterized by macular edema *(1004)*

7. _____ Dangerous drop in blood glucose caused by taking too much insulin, not eating enough food or not eating at the right time *(1006)*

8. _____ Results from inadequate blood supply and is experienced as sharp, stabbing pain in muscles *(1005)*

9. _____ Patient goes into a coma from extremely high glucose levels with no evidence of elevated ketones *(1006)*

10. _____ Nerve tissue involvement affects the sympathetic and parasympathetic nervous systems *(1005)*

A. Retinopathy
B. Nephropathy
C. Mononeuropathy
D. Polyneuropathy
E. Autonomic neuropathy
F. Neuropathic foot ulcers
G. Acute hypoglycemia
H. Diabetic ketoacidosis (DKA)
I. Hyperglycemic hyperosmolar nonketotic syndrome (HHNKS)

**C. Complications of Diabetes.** Complete the statement in the numbered column with the most appropriate term in the lettered column. Some terms may be used more than once, and some terms may not be used. *(1004)*

1. Diabetes is the leading cause of _____.

2. With diabetic retinopathy, the vitreous humor becomes cloudy and vision is lost as a result of _____.

3. A symptom of eye problems for patients with diabetes is the presence of spots, which are called _____.

4. People with diabetes account for a large percentage of patients with renal disease, which is called _____.

5. Elevated insulin levels circulating in the blood of patients with diabetes contribute to the premature development of _____.

A. "Floaters"
B. Neuropathy
C. Polyuria
D. Hemorrhage
E. Atherosclerosis
F. Capillary permeability
G. "Cobwebs"
H. Nephropathy
I. End-stage renal disease (ESRD)

**D. Ketoacidosis.** Complete the statement in the numbered column with the most appropriate term in the lettered column. Some terms may be used more than once, and some terms may not be used. *(1007)*

1. Treatment of ketoacidosis is aimed at correction of three main problems, which are acidosis, dehydration, and _____.

2. The patient with ketoacidosis may have lost a large volume of fluid as the result of vomiting, hyperventilation, and _____.

3. Replacement of potassium is vital in patients with ketoacidosis because hypokalemia can lead to severe _____.

4. A life-threatening emergency caused by lack of insulin or inadequate amounts of insulin is called diabetic _____.

5. Air hunger, seen in patients with ketoacidosis, is observed as _____.

6. The movement of potassium from the extracellular compartment into the cells is enhanced by _____.

7. Ketoacidosis results in disorders in the metabolism of carbohydrates, fats, and _____.

8. The electrolyte of primary concern in ketoacidosis is _____.

A. Glucose
B. Ketoacidosis
C. Insulin
D. Electrolyte imbalance
E. Potassium
F. Cardiac dysrhythmias
G. Kussmaul respirations
H. Protein
I. Sodium
J. Polyuria

E. **Insulin.** Indicate for each of the following actions or conditions whether insulin (A) increases or (B) decreases it.

1. _____ Rate of metabolism of carbohydrates *(1002)*
2. _____ Conversion of glucose to glycogen *(1002)*
3. _____ Conversion of glycogen to glucose *(1002)*
4. _____ Fatty acid synthesis and conversion of fatty acids into fat *(1002)*
5. _____ Breakdown of adipose tissue *(1002)*
6. _____ Rate of glucose utilization *(1002)*
7. _____ Mobilization of fat *(1002)*
8. _____ Conversion of fats to glucose *(1002)*
9. _____ Protein synthesis in tissue *(1003)*
10. _____ Conversion of protein into glucose *(1003)*

F. **Insulin.** Which organs of the body do not depend on insulin for the transport of glucose into them? Select all that apply. *(1002)*

1. _____ Kidneys
2. _____ Brain and nerve cells
3. _____ Lens of the eye
4. _____ Lungs
5. _____ Heart
6. _____ Exercising muscles

G. **Risk Factors.** Which are risk factors for type 2 diabetes mellitus? Select all that apply. *(1003)*

1. _____ People who are overweight
2. _____ Family history of diabetes
3. _____ People under the age of 40
4. _____ Latin American/Hispanic
5. _____ Asian
6. _____ African-American
7. _____ Native American

H. **Foot Problems.** Which are causes of foot problems in the person with diabetes? Select all that apply. *(1005)*

1. _____ Impaired hormone supply
2. _____ Impaired blood supply
3. _____ Impaired nerve supply

I. **Foot Complications.** Explain why the patient with diabetes may have an ulcer or necrotic area in the foot and may be unaware of the problem. *(1005-1006)*

**J.   Foot Complications.** List changes that occur in the three items below when the foot's nerve supply is impaired and when the foot's blood supply is impaired. *(1005)*

|  | Impaired Nerve Supply | Impaired Blood Supply |
|---|---|---|
| 1.  Color and temperature |  |  |
| 2.  Pulses |  |  |
| 3.  Sensation |  |  |

**K.   Ketoacidosis.** Which situations put the patient with diabetes at risk for ketoacidosis? Select all that apply. *(1007)*

1. _____     When patient eats too much food and does not take enough insulin
2. _____     When the patient does not get enough exercise
3. _____     When the patient experiences stress such as infection or surgery
4. _____     When diabetes mellitus has not been diagnosed

**L.   HHNKS.** Which statements explain why patients receiving total parenteral nutrition or dialysis are likely to have hyperosmolar nonketotic coma? Select all that apply. *(1008)*

1. _____     IV solutions containing large amounts of glucose are administered to the patient.
2. _____     The digestive system is bypassed.
3. _____     There is no stimulus to trigger the pancreas to release insulin.
4. _____     Patients can go into a coma from extremely low glucose levels.

**M.   Insulin Administration.**

1.   What are areas of injection sites for insulin? Select all that apply. *(1014)*

   1. _____     Buttocks
   2. _____     Upper arm
   3. _____     Abdomen
   4. _____     Thighs

2.   Which statements are true regarding the administration of insulin? Select all that apply. *(1014)*

   1. _____     It is best to rotate sites from one area of the body to another.
   2. _____     The site with the fastest absorption rate is the abdomen.
   3. _____     Exercise decreases the absorption rate of insulin.
   4. _____     Heat and massage increase the absorption rate

N.  **Serum Glucose Levels.** Indicate whether (A) too much or (B) not enough of the following factors causes serum glucose levels to drop. *(1017)*

1. _____  Insulin

2. _____  Food

3. _____  Exercise

O.  **Hypoglygemia.** Which are initial signs and symptoms of hypoglycemia? Select all that apply. *(1023)*

1. _____  Blurred vision

2. _____  Slurred speech

3. _____  Shakiness

4. _____  Nervousness

5. _____  Bradycardia

6. _____  Anxiety

7. _____  Lightheadedness

8. _____  Hunger

9. _____  Drowsiness

10. _____  Tingling or numbness of the lips or tongue

11. _____  Diaphoresis

12. _____  Disorientation

P.  **Diagnostic Tests.** Match the description in the numbered column with the diagnostic test in the lettered column.

1. _____  A reading greater than 200 mg/dL indicates a diagnosis of diabetes mellitus. *(1017)*

    A.  Serum glucose levels

    B.  Oral glucose tolerance test (OGTT)

    C.  Glycosylated hemoglobin (HbA1C) levels

2. _____  Reflects glucose levels over the past few months. *(1017)*

3. _____  Blood is drawn at 30 minutes and 1 hour after the ingestion of glucose and then hourly for 3 to 5 hours when patient is suspected of having DM. *(1009)*

**Q. Insulin.** Match the description in the numbered column with the drug in the lettered column. Refer to Drug Therapy Table, p. 1013 in the textbook. *(1013)*

1. _____   Category that includes NPH and Lente insulin

2. _____   Category that includes Ultralente and insulin glargine (Lantus)

3. _____   Category that includes Exubera (insulin human rDNA origin)

4. _____   Category that includes Humalog and NovoLog

5. _____   Category that includes Regular insulin

6. _____   Onset occurs in less than 15 minutes

7. _____   The peak occurs in 2–3 hours

8. _____   The peak occurs in 30–90 minutes

9. _____   Duration is 20–36 hours

10. _____   The onset is 30 minutes– 1 hour

11. _____   Can be given IV

A.   Rapid-acting
B.   Short-acting
C.   Intermediate-acting
D.   Long-acting
E.   Inhaled rapid short-acting

**R. Insulin.**

1.   Which insulins are clear in appearance? *(1011)*

2.   Why can insulin not be given orally? *(1012)*

**S. Drug Therapy.** Refer to Drug Therapy Table in the textbook, Oral Hypoglycemics for Type 2 Diabetes, p. 1016 in the textbook. Match the descriptions in the numbered column with the drug in the lettered column. Answers may be used more than once.

1. _____ Drugs in this category include Actos and Avandia *(1016)*

2. _____ Drugs in this category include glipizide (Glucotrol) and glyburide (Diabeta) *(1015)*

3. _____ The main drug in this category is metformin (Glucophage) *(1016)*

4. _____ Drugs in this category include acarbose and miglitol *(1015)*

5. _____ Drugs in this category include Prandin and Starlix *(1015)*

6. _____ Two categories that stimulate pancreatic secretion of insulin *(1015, 1016)*

7. _____ Action is to delay absorption of carbohydrates in the intestine *(1015)*

8. _____ Action is to inhibit hepatic glucose production and increase insulin sensitivity *(1016)*

9. _____ Action is to increase sensitivity in the tissues *(1015)*

A. Sulfonylureas (three generations)
B. Biguanides
C. Meglitinides/D-phenylalanines
D. Thiazolinediones
E. Alpha-glucosidase inhibitors

**T. Hypoglycemia.** Refer to Table 46-1, p. 1027 in the textbook.

1. Which are exogenous causes of hypoglycemia? Select all that apply. *(1027)*
   1. _____ Tumors
   2. _____ Insulin
   3. _____ Alcohol
   4. _____ Exercise
   5. _____ Severe liver deficiency
   6. _____ Oral hypoglycemic drugs

2. What is the most frequent cause of hypoglycemia? *(1017)*
   1. Liver deficiency
   2. Alcohol
   3. Oral hypoglycemic agents
   4. Insulin

## MULTIPLE-CHOICE QUESTIONS

**U.** Choose the most appropriate answer.

1. Which of the following inhibits the conversion of glycogen to glucose? *(1002)*
   1. Fatty acids
   2. Insulin
   3. Triglycerides
   4. Ketones

2. Which herbal supplement can lower blood glucose? *(1007)*
   1. Ginseng
   2. Ginkgo
   3. Kava kava
   4. Ephedra

3. The diagnosis of diabetes is based on serum: *(1008)*
   1. amylase levels.
   2. red blood cell count.
   3. hemoglobin.
   4. serum glucose levels.

4. Which of the following represents normal fasting serum glucose levels? *(1008)*
   1. 30–50 mg/dL
   2. 70–120 mg/dL
   3. 150–200 mg/dL
   4. 205–300 mg/dL

5. The American Diabetes Association recommends that 60–70% of the total daily calories should come from: *(1010)*
   1. protein.
   2. saturated fats.
   3. carbohydrates and monounsaturated fats.
   4. polyunsaturated fats.

6. The most commonly used insulin concentration is: *(1012)*
   1. U-40.
   2. U-80.
   3. U-100.
   4. U-500.

7. The prescription for insulin, including schedule for dosages, type, and amount, is written to mimic the action of a normal: *(1012)*
   1. stomach.
   2. liver.
   3. gallbladder.
   4. pancreas.

8. Regular insulin should be given: *(1013)*
   1. at bedtime.
   2. before meals.
   3. during meals.
   4. after meals.

9. Which injection site has the fastest rate of absorption for insulin? *(1013)*
   1. Upper arm
   2. Upper buttocks
   3. Abdomen
   4. Thighs

10. The two oral sulfonylurea hypoglycemic agents that are recommended for older patients are glipizide (Glucotrol) and: *(1015)*
    1. chlorpropamide (Diabinese).
    2. glyburide (DiaBeta, Micronase).
    3. tolbutamide (Orinase).
    4. acetohexamide (Dymelor).

11. When mixing Regular and longer-acting insulins, which should be drawn into the syringe first? *(1014)*
    1. Regular insulin
    2. Protamine zinc insulin
    3. Ultralente U insulin
    4. Lente L insulin

12. A reason for avoiding long-acting oral sulfonylurea hypoglycemic agents in older patients is that decreased renal function in older adults makes them more prone to: *(1015)*
    1. hyponatremia.
    2. hypernatremia.
    3. hypoglycemia.
    4. hyperglycemia.

13. Which is a side effect of sulfonylureas used in the treatment of diabetes mellitus? *(1015)*
    1. Hyperglycemia
    2. Hypoglycemia
    3. Hyperkalemia
    4. Hypokalemia

14. Patients who require insulin injections need to self-monitor levels of: *(1017)*
    1. serum cholesterol.
    2. red blood cells.
    3. amylase.
    4. blood glucose.

15. Late signs of hypoglycemia include: *(1023)*
    1. palpitations and dyspnea.
    2. oliguria and hypotension.
    3. peripheral edema and tachypnea.
    4. confusion and unconsciousness.

16. To detect possible changes in the eyes associated with diabetes mellitus, the nurse inquires whether the patient has had floaters, blurred vision, or: *(1020)*
    1. hemorrhage.
    2. infection.
    3. diplopia.
    4. conjunctivitis.

17. During the physical assessment of the diabetic patient, the nurse inspects the feet carefully for lesions, discoloration, and: *(1020)*
    1. edema.
    2. ability to dorsiflex.
    3. ability to evert.
    4. dehydration.

18. A nursing diagnosis for patients with diabetes is chronic pain related to: *(1019)*
    1. abnormal blood glucose levels.
    2. adverse effects of drugs.
    3. neuropathy.
    4. alterations in urine output.

19. Patients with diabetes may have disturbed sensory perception related to: *(1019)*
    1. dietary restrictions.
    2. anxiety and fear.
    3. imbalance between food intake and activity expenditure.
    4. neurologic and circulatory changes.

20. Alterations in tactile sensations in diabetic patients may result in: *(1022)*
    1. burns or frostbite.
    2. floaters or diplopia.
    3. altered urine output or oliguria.
    4. abnormal blood glucose levels.

21. Disturbed thought processes in diabetic patients, including confusion, anger, and decreased level of consciousness, may be due to: *(1022)*
    1. neuropathy.
    2. nephropathy.
    3. ketoacidosis.
    4. hyperglycemia.

22. Hypoglycemia is defined as a syndrome that develops when the blood glucose level falls to less than: *(1023)*
    1. 10–15 mg/dL.
    2. 45–50 mg/dL.
    3. 80–120 mg/dL.
    4. 200–300 mg/dL.

23. Endogenous hypoglycemia occurs when internal factors cause an excessive secretion of insulin or an increase in the metabolism of: *(1023)*
    1. protein.
    2. fats.
    3. calcium.
    4. glucose.

24. When blood glucose levels fall rapidly, the four substances that are secreted by the body in an attempt to increase glucose levels are cortisol, glucagon, growth hormone, and: *(1023)*
    1. antidiuretic hormone.
    2. epinephrine.
    3. aldosterone.
    4. thyroxine.

25. Early signs of hypoglycemia include: *(1023)*
    1. bradycardia and edema.
    2. oliguria and constipation.
    3. infection and red skin.
    4. weakness and hunger.

26. Which group of oral antidiabetic agents does not cause hypoglycemia as a side effect? *(1015)*
    1. Biguanides (metformin)
    2. Alpha-glucosidase inhibitors (Precose)
    3. Sulfonylureas
    4. Thiazolidinediones (Avandia)

27. Patients with hypoglycemia are at risk for injury related to: *(1025)*
    1. oliguria and nephropathy.
    2. polydipsia and polyphagia.
    3. dizziness and weakness.
    4. retinopathy and hypotension.

28. Hyperosmolar nonketotic coma is loss of consciousness caused by extremely high serum: *(1008)*
    1. ketones.
    2. glucose.
    3. calcium.
    4. potassium.

29. When a patient is given insulin for diabetic ketoacidosis, the nurse should monitor the patient for: *(1008)*
    1. hyperglycemia.
    2. hypoglycemia.
    3. hypokalemia.
    4. thrombocytopenia.

30. When a patient's serum glucose is 260 mg/dL and ketoacidosis is present, the patient should: *(1011)*
    1. administer glucagon.
    2. drink 8 ounces of skim milk.
    3. drink 4 ounces of concentrated orange juice.
    4. avoid exercise.

31. Your patient has taken NPH insulin at 8:00 am. At what time of day should he avoid exercise in order to prevent hypoglycemia? *(1013)*
    1. 9:00 AM
    2. 10:00 AM
    3. 12:00 PM
    4. 4:00 PM

32. Which type of insulin is a clear solution? *(1011)*
    1. Ultralente
    2. NPH insulin
    3. Lente insulin
    4. Insulin glargine (Lantus)

33. The goal of the diabetic diet is to: *(1009)*
    1. limit carbohydrate intake.
    2. increase protein intake.
    3. limit total calorie intake.
    4. normalize plasma glucose levels.

V. **Nursing Care Plan.** Refer to Nursing Care Plan, The Patient with Type 1 Diabetes Mellitus, on p. 1024 in the textbook.

1. What is the priority nursing diagnosis for this patient? *(1024)*

2. What data collected in the health history and physical examination indicate the presence of type I DM? *(1024)*

W. **Nursing Care Plan.** Refer to Nursing Care Plan, The Patient with Type 2 Diabetes Mellitus, on p. 1026 in the textbook.

1. What is the priority diagnosis for this patient? *(1026)*

2. What data collected in the health history and physical examination are related to the presence of type 2 DM? *(1026)*

# CHAPTER 47

# Female Reproductive Disorders

---

## OBJECTIVES

1. List data to be collected when assessing the female reproductive system.

2. Describe the nursing interventions for women who are undergoing diagnostic tests and procedures for reproductive system disorders.

3. Identify the nursing interventions associated with douche, cauterization, heat therapy, and topical medications used to treat disorders of the female reproductive system.

4. Explain the pathophysiology, signs and symptoms, complications, diagnostic procedures, and medical or surgical treatment for selected disorders of the female reproductive system.

5. Assist in developing a nursing care plan for the patient with common disorders of the female reproductive system.

6. Describe the nursing interventions for the patient who is menopausal.

---

## LEARNING ACTIVITIES

A. **Key Terms.** Match the definition in the numbered column with the most appropriate term in the lettered column.

1. _____ Surgical excision of a fallopian tube and ovary *(1053)*

2. _____ Difficult or painful sexual intercourse in women *(1050)*

3. _____ A condition in which endometrial tissue is located, abnormally, outside the uterus *(1052)*

4. _____ Inflammation of breast tissue *(1048)*

5. _____ Menstrual periods characterized by profuse or prolonged bleeding *(1044)*

6. _____ Herniation of the urinary bladder into the vagina *(1058)*

7. _____ Bleeding or spotting between menstrual periods *(1044)*

8. _____ Surgical removal of the uterus *(1053)*

9. _____ Abnormal cells *(1035)*

10. _____ Cessation of menstruation *(1033)*

11. _____ Herniation of part of the rectum into the vagina *(1058)*

12. _____ Age at which the first menstrual period occurs *(1032)*

13. _____ Painful menstruation *(1053)*

A. Cystocele
B. Menopause
C. Dysmenorrhea
D. Endometriosis
E. Menorrhagia
F. Metrorrhagia
G. Rectocele
H. Dyspareunia
I. Hysterectomy
J. Dysplasia
K. Mastitis
L. Menarche
M. Salpingo-oophorectomy

B. **Diagnostic Procedures.** Match the definition or description in the numbered column with the most appropriate term in the lettered column. Some terms may be used more than once, and some terms may not be used. *(1040)*

1. _____ A type of invasive surgery procedure in which a large amount of cervical tissue is removed to treat cancer

2. _____ An invasive surgical procedure that provides direct visualization of the female pelvic cavity

3. _____ A test for which specimens are collected routinely to detect cervical cancer and dysplasia

4. _____ A procedure that is commonly done before cervical biopsies

5. _____ A type of biopsy done in a physician's office or an outpatient clinic to diagnose cervical cancer

6. _____ Specimens collected to identify infections

7. _____ The procedure that is done to identify ectopic pregnancy or pelvic masses

8. _____ A test performed to diagnose uterine cancer

9. _____ A procedure in which an instrument is used to inspect the cervix under magnification and to identify abnormal and potentially cancerous tissue

10. _____ Deliberate tissue destruction by means of heat, electricity, or chemicals

11. _____ Visualization of abdominal organs in order to perform tubal ligation

A.   Multiple-punch biopsy
B.   Papanicolaou (Pap) smear
C.   Dilation and curettage
D.   Culture and smear
E.   Cone biopsy
F.   Aspiration biopsy
G.   Endometrial biopsy
H.   Culdoscopy
I.   Breast biopsy
J.   Colposcopy
K.   Laparoscopy
L.   Cauterization

**C. Uterine Displacement.** Match the definition or description in the numbered column with the most appropriate term in the lettered column. Some terms may be used more than once, and some terms may not be used. *(1061)*

1. _____ The body of the uterus bends backward on itself

2. _____ A forward tilt of the uterus at a sharp angle to the vagina

3. _____ The uterus bends forward on itself

4. _____ A backward tilt of the uterus with the cervix pointed downward toward the anterior vaginal wall

A. Anteflexion
B. Introversion
C. Retroversion
D. Retroflexion
E. Extraversion
F. Anteversion

**D. Mastectomy.** Complete the statement in the numbered column with the most appropriate term in the lettered column. Some terms may be used more than once, and some terms may not be used.

1. Mastectomy patients are at risk for injury related to _____. *(1066)*

2. The removal of the tumor with a margin of surrounding healthy tissue but preserving most of the breast is called _____. *(1063)*

3. A low-incidence cancer of the nipple and areola is _____. *(1063)*

4. The implantation of a tissue expander injected with saline is a type of _____ *(1064)*

5. The removal of all breast tissue, overlying skin, axillary lymph nodes, and underlying pectoral muscles is called _____. *(1063)*

6. If breast cancer cells removed during surgery need estrogen for cell replication, they are said to be _____. *(1063)*

7. Removal of the entire breast is called _____. *(1063)*

A. Paget's disease
B. ER-negative
C. Radical mastectomy
D. Simple mastectomy
E. Silicone implant
F. ER-positive
G. Lymphedema
H. Breast reconstruction
I. Lumpectomy

**E. Menstruation.** Match the term in the numbered column with the most appropriate numerical range in the lettered column. (These terms refer to the variations within normal menstrual periods.) Some ranges may be used more than once, and some ranges may not be used. *(1031)*

1. _____ Length of cycle (days)

2. _____ Duration of menstruation (days)

3. _____ Amount of blood loss (mL)

A. 2–8
B. 10–14
C. 21–40
D. 40–100
E. 150–200

F. **Sexually Transmitted Infection.** Match the description in the numbered column with the most appropriate term in the lettered column. Some terms may be used more than once, and some terms may not be used.

1. _____ Often seen with diabetes *(1045)*

2. _____ A sexually transmitted infection that is the primary cause of ectopic pregnancy and infertility *(1050)*

3. _____ Includes profuse, frothy, and yellow-gray discharge *(1045)*

4. _____ Includes cottage cheese-like discharge *(1045)*

5. _____ Protozoal infection *(1045)*

6. _____ Fungal infection *(1045)*

7. _____ Infection often caused by disruption of the normal vaginal flora *(1045)*

8. _____ A sexually transmitted infection that causes most pelvic inflammatory disease *(1050)*

9. _____ Associated with mastitis *(1048)*

A. *Trichomonas vaginalis*
B. *Chlamydia trachomatis*
C. *Neisseria gonorrheae*
D. *Candida albicans*
E. *Staphylococcus aureus*

**G.  Uterine Prolapse.** Match the definition or description in the numbered column with the most appropriate term in the lettered column. Some terms may be used more than once, and some terms may not be used. *(1059-1060)*

1.  _____   Level of prolapse if the cervix protrudes from the vaginal opening

2.  _____   A vaginal disorder caused by weakness of supportive structures between the vagina and bladder

3.  _____   Level of prolapse if the vagina is inverted and both the cervix and the body of the uterus protrude from the vaginal opening

4.  _____   Method used to diagnose first-degree uterine prolapse

5.  _____   Nonsurgical treatment of uterine prolapse that is aimed at elevating the uterus

6.  _____   A vaginal disorder caused by weakness of supportive structures between the vagina and rectum

7.  _____   A condition in which the uterus descends into the vagina from its usual position in the pelvis

8.  _____   Method used to diagnose second- and third-degree uterine prolapse

9.  _____   Level of prolapse if the cervix is above the vaginal opening

A.  Pessary
B.  Third-degree
C.  Visual inspection
D.  First-degree
E.  Rectocele
F.  Uterine prolapse
G.  Second-degree
H.  Fourth-degree
I.  Cystocele
J.  Laparoscopy
K.  Pelvic examination

**H. Cystocele/Rectocele.** Match the nursing diagnosis for patients with cystocele and rectocele in the numbered column with the appropriate nursing intervention in the lettered column. Some interventions may be used more than once. *(1058)*

1. _____ Stress incontinence
2. _____ Constipation
3. _____ Risk for infection
4. _____ Acute pain

A. Initial application of cold to reduce pain and swelling
B. Teaching the patient Kegel exercises
C. Emphasizing the need for a high-fiber diet
D. Sitz baths and heat lamps
E. Instructing the patient to report signs of urinary frequency, burning, or foul odor
F. Use of indwelling or suprapubic catheter

**I. Hysterectomy.** Match the preoperative and postoperative nursing diagnoses in the numbered column for a patient with a hysterectomy with the appropriate nursing interventions in the lettered column. *(1056-1057)*

1. _____ Deficient knowledge of information or misinterpretation of effects of HRT
2. _____ Risk for fluid volume deficit related to postoperative bleeding
3. _____ Urinary retention related to surgical manipulation, local tissue edema, temporary sensory or motor impairment
4. _____ Self-esteem disturbance related to perceived potential changes in femininity, effect on sexual relationship
5. _____ Ineffective tissue perfusion related to reduction of cellular components necessary for delivery of oxygen, hypovolemia, reduction of blood flow, intraoperative trauma
6. _____ Constipation related to weakening of abdominal musculature, abdominal pain, decreased physical activity, dietary changes, environmental changes

A. Assist patient to bathroom or commode; use bedpan only if absolutely necessary
B. Instruct and assist with foot and leg exercises while the patient is confined to bed; encourage and assist with ambulation when allowed
C. Explain that positions for sexual intercourse should avoid pressure on the abdominal incision for as long as incisional tenderness persists
D. Check mucous membranes for moisture
E. Auscultate abdomen for bowel sounds
F. Explain that estrogen may increase fluid retention, which may make one "feel fat"

**J.  Drug Therapy.** Refer to Drug Therapy Table on pp. 1041-1043 in the textbook. Match the actions and uses of drugs in the numbered column with the drug used to treat disorders of the female reproductive system in the lettered column. Answers may be used more than once. *(1041-1043)*

1. _____   Enhances bone formation; depresses betalipoprotein and cholesterol plasma levels; used to replace natural hormones after menopause and to treat advanced breast cancer and prostate cancer

2. _____   Promotes secretory function in endometrium; influences contractile activity of the uterus; used with estrogens as oral contraceptives

3. _____   Inhibits production of pituitary gonadotropins; used to treat endometriosis and fibrocystic breast disease

4. _____   Initially increases and then decreases testosterone levels; used to treat endometriosis

5. _____   Suppresses ovulation to prevent pregnancy

6. _____   Prevents implantation of fertilized ovum; used as emergency postcoital contraceptive

7. _____   Stimulates ovarian follicular growth

8. _____   Treats uterine bleeding and endometriosis

9. _____   Used to treat breast cancer

10. _____  Used as fertility drugs

11. _____  Lupron is example

12. _____  Norplant is example

13. _____  Tamoxifen and Evista are examples

14. _____  Danazol (Danocrine) is example

15. _____  Ortho-Novum is example

16. _____  Clomid and Pergonal are examples

A.  Estrogen-progestin combinations
B.  Androgens
C.  Ovulatory stimulants
D.  Conjugated estrogens
E.  GnRH agonists
F.  Progestins
G.  Estrogen only
H.  Selective estrogen receptor modulators (SERMS)

K.  **Pelvic Exam.** Which are parts of the pelvic exam? Select all that apply. *(1034)*
1.  _____ Visual inspection of the kidneys
2.  _____ Visual inspection and palpation of the external genitalia
3.  _____ Visual inspection of the bladder and ureter
4.  _____ Visual inspection of the vagina and uterine cervix
5.  _____ Bimanual palpation of the vagina and abdomen

L.  **Menopause.** Which are signs and symptoms of menopause? Select all that apply. *(1074)*
1.  _____ Vaginal dryness
2.  _____ Drowsiness
3.  _____ Headache
4.  _____ Hot flashes
5.  _____ Depression

M.  **Breast Cancer.** Refer to Box 47-2 in the textbook. Which are established risk factors for breast cancer? Select all that apply. *(1062)*
1.  _____ Age: 40 or older
2.  _____ Age at menarche: 11 years or younger
3.  _____ Age at first childbirth: 30 years or older
4.  _____ Family history: grandmother, mother, aunt, sister, or daughter
5.  _____ BRCA1 or BRCA2 gene mutation

N.  **PID.** Which groups of women are especially prone to developing pelvic inflammatory disease not associated with sexually transmitted infections? Select all that apply. *(1050)*
1.  _____ Women in low socioeconomic groups
2.  _____ Women who are poorly nourished
3.  _____ Women with compromised resistance to infection

O.  **PID.** Which are signs and symptoms of pelvic inflammatory disease? Select all that apply. *(1050)*
1.  _____ Nausea and vomiting
2.  _____ Abdominal pain
3.  _____ Fever and chills
4.  _____ Hypotension
5.  _____ Dysuria
6.  _____ Irregular bleeding
7.  _____ Foul-smelling vaginal discharge
8.  _____ Dyspareunia

P.  **Endometriosis.** Which are common side effects of danazol, which may be given to patients with endometriosis? Select all that apply. *(1053)*
1.  _____ Irregular bleeding
2.  _____ Fever and chills
3.  _____ Voice deepening
4.  _____ Hirsutism
5.  _____ Clitoral enlargement
6.  _____ Vaginal atrophy and dryness
7.  _____ Thromboembolism

Q.  **Endometriosis.** Explain why oral contraceptives may be prescribed for patients with endometriosis. *(1053)*

R.  **Cystocele.** In addition to stress incontinence and incomplete bladder emptying, what are symptoms that women with cystoceles are likely to experience? Select all that apply. *(1058)*
1. _____   Dyspareunia
2. _____   Lower back and pelvic discomfort
3. _____   Irregular bleeding
4. _____   Recurrent bladder infections

S.  **Breast Cancer.** Which of the following influence a person's chance for getting breast cancer? Select all that apply. *(1062)*
1. _____   Female
2. _____   Increased chance if mother or aunt has had breast cancer
3. _____   Increases markedly from the age of 35 on
4. _____   Early menarche
5. _____   Late menopause
6. _____   Mutation of the BRCA genes

T.  **Mastectomy.** What are ways the nurse can intervene to prevent or minimize lymphedema in the patient with a mastectomy? Select all that apply. *(1066)*
1. _____   Keep affected arm below heart level
2. _____   Take blood pressure on the unaffected arm
3. _____   No venipuncture of IV fluid administration in the affected arm
4. _____   Deodorant may be applied in small amounts 3 days after surgery
5. _____   Exercise arm on affected side frequently

U.  **Ovarian Cancer.** What are ways ovarian cancer metastasizes? Select all that apply. *(1068)*
1. _____   Direct invasion
2. _____   Pleural fluid
3. _____   Lymphatic and venous systems
4. _____   Peritoneal fluid

V.  **Internal Radiation.** Internal radiation as a treatment for patients with ovarian cancer poses a nursing challenge. What are conditions related to internal radiation that make nursing interventions a challenge? Select all that apply. *(1070)*
1. _____   Radiation therapy may cause nausea, vomiting, and diarrhea.
2. _____   Movement of the patient is restricted.
3. _____   Total time for nursing care is restricted because nurses should not be exposed to radiation for more than 2 hours in a 24-hour period.

W. **Drug Therapy.** What types of medications may be prescribed for cancer patients receiving internal radiation to moderate radiation side effects and facilitate patient comfort? Select all that apply. *(1071)*

1. _____   Opioids
2. _____   Antiemetics
3. _____   Tranquilizers
4. _____   Diuretics
5. _____   Antidiarrheal medications

X. **Menopause.** How do the following structures change after menopause without estrogen present? Select all that apply. *(1074)*

1. _____   The uterus becomes enlarged.
2. _____   The vagina shortens.
3. _____   Vaginal tissues become drier.
4. _____   Breast tissue becomes more elastic.
5. _____   Pubic and axillary hair become sparse.
6. _____   Bone mass increases and becomes less flexible.
7. _____   Osteoporosis increases.

Y. **Drug Therapy.** Which are contraindications for estrogen replacement therapy? Select all that apply. *(1074)*

1. _____   Certain types of cancer (such as estrogen receptor breast cancer)
2. _____   Hot flashes
3. _____   Undiagnosed uterine bleeding
4. _____   Thromboembolism

Z. **Nursing Diagnoses.** Match the nursing diagnoses in the numbered column with the disorder in the lettered column. Answers may be used more than once.

1. _____ Altered sexuality patterns related to physical and emotional effects of cancer of the reproductive system *(1070)*

2. _____ Risk for injury related to trauma of the exposed uterus *(1060)*

3. _____ Acute pain related to inflammation *(1051)*

4. _____ Sexual dysfunction related to abnormal uterine position *(1060)*

5. _____ Risk for injury (to patient and others) related to effects of radiotherapy, chemotherapy *(1070)*

6. _____ Disturbed body image related to altered appearance, perceived loss of attractiveness *(1066)*

7. _____ Stress incontinence related to pelvic muscle weakness *(1058)*

8. _____ Risk for injury related to lymphedema secondary to excision of lymph nodes *(1060)*

9. _____ Situational low self-esteem related to inability to conceive or feeling of failure *(1073)*

10. _____ Risk for injury related to possible abscess formation *(1049)*

11. _____ Sexual dysfunction related to painful intercourse *(1058)*

12. _____ Impaired physical mobility of affected arm related to axillary lymph node dissection *(1066)*

A. Mastitis
B. PID
C. Cystocele and rectocele
D. Uterine prolapse
E. Postoperative mastectomy
F. Cancer of the cervix, ovaries, vulva, or vagina
G. Infertility

**AA. External Female Genitalia.** Using Figure 47-1 (p. 1031) below, label the external female genitalia (A–L) from the terms (1–12) below. *(1031)*

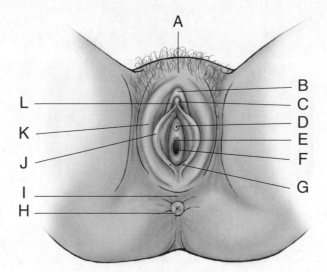

1. _____   Labia minora
2. _____   Hymen
3. _____   Labia majora
4. _____   Clitoris body
5. _____   Clitoris glans
6. _____   Mons pubis

7. _____   Vaginal orifice (introitus)
8. _____   Urethral meatus
9. _____   Perineum
10. _____   Prepuce
11. _____   Anus
12. _____   Bartholin's glands

**BB. Internal Female Genitalia.** Using Figure 47-2 (p. 1032) below, label the sites of endometriosis (A–L) from the terms provided (1–12) below. *(1032)*

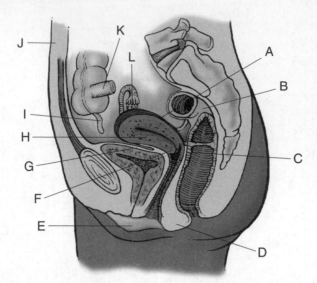

1. _____    Anterior cul-de-sac and bladder
2. _____    Ileum
3. _____    Ovary
4. _____    Cervix
5. _____    Perineum
6. _____    Vulva

7. _____    Posterior surface of uterus
8. _____    Umbilicus
9. _____    Pelvic colon
10. _____   Uterine wall
11. _____   Rectovaginal septum
12. _____   Appendix

## MULTIPLE-CHOICE QUESTIONS

**CC.** Choose the most appropriate answer.

1. The two main hormones produced by the ovaries are: *(1031)*
   1. estrogen and progesterone.
   2. testosterone and prolactin.
   3. thyroxine and oxytocin.
   4. follicle-stimulating hormone and luteinizing hormone.

2. When a patient comes to a clinic with a female reproductive system problem, the opening question the nurse should ask is: *(1032)*
   1. "What is wrong with you today?"
   2. "What is the problem that made you come in?"
   3. "Why did you come to the clinic today?"
   4. "What is the reason for your visit?"

3. The physical examination of women with reproductive system problems includes the assessment for the presence of Homans' sign in order to detect possible: *(1035)*
   1. vaginal infection.
   2. thrombophlebitis.
   3. abdominal distention.
   4. breast lumps.

4. In which position is the patient placed for a pelvic exam? *(1034)*
   1. Lithotomy
   2. Right side-lying
   3. Knee-chest
   4. Supine

5. Advise the patient that air entering the pelvic cavity during the culdoscopy procedure may cause pain in the: *(1037)*
   1. abdomen.
   2. heart.
   3. thigh.
   4. shoulder.

6. A method of deliberate tissue destruction through use of heat, electricity, or chemicals is called: *(1039)*
   1. culdoscopy.
   2. colposcopy.
   3. cauterization.
   4. dilation and curettage.

7. A particularly helpful type of heat application for small areas such as the vulva or perineum is: *(1040)*
   1. sitz baths.
   2. an electric heating pad.
   3. Aquathermia (K-pad).
   4. hot compresses.

8. Three signs for which the nurse must observe in patients taking sitz baths are severe pain, shock, and: *(1040)*
   1. dyspnea.
   2. faintness.
   3. dermatitis.
   4. headache.

9. Dilation of large pelvic vessels during sitz baths may cause: *(1040)*
   1. hypertension.
   2. hypotension.
   3. pneumonia.
   4. seizures.

10. Following the administration of vaginal suppositories, the patient is asked to remain in which position for at least 15 minutes to allow the medication to be absorbed? *(1040)*
    1. Prone
    2. Supine
    3. Sitting
    4. Right side-lying

11. Deviations from normal menstrual cycles are viewed as: *(1044)*
    1. uterine bleeding disorders.
    2. vaginal hemorrhage problems.
    3. endometrial cancers.
    4. pelvic inflammatory diseases.

12. The most common characteristics of vulvitis are inflammation and: *(1045)*
    1. bleeding.
    2. pruritus.
    3. cheese-like discharge.
    4. pain.

13. A significant discharge may be seen in: *(1045)*
    1. vulvitis.
    2. cystitis.
    3. vaginitis.
    4. pyelonephritis.

14. Signs and symptoms of vaginitis include local swelling, itching, and: *(1046)*
    1. redness.
    2. pus.
    3. hemorrhage.
    4. ulcers.

15. A potential complication of vulvitis and vaginitis is: *(1046)*
    1. hypotension.
    2. ascending infection.
    3. seizures.
    4. thrombophlebitis.

16. Bartholin's glands are vulnerable to a wide variety of infectious microorganisms due to their: *(1047)*
    1. size.
    2. location.
    3. structure.
    4. secretions.

17. When Bartholin's glands are infected, the resultant edema and pus formation occlude the duct and form: *(1047)*
    1. tumors.
    2. cysts.
    3. warts.
    4. abscesses.

18. The most noticeable symptom of bartholinitis, which causes patients to seek medical attention, is: *(1047)*
    1. edema.
    2. pain.
    3. discharge.
    4. itching.

19. The most serious complication of a Bartholin's gland abscess is: *(1047)*
    1. hypertension.
    2. dyspnea.
    3. systemic infection.
    4. kidney failure.

20. Conservative treatment of bartholinitis is sitz baths and oral: *(1048)*
    1. diuretics.
    2. anticholinergics.
    3. antispasmodics.
    4. analgesics.

21. Cervicitis related to menopause is treated by: *(1048)*
    1. estrogens.
    2. antiemetics.
    3. diuretics.
    4. analgesics.

22. The portal of entry for organisms that cause mastitis is the: *(1048)*
    1. areola.
    2. mammary gland.
    3. nipple.
    4. lactating duct.

23. The most serious complication of pelvic inflammatory disease is: *(1050)*
    1. peritonitis.
    2. pneumonia.
    3. hemorrhage.
    4. hypertension.

24. Treatment of pelvic inflammatory disease includes rest, application of heat, and administration of: *(1051)*
    1. antiemetics.
    2. antibiotics.
    3. diuretics.
    4. antispasmodics.

25. The major symptom of endometriosis is: *(1053)*
    1. hemorrhage.
    2. pain.
    3. fever.
    4. tachycardia.

26. Because the uterine endometrial tissue is bleeding simultaneously in endometriosis, pain appears as dysmenorrhea and may extend to a feeling of: *(1053)*
    1. stabbing pain.
    2. sudden weakness.
    3. difficulty breathing.
    4. pelvic heaviness.

27. Women who are given androgenic steroids for treatment of endometriosis often experience the common side effect of: *(1053)*
    1. masculinizing characteristics.
    2. palpitations.
    3. insomnia.
    4. diuresis.

28. Surgical management is commonly employed for patients with endometriosis and includes: *(1053)*
    1. colposcopy.
    2. culdoscopy.
    3. laparoscopy.
    4. dilation and curettage.

29. Severe and sudden abdominal pain may occur as a complication of follicular ovarian cysts due to: *(1054)*
    1. infection.
    2. rupture.
    3. muscle spasms.
    4. vaginitis.

30. The only procedure for making a definitive diagnosis of cancer from breast cysts is: *(1063)*
    1. surgical biopsy.
    2. mammography.
    3. palpation.
    4. ultrasound.

31. A serious complication of a very large fibroid tumor is that it may compress the urethra, obstructing urine flow and causing secondary: *(1055)*
    1. vaginitis.
    2. pelvic inflammatory disease.
    3. hydronephrosis.
    4. diuresis.

32. For women with fibroid tumors who desire to become pregnant, a procedure that can be done by laser surgery to remove only the tumor is: *(1055)*
    1. hysterectomy.
    2. myomectomy.
    3. dilation and curettage.
    4. culdoscopy.

33. Women at risk for developing rectoceles and cystoceles are those who have experienced a weakened pubococcygeal muscle due to: *(1058)*
    1. extended antibiotic treatment.
    2. repeated pregnancies.
    3. effects of herpes infection.
    4. poor nutrition.

34. A treatment of small cystoceles that is aimed at improving the tone of the pubococcygeal muscle is: *(1058)*
    1. pelvic floor (Kegel) exercises.
    2. surgical intervention (A and P repair).
    3. vaginal hysterectomy.
    4. increased fluid intake.

35. The most common surgical treatment for uterine prolapse is: *(1059)*
    1. vaginal hysterectomy.
    2. lithotripsy.
    3. culdoscopy.
    4. dilation and curettage.

36. Nearly one-half of all malignant breast tumors are located in the: *(1062)*
    1. nipple-areolar complex.
    2. lower outer quadrant.
    3. upper outer quadrant.
    4. lower inner quadrant.

37. Which of the following is an established risk factor for breast cancer? *(1062)*
    1. Age of first baby 24 years or older
    2. Age 12 years or older at menarche
    3. Radiation exposure
    4. Age over 50

38. It is recommended that yearly mammograms be done every year beginning at age: *(1063)*
    1. 35.
    2. 40.
    3. 50.
    4. 65.

39. A synthetic nonsteroidal antiestrogen that acts as an estrogen antagonist and blocks circulating estrogen from reaching the cancer receptor cells is: *(1063)*
    1. progesterone.
    2. tamoxifen.
    3. prednisone.
    4. doxorubicin (Adriamycin).

40. A common nursing diagnosis for mastectomy patients is: *(1066)*
    1. Disturbed sleep pattern.
    2. Decreased cardiac output.
    3. Functional incontinence.
    4. Disturbed body image.

41. An important aspect of postoperative care after mastectomy is directed toward the prevention and minimization of: *(1066)*
    1. lymphedema.
    2. hemorrhage.
    3. hypertension.
    4. nausea.

42. Most types of cervical cancer are associated with microbes such as human papillomavirus and herpes simplex virus; therefore, it is thought that cervical cancer is related to: *(1067)*
    1. high-fat diets.
    2. diabetes mellitus.
    3. sexually transmitted infections.
    4. multiple pregnancies.

43. The high mortality from ovarian cancer is due to the fact that: *(1068)*
    1. symptoms are multiple and serious.
    2. it is asymptomatic in early stages.
    3. abnormal cell growth occurs in one ovary.
    4. it is diagnosed around the time of menopause concurrent with ascites.

44. Diminished ovarian function associated with aging causes cessation of ovulation as well as decreased production of: *(1074)*
    1. thyroxine.
    2. estrogen.
    3. epinephrine.
    4. prolactin.

45. With natural menopause, the woman's first sign may be: *(1074)*
    1. increased temperature.
    2. loss of memory.
    3. menstrual irregularity.
    4. bone pain.

46. A women is said to be postmenopausal when she has not had a menstrual period for: *(1074)*
    1. 3 months.
    2. 1 year.
    3. 2 years.
    4. 5 years.

47. Some women experience surgical menopause, which occurs as a result of surgical removal of the: *(1074)*
    1. ovaries.
    2. uterus.
    3. vagina.
    4. cervix.

48. The type of drug therapy prescribed promptly for surgical menopause to decrease menopausal symptoms is: *(1074)*
    1. diuretics.
    2. steroids.
    3. estrogen.
    4. analgesics.

49. The symptom of hot flashes that may accompany menopause is due to: *(1074)*
    1. increased menstrual bleeding.
    2. vasodilation.
    3. abdominal cramps.
    4. increased body temperature.

50. Progesterone is added to estrogen replacement therapy in postmenopausal patients to decrease the risk of: *(1074)*
    1. breast cancer.
    2. hot flashes.
    3. endometrial cancer.
    4. insomnia.

51. The treatment of choice for large and symptomatic cystoceles and rectoceles is: *(1058)*
    1. hysterectomy.
    2. myomectomy.
    3. Kegel exercises.
    4. A and P repair.

52. The incidence of fibroid tumors is increased among women who are: *(1054)*
    1. African-American.
    2. Caucasian.
    3. Asian.
    4. Hispanic.

53. Recent findings from the Women's Health Initiative (2002) indicate that combination estrogen–progestin therapy increases the risk of breast cancer and: *(1074)*
    1. osteoporosis.
    2. endometriosis.
    3. coronary heart disease.
    4. amenorrhea.

**DD. Nursing Care Plan.** Refer to the Nursing Care Plan on pp. 1056-1057 of the textbook.

1. What is the priority postoperative nursing diagnosis for this patient? *(1056-1057)*

2. What are data collected from the health history and physical examination that indicate a need for hysterectomy? *(1056-1057)*

# Male Reproductive Disorders

---

## OBJECTIVES

1. Describe the major structures and functions of the normal male reproductive system.

2. Identify data to be collected when assessing a male patient with a reproductive system disorder.

3. Discuss commonly performed diagnostic tests and procedures and the nursing implications of each.

4. Identify common therapeutic measures used to treat disorders of the male reproductive system and the nursing implications of each.

5. For selected disorders of the male reproductive system, explain the pathophysiology, signs and symptoms, complications, medical diagnosis, and medical treatment.

6. Assist in developing a nursing care plan for a male patient with a reproductive system disorder.

---

## LEARNING ACTIVITIES

**A. Anatomy and Physiology.** Match the description or definition in the numbered column with the most appropriate term in the lettered column. Some terms may be used more than once, and some may not be used.

1. _____ Male reproductive organs *(1077)*

2. _____ Extends from the bladder to the urinary meatus at the end of the penis *(1078)*

3. _____ The production of sperm *(1079)*

4. _____ Produces alkaline liquid that enhances motility and fertility of sperm *(1078)*

5. _____ A hormone necessary for the development of male reproductive organs, descent of the testicles, and production of sperm *(1077)*

6. _____ Provides outflow for semen during ejaculation *(1078)*

7. _____ The condition when the testes are located outside a dependent scrotal position *(1079)*

8. _____ The surgical removal of a portion of the vas deferens *(1098)*

A. Testosterone
B. Cryptorchidism
C. Urethra
D. Prostate
E. Vasectomy
F. Spermatogenesis
G. Testes

**B. Erectile Dysfunction.** Complete the statement in the numbered column with the most appropriate term in the lettered column. Some terms may be used more than once, and some may not be used.

1. In erectile dysfunction, arteriosclerosis compromises the ability to fill with blood because of _____. *(1093)*

2. Two conditions in patients with diabetes mellitus that may contribute to erectile dysfunction are autonomic neuropathy and _____. *(1093)*

3. The type of erectile dysfunction likely to be caused by high blood pressure and its treatment is _____. *(1095)*

4. Two treatments that may be recommended for treating erectile dysfunction in the diabetic patient are papaverine self-injection and _____. *(1093)*

5. Spinal cord injuries that are more complete and more likely to cause erectile dysfunction are those injuries that are _____. *(1095)*

6. The most likely drugs to cause erectile dysfunction are: _____. *(1095)*

A. Failure to store
B. Low
C. Antihypertensives
D. Failure to initiate
E. Atherosclerosis
F. Penile implant
G. Vascular surgery
H. High
I. Failure to fill
J. Antibiotics
K. Reduced blood flow
L. Neurologic disorders

C. **Male Reproductive Disorders.** Match the description or definition in the numbered column with the most appropriate term in the lettered column. Some terms may be used more than once, and some may not be used.

1. _____ May be caused by infections, trauma, or the reflux of urine from the urethra through the vas deferens *(1087)*

2. _____ May be caused by injury to the penis, sickle cell crisis, medications, or papaverine injections *(1097)*

3. _____ Inflammation of one or both testes *(1087)*

4. _____ Enlargement of the prostate *(1088)*

5. _____ The development of a hard, nonelastic fibrous tissue just under the skin of the penis *(1096)*

6. _____ Inflammation of the prostate gland *(1085)*

7. _____ Treated with bed rest, ice packs, sitz baths, analgesics, antibiotics, anti-inflammatory drugs, and scrotal support *(1087)*

8. _____ Signs and symptoms include fever, tenderness, and scrotal redness *(1087)*

9. _____ A prolonged penile erection not related to sexual desire *(1097)*

10. _____ Signs and symptoms may include dysuria, frequency, hematuria, and foul-smelling urine *(1085)*

11. _____ Treated with antibiotics, analgesics, and sitz baths *(1087)*

12. _____ Treatment may include topical or oral medications with vitamin E, oral aminobenzoic acid, radiation, surgical removal, and colchicine *(1096)*

13. _____ Signs and symptoms include painful scrotal edema, nausea, vomiting, chills, and fever *(1087)*

14. _____ Signs and symptoms include decreasing size and force of the urinary stream, urine retention, and post-void dribbling *(1088)*

A. Orchitis
B. Prostatitis
C. Phimosis
D. Epididymitis
E. Benign prostatic hypertrophy
F. Priapism
G. Prostate cancer
H. Peyronie's disease

**D. Testicular Cancer.** Match the nursing diagnosis for the patient with testicular cancer in the numbered column with the "related to" statement in the lettered column. *(1100)*

1. _____   Anxiety
2. _____   Acute pain
3. _____   Impaired urinary elimina-
                   tion
4. _____   Risk for injury
5. _____   Constipation
6. _____   Situational low self-esteem

A.   Diminished or absent peristalsis caused by bowel manipulation during surgery
B.   Effects of anesthesia and abdominal surgery
C.   Diagnosis of cancer or anticipation of side effects of treatments
D.   Potential loss of reproductive capacity
E.   Surgical incision
F.   Surgery

**E. Epididymitis.** Which are treatment methods for a patient with epididymitis? Select all that apply. *(1087)*

1. _____   Bed rest
2. _____   Local heat
3. _____   Ice packs
4. _____   Sitz baths
5. _____   Analgesics
6. _____   Scrotal support

**F. Benign Prostatic Hypertrophy (BPH).** Which are factors that may trigger urinary retention in a patient with BPH? Select all that apply. *(1088)*

1. _____   Infections
2. _____   Delayed voiding
3. _____   Bed rest
4. _____   Anti-inflammatory agents
5. _____   Antihistamines
6. _____   Chilling

G. **Prostatectomy.** Match the nursing interventions for a patient with a prostatectomy in the numbered column with the nursing diagnosis in the lettered column. Some diagnoses may be used more than once, and some may not be used. *(1091)*

1. _____ Reposition tubing

2. _____ Inspect urine, dressing, and wound drainage for excess bleeding

3. _____ Use isotonic fluid for irrigation

4. _____ Use strict aseptic technique

5. _____ Maintain urine flow

6. _____ Assess bladder for distention

7. _____ Watch for water intoxication

8. _____ Keep closed urinary drainage systems intact

9. _____ Monitor output

10. _____ Monitor for signs of infection [temperature above 101° F (38.3° C)]; purulent wound drainage, and confusion)

11. _____ Give antispasmodics and analgesics

12. _____ Irrigate bladder as ordered; notify surgeon if you cannot clear tubing

A. Risk for deficient fluid volume related to hemorrhage

B. Acute pain related to urinary obstruction, bladder spasms, and surgical trauma

C. Risk for infection related to invasive procedures of the urinary tract or catheterization

D. Risk for injury related to obstructed urine flow, excessive absorption of irrigating fluids, or trauma to urinary sphincter

H. **Drug Therapy for Urinary Retention.** Match the drug actions in the numbered column with the drugs in the lettered column. Answers may be used more than once. *(1088)*

1. _____ Relax smooth muscle in the bladder neck and prostate

2. _____ Decrease testosterone levels

3. _____ Suppress prostatic tissue growth

4. _____ Reduce obstruction to urinary flow

A. Finasteride (Proscar) and Duagen (5-alpha-reductase inhibitors)

B. Tamsulosin (Flomax) and Cardura (alpha-adrenergic blocking agents)

I.  **Cancer.** What are the three most common parts of the male reproductive system that may be affected by cancer? *(1103)*

    1. _____     Epididymitis

    2. _____     Penis

    3. _____     Testicles

    4. _____     Scrotum

    5. _____     Prostate gland

J.  **Drug Therapy.** Match characteristics of drugs used to treat disorders of the male reproductive system in the numbered column with the drugs in the lettered column. *(1089)*

    1. _____     Prescribed for failure to fill or store

    2. _____     Replacement for low hormone levels in men

    3. _____     Decreases testosterone level; used to treat prostate cancer

    4. _____     Examples are Viagra (sildenafil), Levitra (vardenafil) and Cialis (tadalafil)

    5. _____     Relaxes smooth muscle in corpus cavernosum, increasing blood flow

    6. _____     Used with luteinizing-releasing hormone (LHRH) to treat prostate cancer, decreasing testosterone level

    A.  Testosterone
    B.  Agents used to treat erectile dysfunction
    C.  Estrogen products (Tace)
    D.  Testosterone inhibitors

**K. Male Reproductive System.** Using Figure 48-1 (p. 1078) below, label the parts of the male reproductive system (A–Q) from the terms (1–17) below. *(1078)*

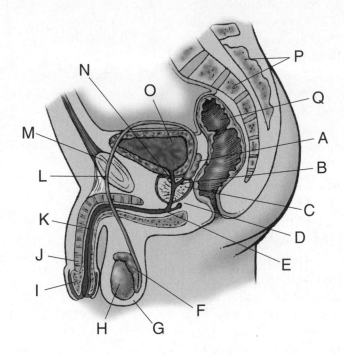

| | | | | |
|---|---|---|---|---|
| 1. | _____ | Sacrum | 10. _____ | Rectum |
| 2. | _____ | Corpus cavernosum penis | 11. _____ | Pubic symphysis |
| 3. | _____ | Scrotum | 12. _____ | Testis |
| 4. | _____ | Seminal vesicle | 13. _____ | Prostate gland |
| 5. | _____ | Prostatic urethra | 14. _____ | Penile urethra |
| 6. | _____ | Glans penis | 15. _____ | Epididymis |
| 7. | _____ | Bladder | 16. _____ | Bulbourethral (Cowper's) glands |
| 8. | _____ | Vas deferens | 17. _____ | Ejaculatory duct |
| 9. | _____ | Membranous urethra | | |

**L. Diagnostic Procedures.** Refer to DTP 48-1, Diagnostic Procedures, p. 1086 in the textbook. Match the numbered descriptions with the diagnostic procedure in the lettered column.

1. _____ Detects elevations associated with metastatic prostate cancer and is used to assess effects of treatment for prostate cancer *(1086)*

2. _____ Uses a lighted instrument inserted through the urethra to detect prostatic hypertrophy and bladder tumors *(1086)*

3. _____ Uses radioactive substances to asses testicular abnormalities (tumors, abscesses, epididymitis) *(1087)*

4. _____ Assess level of hormones needed for sexual development and function (luteinizing hormone, prolactin, follicle-stimulating hormone, testosterone) *(1086)*

5. _____ Examines a specimen to assess male fertility or to document sterilization after vasectomy *(1086)*

6. _____ An antigen is injected intradermally; site is examined after 48 hours to determine an immune response; used in patients with infertility problems *(1086)*

7. _____ Material is examined microscopically to detect sexually transmitted infections and identify pathogens. *(1086)*

8. _____ Detects increases that may be associated with prostatic cancer, prostatic hypertrophy by drawing a blood sample *(1086)*

A. Mumps test
B. Cystoscopy
C. Urethral smears
D. Serum acid phosphatase
E. Semen analysis
F. Endocrinologic studies
G. Tumor markers (PSA, serum prostate-specific antigen)
H. Radionuclide imaging

**M. Nursing Diagnoses.** Match the nursing diagnosis in the numbered column with the disorder in the lettered column. Answers may be used more than once.

1. _____ Risk for deficient fluid volume related to hemorrhage *(1091)*

2. _____ Constipation related to diminished or absent peristalsis caused by bowel manipulation during surgery *(1100)*

3. _____ Risk for infection related to invasive procedures of the urinary tract and surgical incision *(1091)*

4. _____ Situational low self-esteem related to impaired sexual function *(1093)*

5. _____ Risk for injury related to obstructed urine flow, trauma to the urinary tract *(1091)*

6. _____ Impaired urinary elimination related to obstruction *(1090)*

7. _____ Acute pain related to tissue trauma and bladder spasms *(1091)*

A. Benign prostatic hypertrophy (BPH)
B. Erectile dysfunction
C. Prostatectomy
D. Testicular cancer, postoperative

## MULTIPLE-CHOICE QUESTIONS

**N.** Choose the most appropriate answer.

1. Three normal changes that may occur in the male reproductive system due to aging are decreased testosterone, a longer refractory period between erections, and: *(1081)*
   1. penile discharge.
   2. pain with urination.
   3. slower arousal.
   4. descent of testicles.

2. Erectile dysfunction related to diabetes mellitus may be caused by: *(1093)*
   1. spinal cord injury.
   2. atherosclerosis.
   3. low hormone levels.
   4. medication side effects.

3. Autonomic neuropathy inhibits muscle relaxation of lacunar spaces of the erectile chambers, which may make: *(1093)*
   1. the patient anxious about performance.
   2. adequate filling of the penis with blood for an erection impossible.
   3. testosterone levels abnormally low.
   4. the patient sterile.

4. Assessment of the male reproductive system may be difficult for some patients because of health beliefs, need for privacy, or: *(1081)*
   1. chronic disease.
   2. advanced age.
   3. defensiveness about sexual behavior.
   4. lack of sexual experience.

5. Which test is done to document sterilization after a vasectomy? *(1083)*
   1. Ultrasonography
   2. Radiography
   3. Analysis of semen
   4. CBC

6. Past medical history helps link the current problem with previous problems and should include information about injuries, diseases, surgeries, allergies, treatments, and: *(1081)*
   1. marital status.
   2. medications.
   3. age and health of siblings.
   4. age and health of parents.

7. The health history should include information about medications the patient is taking because they may: *(1082)*
   1. impair his cognitive abilities.
   2. make him too tired to participate in the assessment.
   3. impair sexual function.
   4. impair gastrointestinal function.

8. Physical examination of the male reproductive system can be accomplished by inspection and: *(1082)*
   1. palpation.
   2. auscultation.
   3. percussion.
   4. radiography.

9. Which drug may cause hypotension and cardiovascular collapse in patients who are taking nitrate vasodilators? *(1089)*
   1. Alprostadil
   2. Sildenafil
   3. Papaverine
   4. Testosterone

10. Transurethral prostatectomy is the most common surgical procedure for benign prostatic hypertrophy. In this procedure: *(1088)*
    1. the prostate is approached through the bladder by way of a low abdominal incision.
    2. portions of the prostate are cut away through a resectoscope inserted into the urethra.
    3. access to the prostate is gained through an incision between the scrotum and the anus.
    4. the surgeon reaches the prostate through a low abdominal incision and opens the front of the prostate

11. Nursing diagnoses for the patient with benign prostatic hypertrophy include: *(1090)*
    1. Risk for infection.
    2. Sexual dysfunction.
    3. Pain.
    4. Impaired urinary elimination.

12. Nursing diagnoses for the patient immediately following a prostatectomy may include: *(1091)*
    1. Anxiety.
    2. Fear.
    3. Risk for deficient fluid volume.
    4. Impaired urinary elimination.

13. Men with low sperm counts should be evaluated for: *(1085)*
    1. congestive heart failure.
    2. anemia.
    3. thyroid function.
    4. renal disease.

14. A common obstructive symptom of BPH is: *(1088)*
    1. urine retention.
    2. nocturia.
    3. frequency.
    4. hematuria.

15. The reason for bladder irrigation following a TURP procedure is to: *(1091)*
    1. decrease postoperative infection.
    2. prevent constriction of the urethra.
    3. prevent clot formation and obstruction.
    4. decrease urinary retention.

16. If postvoid dribbling occurs in a postoperative TURP patient after removal of the catheter, the nurse should: *(1093)*
    1. suggest perineal exercises.
    2. recommend biofeedback.
    3. use isotonic fluid for irrigation.
    4. monitor for signs of infection.

17. Drugs most likely to interfere with erection are: *(1095)*
    1. antihistamines.
    2. decongestants.
    3. analgesics.
    4. antihypertensives.

18. Persistent or rising PSA levels in a patient who has undergone treatment for prostatic cancer indicate: *(1102)*
    1. a normal change that occurs with aging.
    2. an increased risk of infertility.
    3. obstruction of the urethra.
    4. advancing or recurrent tumor growth.

19. Which herb is thought to increase penile blood flow? *(1095)*
    1. Ginkgo biloba
    2. Kava kava
    3. Garlic
    4. Oil of jasmine

20. Which is an established risk factor for testicular cancer? *(1099)*
    1. Multiple sex partners
    2. African-American
    3. Caucasian
    4. High-fat diet

21. A cancer that occurs much more frequently among African-American men than Caucasians is: *(1101)*
    1. prostatic cancer.
    2. testicular cancer.
    3. penile cancer.
    4. bladder cancer.

22. Which is a common symptom of epididymitis? *(1087)*
    1. Hypertension
    2. Fever
    3. Swelling
    4. Fatigue

23. Which intervention is appropriate for a patient with BPH? *(1090)*
    1. Place a rolled towel across the patient's thighs to elevate the scrotum and reduce pain.
    2. Provide bed rest, scrotal support, and local heat to the scrotum.
    3. Drink at least eight glasses of fluids throughout the day.
    4. Eat a high-protein diet.

24. Postprostatectomy teaching includes which of the following? *(1093)*
    1. Consume a low-fiber diet.
    2. Limit fluids to four glasses of fluid each day.
    3. Use an ice bag and scrotal support.
    4. If semen is ejaculated into the bladder, it is not harmful.

25. Which extract relieves urinary symptoms associated with BPH and reduces serum levels of PSA? *(1088)*
    1. Siberian ginseng
    2. Ginkgo biloba
    3. Saw palmetto
    4. Oil of rose

26. Which is an irritative symptom of BPH? *(1088)*
    1. Nocturia
    2. Urine retention
    3. Postvoid dribbling
    4. Decreased force of urinary stream

27. Which drugs may cause urinary retention in patients with BPH? *(1088)*
    1. Smooth muscle relaxants
    2. Cold remedies
    3. Analgesics
    4. Antacids

28. Which drug is given to a postprostatectomy patient to relieve bladder spasms? *(1091)*
    1. Propantheline bromide (Pro-Banthine)
    2. Tansudosin (Flomax)
    3. Phenoxybenzamine HCl (Dibenzyline)
    4. Finasteride (Proscar)

29. Which herb can give a false negative result in patients with prostate cancer? *(1088)*
    1. Garlic
    2. Ginkgo biloba
    3. Siberian ginseng
    4. Saw palmetto

O. **Nursing Care Plan.** Refer to Nursing Care Plan, The Patient with a Prostatectomy, on p. 1092 in the textbook.

1. What is the priority nursing diagnosis? *(1092)*

# Sexually Transmitted Infections

---

## OBJECTIVES

1. List infectious diseases classified as sexually transmitted infections.

2. Explain the importance of the nurse's approach when dealing with patients who have sexually transmitted infections.

3. Discuss tests used to diagnose sexually transmitted infections and the nursing considerations associated with each.

4. Explain why sexually transmitted infections must be reported to the health department.

5. For selected sexually transmitted infections, describe the pathophysiology, signs and symptoms, complications, and medical treatment.

6. Design a teaching plan on the prevention of sexually transmitted infections.

7. List nursing considerations when a patient is on drug therapy for a sexually transmitted infection.

8. Identify data to be collected when assessing a patient with a sexually transmitted infection.

9. Assist in developing a nursing care plan for a patient with a sexually transmitted infection.

---

## LEARNING ACTIVITIES

A. **Key Terms.** Match the definition in the numbered column with the most appropriate term in the lettered column.

1. _____ A papule that breaks down into a painless ulcer at the site of entry of the organism that causes syphilis *(1111)*

2. _____ Disorder of immune system in which the blood has antibodies for the human immunodeficiency virus (HIV), meaning that the individual has been infected with this virus *(1115)*

3. _____ Most common STI in the U.S.; often has no symptoms *(1106)*

4. _____ An infection of the ovaries, fallopian tubes, and pelvic area *(1110)*

5. _____ Dormant; during this period of a disease, there are no signs or symptoms of the disease *(1112)*

6. _____ Burning of tissue *(1111)*

7. _____ A disease that can be transmitted by intimate genital, oral, or rectal contact *(1105)*

8. _____ An infection caused by an organism that usually does not cause a disease but becomes pathogenic when body defenses are impaired *(1115)*

A. Vaginitis
B. Cautery
C. Chlamydial infection
D. HIV-positive
E. Sexually transmitted infection
F. Pelvic inflammatory disease
G. Chancre
H. Latent

**B. Sexually Transmitted Infections.** Complete the statement in the numbered column with the most appropriate term in the lettered column. Some terms may be used more than once, and some terms may not be used.

1. Erythromycin ophthalmic ointment may be ordered for the newborn to prevent eye infection caused by exposure during delivery to _____. *(1108)*

2. A papule that becomes a painless red ulcer within a week is a sign of _____. *(1111)*

3. Treatment with ceftriaxone sodium (Rocephin) and doxycycline calcium (Vibramycin) or tetracycline cures most cases of _____. *(1110)*

4. The disease caused by the spirochete *Treponema pallidum* is _____. *(1111)*

5. If gonorrhea is untreated, the bacteria remain in the body and the person remains _____. *(1110)*

6. When the chancre disappears, patients may erroneously assume that they are cured; in fact, the infecting organism has moved into the _____. *(1111)*

7. Infections that may lead to heart tissue and joint damage are complications of _____. *(1110)*

8. Pustules, fever, sore throat, and generalized aching are symptoms that occur in the secondary stage of _____. *(1111)*

9. A typical lesion, called a *chancre*, is the first sign of _____. *(1111)*

10. If untreated, gonorrhea can cause _____. *(1110)*

A. Gonorrhea
B. Sterility
C. Infectious
D. Digestive system
E. Syphilis
F. *Chlamydia trachomatis*
G. Blood
H. Gonococci
I. Liver failure
J. *Treponema pallidum*

**C. Sexually Transmitted Infections.** Complete the statement in the numbered column with the most appropriate term in the lettered column. Some terms may be used more than once, and some terms may not be used.

1. An eye ointment that is recommended because it is effective against chlamydia as well as gonorrhea is _____. *(1108)*

2. An antibody test called the Herp-Check can detect active _____. *(1113)*

3. In females, venereal warts generally appear around the urethra, vagina, cervix, perineum, anal canal, and _____. *(1114)*

4. A penile discharge that is initially thin and then creamy, accompanied by painful urination, is a symptom of _____. *(1106)*

5. A sexually transmitted infection caused by a protozoan parasite is _____. *(1114)*

6. The drug of choice for the treatment of trichomoniasis is _____. *(1114)*

7. If left untreated, chlamydia can result in _____. *(1106)*

8. A condition caused by the human papillomavirus is _____. *(1114)*

9. There is an increased risk of cervical cancer in women who have _____. *(1113)*

10. The drug of choice for treatment of bacterial vaginosis is _____. *(1115)*

11. Premature births and miscarriages are high among women with _____. *(1113)*

12. The most common STI in the United States is _____. *(1106)*

A. *Chlamydia trachomatis*
B. *Condylomata acuminata* (venereal warts)
C. Erythromycin
D. Metronidazole (Flagyl)
E. Heart damage
F. Vulva
G. Acyclovir (Zovirax)
H. Trichomoniasis
I. Tetracycline
J. Herpes simplex infection (HSV)
K. Sterility

**D.  Sexually Transmitted Infections.** Complete the statement in the numbered column with the most appropriate term in the lettered column. Some terms may be used more than once, and some terms may not be used.

1. Complaints of flu-like symptoms and a burning sensation during urination are symptoms of _____. *(1113)*

2. Venereal warts are generally pink and soft with a _____ mass. *(1114)*

3. A frothy, yellowish vaginal discharge with a foul odor is a sign of _____. *(1113-1114)*

4. Males with venereal warts generally present with warts on the glans, foreskin, urethral opening, penile shaft, or _____. *(1114)*

5. An infection transmitted by contact with the mucous membranes in the mouth, eyes, urethra, vagina, or rectum is _____. *(1106)*

6. Painful, itchy sores on or around the genitals that appear about 2–20 days after infection are symptoms of _____. *(1113)*

7. Genital irritation; a thin, gray discharge; and a fishy odor are symptoms of _____. *(1115)*

8. Newborns with eye damage or infant pneumonia may have been exposed to _____. *(1106)*

9. A drug that is helpful in minimizing symptoms of herpes simplex virus is the antiviral drug called _____. *(1109)*

10. Cryosurgery may be used in the treatment of _____. *(1114)*

A.  Acyclovir (Zovirax)
B.  Trichomoniasis
C.  *Chlamydia trachomatis*
D.  Strawberry-like
E.  Metronidazole (Flagyl)
F.  Herpes simplex infection (HSV)
G.  Bacterial vaginosis
H.  Cauliflower-like
I.  Anus
J.  *Condylomata acuminata* (venereal warts)
K.  Scrotum

**E.  Drug Therapy.** Refer to Table 49-1 in the textbook. Match the description in the numbered column with the drug classification in the lettered column. Answers may be used more than once.

1. _____   Example is Cipro, which is effective against gonorrhea. *(1108)*

2. _____   Example is Bactrim, which is used to treat urinary tract infections and *Pneumocystis carinii* infections. *(1108)*

3. _____   Used to treat HIV infection. *(1109)*

4. _____   Example is penicillin G, which is effective against organisms that cause gonorrhea and syphilis. *(1107)*

5. _____   Example is erythromycin, which is used to treat chlamydial infections, syphilis, and gonorrhea. *(1108)*

6. _____   Example is Rocephin, used to treat gonorrhea. Side effects include allergic reactions in patients allergic to cephalosporins or penicillin, nephrotoxicity, and superinfections. *(1107)*

7. _____   Example is Achromycin, used to treat gonorrhea, syphilis, and chlamydial infections. Side effects include discoloration of developing teeth. *(1107)*

8. _____   Example is Flagyl, used to treat trichomonas. *(1108)*

9. _____   Example is acyclovir, used to treat genital herpes infections. *(1109)*

10. _____   Topical agents used to remove genital warts. *(1109)*

A.   Antibacterials
B.   Tetracyclines
C.   Macrolides
D.   Fluoroquinolones
E.   Sulfonamides
F.   Miscellaneous anti-infectives
G.   Antivirals
H.   HAART
I.   Dermatologic agents

F.  **Diagnostic Tests.** Which of the following STIs involve a vaginal or penile discharge for which smears and cultures are taken for diagnosis? Select all that apply. *(1106)*

   1. _____  Gonococcal infection

   2. _____  Chlamydial infection

   3. _____  Herpes simplex (HSV)

   4. _____  Trichomoniasis

   5. _____  Syphilis

   6. _____  Venereal warts

   7. _____  HIV infection

G.  **Reporting.** Which sexually transmitted infections (confirmed cases) must be reported to the local health department? Select all that apply. *(1106)*

   1. _____  HIV

   2. _____  Herpes simplex

   3. _____  Gonorrhea

   4. _____  Syphilis

   5. _____  Trichomonas infections

   6. _____  Chlamydia

H.  **Treatment of STIs.**

  1. Which of the following manifestations may occur during the first 24 hours in patients with syphilis who are treated with penicillin? Select all that apply. *(1107)*

    1. _____  Numbness of the extremities

    2. _____  Sore throat

    3. _____  Headache

    4. _____  Fever

    5. _____  Muscle aches

  2. Which treatments may be used for a patient with genital warts? Select all that apply. *(1114)*

    1. _____  Administration of penicillin

    2. _____  Cryotherapy

    3. _____  Surgical removal

    4. _____  Injection of interferon into the lesions

  3. Which STIs can be cured with drug therapy? Select all that apply. *(1106-1108)*

    1. _____  Herpes simplex (HSV-2)

    2. _____  Chlamydia

    3. _____  Venereal warts

    4. _____  Gonorrhea

    5. _____  Syphilis

I. **Patient Teaching.** Which of the following are ways to reduce the risk of gonorrhea? Select all that apply. *(1111)*

1. _____  Have all sexual partners treated.

2. _____  Take complete prescription of Cipro or tetracycline, even if symptoms disappear.

3. _____  Avoid unprotected sex until patient and sexual partners have been treated.

4. _____  Ensure that VDRL blood studies are done.

J. **Prevention.** Refer to Box GB 49-2. Which are considered unsafe sexual practices in preventing transmission of infection? Select all that apply. *(1119)*

1. _____  Oral sex without condom

2. _____  Mutual masturbation

3. _____  Vaginal or anal intercourse with properly used condom

4. _____  Ingestion of urine or semen

5. _____  Open-mouthed kissing

K. **Signs and Symptoms of STIs.**

1. Which are signs and symptoms of chlamydia infection? Select all that apply. *(1106)*

   1. _____  Greenish yellow urethral discharge

   2. _____  May be no signs or symptoms

   3. _____  Painful, frequent urination in males

   4. _____  Lower abdominal pain in females

   5. _____  Enlarged lymph nodes

2. Which are signs and symptoms of syphilis? Select all that apply. *(1111)*

   1. _____  Round ulcer with well-defined margin (chancre) is present

   2. _____  Sore throat

   3. _____  Regional lymphadenopathy

   4. _____  Profuse, watery vaginal discharge

L. **Nursing Diagnoses.** Which of the following are common nursing diagnoses for a patient with a sexually transmitted infection? Select all that apply. *(1116)*

1. _____  Deficient fluid volume related to anorexia

2. _____  Imbalanced nutrition: less than body requirements related to vomiting

3. _____  Sexual dysfunction related to fear of transmission

4. _____  Situational low self-esteem related to diagnosis

5. _____  Risk for injury related to disease process

6. _____  Acute pain related to lesions and inflammation

7. _____  Activity intolerance related to prescribed bed rest

8. _____  Excess fluid volume related to renal dysfunction

## MULTIPLE-CHOICE QUESTIONS

**M.** Choose the most appropriate answer.

1. What percentage of all cases of sexually transmitted infections involve people between the ages of 15 and 24? *(1105)*
   1. 50%
   2. 65%
   3. 75%
   4. 85%

2. Serologic tests for STIs are designed to detect infectious diseases by measuring: *(1105-1106)*
   1. white blood cells.
   2. red blood cells.
   3. clotting factors.
   4. antigens or antibodies.

3. Patients with gonococcal, chlamydial, herpes simplex, trichomonal, or yeast infections often have: *(1106)*
   1. vaginal or penile discharge.
   2. increased temperature or tachycardia.
   3. generalized infection and rash.
   4. mouth sores and pharyngitis.

4. When collecting a sample of vaginal discharge for culture and sensitivity tests, the person collecting the sample always wears: *(1106)*
   1. goggles.
   2. a mask.
   3. gloves.
   4. a gown.

5. If males have a whitish or greenish colored discharge from the penis and complain of a burning sensation during urination, this is suggestive of: *(1110)*
   1. HSV infection.
   2. chlamydia.
   3. gonorrhea.
   4. syphilis.

6. Female patients with gonorrhea are likely to have vaginal discharge, a burning sensation during urination, abnormal menstruation, and: *(1110)*
   1. dyspnea.
   2. abdominal pain.
   3. hypotension.
   4. edema.

7. Paralysis, mental illness, blindness, and heart disease may occur as complications of: *(1112)*
   1. HSV infection.
   2. cervicitis.
   3. syphilis.
   4. gonorrhea.

8. Two screening tests for syphilis include the rapid plasma reagin (RPR) and the: *(1112)*
   1. VDRL.
   2. RBC.
   3. WBC.
   4. BUN.

9. The treatment of choice for syphilis is: *(1112)*
   1. doxycycline calcium (Vibramycin).
   2. erythromycin.
   3. tetracycline.
   4. penicillin.

10. After completing treatment for primary or secondary syphilis, the patient is advised not to engage in sexual activity for: *(1112)*
    1. 5 days.
    2. 2 weeks.
    3. 1 month.
    4. 6 months.

11. If untreated, sterility, prostatitis in males, and pelvic inflammatory disease in females may result from: *(1110)*
    1. syphilis.
    2. gonorrhea.
    3. HSV infection.
    4. venereal warts.

12. Which STI can be transmitted through the placenta, causing an infant to be born with the disease? *(1111)*
    1. HSV infection
    2. gonorrhea
    3. syphilis
    4. chlamydia

13. A discussion of sexual behavior can be awkward for the nurse and the patient. Before nurses can deal with patients' sexuality, they must: *(1116)*
    1. present the patient with written information.
    2. be aware of their own values.
    3. ask the patient to demonstrate understanding of the material presented by stating information in his/her own words.
    4. check the patient's chart to see whether he/she has an STI.

14. With a sexually transmitted infection, common reasons that patients give for seeking medical care include pain, fever, lesions, or genital: *(1106)*
    1. itching.
    2. edema.
    3. bleeding.
    4. discharge.

15. Specimens collected during a pelvic exam are handled as: *(1118)*
    1. infective material.
    2. clean specimens.
    3. sterile specimens.
    4. chemically unstable material.

16. A nursing diagnosis related to lesions or inflammation for patients with STIs is: *(1117)*
    1. Anxiety.
    2. Acute pain.
    3. Situational low self-esteem.
    4. Ineffective management of therapeutic regimen: noncompliance.

17. A nursing diagnosis related to possible effects of STI or partner reaction to the STI is: *(1117)*
    1. Pain.
    2. Risk for injury.
    3. Anxiety.
    4. Impaired tissue integrity.

18. A nursing diagnosis related to stigma associated with STIs, shame, or anger is: *(1117)*
    1. Sexual dysfunction.
    2. Pain.
    3. Ineffective coping.
    4. Risk for infection.

19. Some STIs are painless, but patients may have pain associated with oral lesions, rectal lesions, or: *(1118)*
    1. vaginal bleeding.
    2. genital edema.
    3. nerve irritation.
    4. pelvic infection.

20. Untreated STIs can lead to serious complications such as pelvic inflammatory disease and: *(1105)*
    1. edema.
    2. sterility.
    3. shock.
    4. kidney failure.

21. Emergency drugs for possible hypersensitivity reactions that need to be kept on hand when administering drug therapy to patients with STIs include epinephrine, corticosteroids, and: *(1118)*
    1. acyclovir (Zovirax).
    2. diphenhydramine hydrochloride (Benadryl).
    3. didanosine (Videx).
    4. pentamidine isethionate (Pentam).

22. Chronic infections, such as HSV and HIV, require permanent alterations in: *(1119)*
    1. sexual activity.
    2. menstrual periods.
    3. skin integrity.
    4. nutritional habits.

23. Related to altered sexuality patterns in patients with STIs, the nurse explains that sexual dysfunction may be overcome by dealing with: *(1119)*
    1. the adverse drug effects of prescribed medications.
    2. the need for more exercise.
    3. emotional reactions to the disease.
    4. conflict resolution.

24. Females with HSV infections are advised to have annual Papanicolaou smears because they are at increased risk of: *(1119)*
    1. pyelonephritis.
    2. cervical cancer.
    3. kidney failure.
    4. AIDS.

25. The herpes simplex virus can be transmitted by sexual contact, but unlike most other STIs, it can also be transmitted by: *(1113)*
    1. air droplets.
    2. mouth-to-nose contact.
    3. fecal contamination.
    4. hand contact.

26. Most STIs respond to antimicrobial agents, but an exception is HSV, which is minimized but not cured by: *(1113)*
    1. penicillin G.
    2. tetracycline hydrochloride (Achromycin).
    3. acyclovir (Zovirax).
    4. metronidazole (Flagyl).

27. Which STI has symptoms similar to those of gonorrhea? *(1106)*
    1. Syphilis
    2. Herpes simplex
    3. Chlamydia
    4. HIV

28. In order to identify and treat infected individuals so that transmission of the STI can be slowed, partners may be notified and confirmed cases of certain STIs must be reported to the: *(1106)*
    1. United States Department of Health.
    2. hospital administrator.
    3. Department of Public Safety.
    4. local public health department.

29. How many new cases of gonorrhea occur in the United States each year? *(1110)*
    1. 100,000
    2. 500,000
    3. 700,000
    4. 1,000,000

30. Gonorrhea can be found in the pharynx, urethra, uterus, and: *(1110)*
    1. kidney.
    2. rectum.
    3. heart.
    4. lungs.

31. Gonorrhea is transmitted most often by: *(1110)*
    1. infected mothers to newborn infants.
    2. direct sexual contact.
    3. skin lacerations of medical personnel.
    4. toilet seats and doorknobs.

32. The heart, joints, skin, and meninges may become involved with which systemic infection? *(1111)*
    1. Gonorrhea
    2. Syphilis
    3. Chlamydia
    4. Genital warts

33. The treatment for gonorrhea is a single dose of IM ceftriaxone sodium (Rocephin), followed by 7 days of oral: *(1110)*
    1. erythromycin.
    2. Vibramycin.
    3. penicillin.
    4. tetracycline.

34. What is the correct treatment for a patient who has trichomoniasis? *(1114)*
    1. Penicillin
    2. Metronidazole (Flagyl)
    3. Acyclovir
    4. Tetracycline

35. An antiviral drug used to treat symptoms of herpes simplex is: *(1113)*
    1. acyclovir.
    2. erythromycin.
    3. penicillin.
    4. metronidazole (Flagyl).

36. Which of the following is the cause of vene-
    real warts? *(1114)*
    1. Human papilloma virus (HPV)
    2. Herpes simplex virus (HSV)
    3. *Chlamydia trachomatis*
    4. *Neisseria gonorrhoeae*

37. What do Papanicolaou's smears detect?
    *(1119)*
    1. Syphilis
    2. Gonorrhea
    3. Cancer of the cervix
    4. Herpes simplex infection

38. Which sexually transmitted infection is the
    most common bacterial STI because people
    have no symptoms? *(1106)*
    1. Syphilis
    2. Gonorrhea
    3. Venereal warts
    4. Chlamydia

N. **Nursing Care Plan.** Refer to Nursing Care Plan,
   The Patient with Gonorrhea, p. 1117 in the
   textbook.

1. What is the priority nursing diagnosis?
   *(1117)*

2. What are risk factors for this patient who
   has gonorrhea? *(1117)*

3. What data collected in the health history
   and physical examination indicate the presence of a gonococcal infection? *(1117)*

4. What are five complications this patient
   with gonorrhea may face if not treated?
   *(1117)*

# CHAPTER 50

# Skin Disorders

---

## OBJECTIVES

1. Describe the structure and functions of the skin.

2. List the components of the nursing assessment of the skin.

3. Define terms used to describe the skin and skin lesions.

4. Explain the tests and procedures used to diagnose skin disorders.

5. Explain the nurse's responsibilities regarding the tests and procedures for diagnosing skin disorders.

6. Explain the therapeutic benefits and nursing considerations for patients who receive dressings, soaks and wet wraps, phototherapy, and drug therapy for skin problems.

7. For selected skin disorders, describe the pathophysiology, signs and symptoms, diagnostic tests, and medical treatment.

8. Assist in developing a nursing care plan for the patient with a skin disorder.

---

## LEARNING ACTIVITIES

A. **Key Terms.** Complete the statement in the numbered column with the most appropriate term in the lettered column. Some terms may be used more than once, and some terms may not be used.

1. The secretion that coats the skin and creates an oily barrier that holds in water is ____C____. *(1123)*

2. A result of the thinning of the skin layers and degeneration of elastin fibers is ____H____. *(1123)*

3. The dissipation of heat from the skin occurs through ____E____. *(1122)*

4. Sweating helps cool the body through ____A____. *(1123)*

5. Ultraviolet rays in sunlight activate a substance in the skin that is eventually converted into ____D____. *(1123)*

6. Heat is retained through ____B____. *(1122)*

7. Two skin secretions are sweat and ____C____. *(1123)*

8. The skin is endowed with sensory receptors for touch, pain, temperature, and ____I____. *(1123)*

A. Evaporation
B. Vasoconstriction
C. Sebum
D. Melanin
E. Vasodilation
F. Sweat
G. Lymph
H. Wrinkling
I. Pressure
J. Lactic acid
K. Vitamin D

**B.  Diagnostic Tests.**

1.  Match the description or definition in the numbered column with the most appropriate term in the lettered column. Some terms may be used more than once, and some terms may not be used.

1.  ___I___   A test used to diagnose viral skin infections *(1129)*

2.  ___L___   Used to diagnose fungal infections by studying a skin specimen *(1129)*

3.  ___F___   An examination in which the patient's skin is inspected under a black light in a darkened room *(1129)*

4.  ___J___   A test used to identify allergens in which common irritants are applied to the skin *(1127)*

5.  ___A___   The removal of skin for microscopic examination *(1127)*

6.  ___G___   A specimen no deeper than the dermis is obtained with a scalpel *(1127)*

7.  ___D___   The type of biopsy in which a circular tool cuts around the lesion, which is then lifted and severed *(1127)*

8.  ___H___   The type of biopsy indicated for deep specimens in which sutures are required to close the site *(1127)*

9.  ___K___   Used to detect mites *(1127)*

A.  Biopsy
B.  Aspiration biopsy
C.  Scalpel
D.  Punch biopsy
E.  Gram's stain
F.  Wood's light
G.  Shave biopsy
H.  Surgical excision
I.  Tzanck's smear
J.  Patch testing
K.  Scabies scraping
L.  KOH examination

2. **Skin Biopsy.** Answer the numbered questions below using the letters in Figure 50-5 (p. 1128) below. Answers may be used more than once. *(1128)*

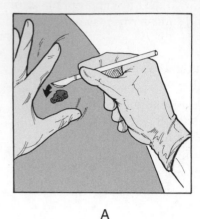 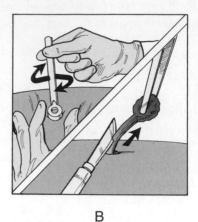 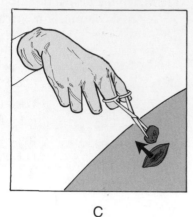

A                              B                              C

1.   What do these pictures show?

2.   ___B___          Which figure shows a punch biopsy?
3.   ___C___          Which figure shows surgical excision?
4.   ___B___          Which figure is a relatively shallow excision in which pressure or chemicals usu-
                      ally control bleeding?
5.   ___C___          Which figure require sutures?
6.   ___A___          Which procedure involves minimal bleeding that is controlled with pressure,
                      cautery, or chemicals?

C.  **Candidiasis Infections.** Complete the statement in the numbered column with the most appropriate term in the lettered column. Some terms may be used more than once, and some terms may not be used. *(1137)*

1.   Candidiasis infections, which are mani-
     fested as red lesions with white plaques, are
     found on the ___E___ .

2.   Infection with lesions of scaly patches
     and raised borders along with pruritus is
     ___H___

3.   Three common sites for candidiasis include
     the mouth, skin, and ___B___ .

4.   Moist red lesions associated with *Candida
     albicans* are seen on the ___F___ .

5.   A yeast infection caused by *C. albicans* is
     known as ___C___ .

6.   Oral candidiasis is treated with
     ___A___ .

7.   In addition to the mouth and vagina, an
     area that is susceptible to candidiasis, ow-
     ing to the constant moisture found there, is
     ___G___ .

A.   Nystatin
B.   Vagina
C.   Candidiasis
D.   Toes
E.   Mucous membranes
F.   Skin
G.   Ostomy site
H.   Tinea
I.   Scalp

**D. Acne Skin Disorders.** Complete the statement in the numbered column with the most appropriate term in the lettered column. Some terms may be used more than once, and some terms may not be used. *(1138)*

1. Mild cases of acne respond well to antibiotics and ___C___.

2. A serious adverse effect of isotretinoin (Accutane) is ___G___.

3. A drug that may be prescribed to counteract the effects of androgenic hormones in acne patients is ___E___.

4. Comedones (whiteheads and blackheads), pustules, and cysts are characteristics of ___B___.

5. Two oral antibiotics that are frequently given for acne are tetracycline and ___F___.

6. Drug prescribed for patient if acne is severe and unresponsive to antibiotics is ___H___.

7. A condition in which androgenic hormones cause increased sebum production and bacteria proliferation, causing hair follicles to block and become inflamed, is ___B___.

8. Drug prescribed for acne that can cause mental depression, possibly leading to suicidal ideation is ___H___.

A. Herpes simplex
B. Acne
C. Tretinoin (Retin-A)
D. Acyclovir (Zovirax)
E. Estrogen
F. Erythromycin
G. Fetal deformities
H. Isotretinoin (Accutane)

E. **Herpes Infections.** Complete the statement in the numbered column with the most appropriate term in the lettered column. Some terms may be used more than once, and some terms may not be used.

1. Older adults are especially susceptible to complications, including ophthalmic involvement, from _____F_____. *(1140)*

2. The first symptoms of heightened sensitivity along a nerve pathway, pain, and itching occur in patients with _____H_____. *(1140)*

3. Cold sores or fever blisters are oral lesions caused by _____E_____. *(1139)*

4. Sites most often infected are the nose, lips, cheeks, ears, and genitalia _____E_____. *(1139)*

5. Wet dressings soaked in Burow's solution may be used to treat lesions associated with _____H_____. *(1140)*

6. Diagnostic tests used to identify herpes infections include _____G_____. *(1140)*

7. Formed when the mucous membranes are affected with the varicella-zoster virus _____D_____. *(1140)*

8. Herpes simplex infections are treated with _____B_____. *(1139)*

9. Herpes zoster infection is commonly called _____H_____. *(1140)*

10. When the skin is infected with the varicella-zoster virus, _____A_____ form. *(1140)*

A. Crusts
B. Acyclovir (Zovirax)
C. Itching
D. Ulcers
E. Herpes simplex virus (HSV)
F. Herpes zoster virus
G. Tzanck's smear
H. Shingles

F. **Skin Cancers.** Complete the statement in the numbered column with the most appropriate term in the lettered column.

1. Squamous cell carcinomas, unlike basal cell carcinomas, grow rapidly and __D__. *(1143)*

2. A chronic autoimmune condition in which bullae (blisters) develop on the face, back, chest, groin, and umbilicus is __I__. *(1142)*

3. The use of liquid nitrogen to freeze and destroy lesions found in actinic keratosis is called __F__. *(1143)*

4. A condition with painless, nodular lesions that have a pearly appearance is __L__. *(1143)*

5. The drug of choice for actinic keratosis is __H__. *(1143)*

6. Disorder that arises from the pigment-producing cells in the skin __A__. *(1143)*

7. Scaly ulcers or raised lesions are characteristics of __E__. *(1143)*

8. Although basal cell carcinomas grow slowly and rarely metastasize, they should be removed because they can cause local __K__. *(1143)*

9. A malignancy of the blood vessels with red, blue, or purple macules is __C__. *(1144)*

10. A precancerous lesion most often found on areas exposed to sunlight, such as the face, neck, forearms, and backs of the hands, is __G__. *(1143)*

11. A condition in which malignant T cells migrate to the skin is __M__. *(1144)*

12. Skin cancers are most common among light-skinned people who have had repeated __B__ exposure. *(1143)*

13. Squamous cell carcinomas are usually caused by overuse of alcohol and __J__. *(1143)*

14. Mohs' surgery is used to determine margins of malignancy for __A__. *(1143)*

A. Melanoma
B. Sun
C. Kaposi's sarcoma
D. Metastasize
E. Squamous cell carcinoma
F. Cryotherapy
G. Actinic keratosis
H. 5-FU
I. Pemphigus
J. Tobacco
K. Tissue destruction
L. Basal cell carcinoma
M. Cutaneous T-cell lymphoma

**G. Burns.** Match the description in the numbered column with the type of burn in the lettered column. Answers may be used more than once. *(1146)*

1. _____A_____    Pink to red and painful, like a sunburn

2. _____C_____    Large, thick-walled blisters or edema

3. _____D_____    Burned tissue lacking sensation

4. _____A_____    Burn affecting only the epidermis

5. _____D_____    Burn involving the epidermis, dermis, and underlying tissues, including fat, muscle, and bone

6. _____C_____    Burned tissue is painful and sensitive to cold air

7. _____B_____    Blistered, weepy, and pale to red or pink

8. _____D_____    Dry, leathery, and sometimes red, white, brown, or black

9. _____C_____    Weeping, cherry-red, exposed dermis

10. _____B_____   A severe sunburn

A.   Superficial burn
B.   Superficial partial-thickness burn
C.   Deep partial-thickness burn
D.   Full-thickness burn

## H.  Skin Lesions.

1.  Match the characteristics and examples of common skin lesions in the numbered column with the letters in Figure 50-3 (p. 1126) below. *(1125)*

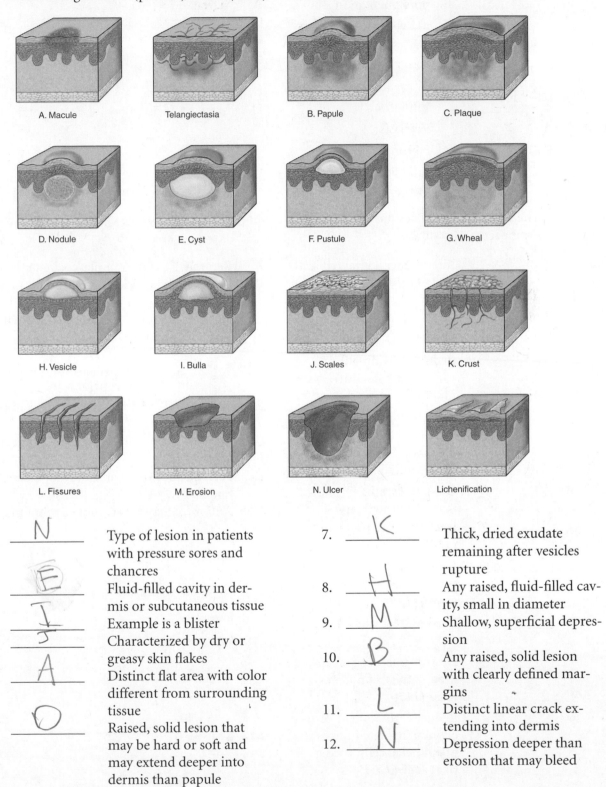

A. Macule    Telangiectasia    B. Papule    C. Plaque

D. Nodule    E. Cyst    F. Pustule    G. Wheal

H. Vesicle    I. Bulla    J. Scales    K. Crust

L. Fissures    M. Erosion    N. Ulcer    Lichenification

1.  ___N___ Type of lesion in patients with pressure sores and chancres

2.  ___E___ Fluid-filled cavity in dermis or subcutaneous tissue

3.  ___I___ Example is a blister

4.  ___J___ Characterized by dry or greasy skin flakes

5.  ___A___ Distinct flat area with color different from surrounding tissue

6.  ___D___ Raised, solid lesion that may be hard or soft and may extend deeper into dermis than papule

7.  ___K___ Thick, dried exudate remaining after vesicles rupture

8.  ___H___ Any raised, fluid-filled cavity, small in diameter

9.  ___M___ Shallow, superficial depression

10.  ___B___ Any raised, solid lesion with clearly defined margins

11.  ___L___ Distinct linear crack extending into dermis

12.  ___N___ Depression deeper than erosion that may bleed

2. Match the example or description in the numbered column with the appropriate type of lesion in the lettered column. *(1125)*

1. ___H___   Freckle, petechia, hy-popigmentation

2. ___C___   Mole, wart

3. ___F___   Herpes simplex, herpes zoster

4. ___E___   Acne, impetigo

5. ___D___   Vitiligo

6. ___Scale___   Psoriasis

7. ___G___   Fibroma

8. ___B___   Allergic response, insect bite, hives

A.   Plaque
B.   Wheal
C.   Papule
D.   Patch
E.   Pustule
F.   Vesicle
G.   Nodule
H.   Macule

**I.   Drug Therapy.**  Match the actions and uses in the numbered column with the appropriate drug classification in the lettered column.

1. ___C___   Interfere with viral replication *(1130)*

2. ___D___   Decrease proliferation of epidermal cells in psoriasis *(1131)*

3. ___F___   Reduce inflammation in various skin disorders *(1130)*

4. ___H___   Kill parasites and their eggs; used to treat pediculosis (lice) and scabies (mite) infestations *(1131)*

5. ___A___   Dissolve keratin and slow bacterial growth; used to treat acne and psoriasis *(1130)*

6. ___E___   Effective against fungi; used to treat fungal infections *(1130)*

7. ___I___   Used to treat psoriasis *(1131)*

8. ___B___   Destroy microorganisms; used to treat skin infections *(1130)*

9. ___G___   Reduce formation of comedones; increase mitosis of epithelial cells; used to treat acne *(1131)*

A.   Keratolytics (for example, coal tar)
B.   Topical antibacterials (for example, bacitracin)
C.   Antiviral agents (for example, acyclovir)
D.   Photosensitivity drugs (for example, methoxsalen)
E.   Topical antifungal agents (for example, nystatin)
F.   Topical anti-inflammatories (for example, hydrocortisone)
G.   Vitamin A derivatives (for example, tretinoin [Retin-A])
H.   Pediculicides and scabicides (for example, lindane [Kwell])
I.   Antipsoriatics (for example, anthralin)

**J.  Skin Infections.**

1.  Match the signs or symptoms in the numbered column with the most appropriate skin infection in the lettered column. Answers may be used more than once. *(1141)*

| 1. __E__ | Vesicle or pustule that ruptures, leaving a thick crust | A. | Furuncle (boil) |
|---|---|---|---|
| 2. __C__ | Inflamed hair follicles with white pustules | B. | Verruca (wart) |
| 3. __A__ | Inflamed skin and subcutaneous tissue with deep, inflamed nodules | C. | Folliculitis |
| 4. __F__ | Clustered, interconnected furuncles | D. | Cellulitis |
| 5. __D__ | Local tenderness and redness at first, then malaise, chills, and fever; site becomes more erythematous; nodules and vesicles may form; vesicles may rupture, releasing purulent material | E. | Impetigo |
| 6. __B__ | At first, small shiny lesions; they enlarge and become rough | F. | Carbuncle |
| 7. __E__ | Treated with antibiotic therapy: erythromycin or dicloxacillin | | |
| 8. __B__ | Treated with electrical current to destroy lesion followed by removal with curette, cryotherapy (freezing), topical medications | | |

2.  Which types of lesions require contact precautions? Select all that apply. *(1125)*

1.  __X__  Wart lesions
2.  __X__  Infected lesions
3.  __X__  Plaque lesions
4.  __X__  Draining lesions
5.  __X__  Weeping lesions
6.  __X__  Scaly lesions

**K.** **Burns.** Match the appearance characteristics in the numbered column with the sensations experienced (in the same depth of burn) in the lettered column. *(1146)*

1. ___B___   Large, thick-walled blisters covering extensive areas (vesiculation); edema; mottled red base; broken epidermis; wet, shiny, weeping surface

2. ___A___   Variable, for example, deep red, black, white, brown; dry surface; edema; fat exposed; tissue disrupted

3. ___C___   Mild to severe erythema; skin blanches with pressure

A. Little pain; insensate
B. Painful; sensitive to cold air
C. Painful; hyperesthetic; tingling; pain eased by cooling

**L.** **Treatment Of Burns.** Match the definition or description in the numbered column with the most appropriate term in the lettered column. Some terms may be used more than once, and some terms may not be used. *(1148)*

1. ___C___   Removal of necrotic tissue from a wound

2. ___A___   Covering a wound with skin

3. ___B___   Can be reduced by use of pressure dressings in early stages of care

4. ___C___   May be accomplished by mechanical means, surgical excision, or enzymes

5. ___B___   Can be reduced by use of custom-fitted garments that apply continuous pressure 24 hours a day

A. Skin grafting
B. Scarring
C. Débridement

**M.** **Nursing Diagnoses of Patients with Burns.**

1. Which nursing diagnoses are most likely to occur in the emergent stage? Select all that apply. *(1149)*
   1. _____   Risk for infection
   2. _____   Risk for imbalanced nutrition
   3. ___X___   Decreased cardiac output
   4. ___X___   Excess fluid volume

2. Which of the following nursing diagnoses are related to patients with burns? Select all that apply. *(1149)*
   1. ___X___   Acute pain related to tissue trauma
   2. ___X___   Risk for infection related to loss of protective skin barrier
   3. _____   Impaired skin integrity related to scratching
   4. ___X___   Hypothermia related to impaired heat-regulating ability of injured skin
   5. ___X___   Impaired physical mobility related to contractures, pain
   6. _____   Impaired skin integrity related to inflammation

**N. Plastic Surgery.** Match the conditions treated with plastic surgery in the numbered column with the type of surgery used in the lettered column. Answers may be used more than once. *(1152)*

1. _____ B _____ Birthmarks
2. _____ A _____ Excess tissue around the eyes
3. _____ B _____ Developmental defects
4. _____ B _____ Disfiguring scars
5. _____ B _____ Receding chin
6. _____ A _____ Facial wrinkles

A. Aesthetic surgery
B. Reconstructive surgery

**O. Skin Infestations.** Match the signs and symptoms of skin infestations in the numbered column with infestation in the lettered column. *(1142)*

1. _____ B _____ Thin, red lines on skin; itching
2. _____ A _____ Itching of hairy areas of body (head, pubis); nits (eggs) seen as tiny white particles attached to hair shafts

A. Lice
B. Scabies

**P. Parts of the Skin.** Using Figure 50-1 (p. 1123) below, label the parts of the skin (A–L) from the terms provided (1–12). *(1123)*

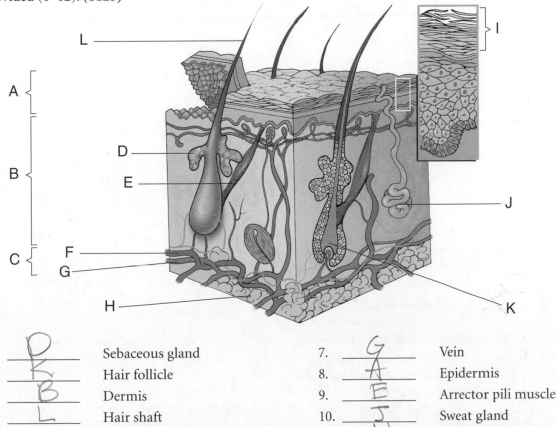

1. _____ D _____ Sebaceous gland
2. _____ K _____ Hair follicle
3. _____ B _____ Dermis
4. _____ L _____ Hair shaft
5. _____ I _____ Stratum corneum
6. _____ F _____ Artery
7. _____ G _____ Vein
8. _____ A _____ Epidermis
9. _____ E _____ Arrector pili muscle
10. _____ J _____ Sweat gland
11. _____ H _____ Adipose tissue
12. _____ C _____ Subcutaneous tissue

**Q. Nursing Diagnoses.** Match the nursing diagnosis in the numbered column with the skin disorder in the lettered column. Answers may be used more than once.

1. ___B___   Impaired skin integrity related to excessive dryness, scratching *(1133)*

2. ___E___   Risk for infection related to moist environment, broken skin *(1136)*

3. ___F___   Disturbed body image related to comedones, pustules, and cysts *(1138)*

4. ___K___   Risk for infection related to surgical incision *(1153)*

5. ___I___   Risk for injury related to improper nail trimming, poor peripheral circulation *(1144)*

6. ___L___   Decreased cardiac output related to hypovolemia secondary to shift of fluid from vascular to extracellular compartment *(1149)*

7. ___H___   Acute pain related to lesions or postherpetic neuralgia *(1140)*

8. ___J___   Risk for deficient fluid volume related to effects of liposuction *(1153)*

9. ___L___   Excess fluid volume related to changes in capillary permeability and accumulation of fluid in body tissues *(1149)*

10. ___J___   Anxiety related to uncertain outcome, anticipated changes in appearance, surgical procedure affecting body image *(1152)*

11. ___B___   Impaired skin integrity related to excessive dryness and scratching *(1133)*

12. ___C___   Disturbed body image related to lesions and scales on skin *(1135)*

13. ___A___   Impaired skin integrity related to intense itching and scratching *(1132)*

A. Pruritus
B. Atopic dermatitis
C. Psoriasis
D. Intertrigo
E. Fungal infection
F. Acne
G. Herpes simplex
H. Herpes zoster
I. Nail disorder
J. Plastic surgery, preoperative
K. Plastic surgery, postoperative
L. Burns

14. ___C___    Social isolation related to embarrassment about flaky skin lesions *(1135)*

15. ___E___    Altered oral mucous membrane related to oral candidiasis *(1137)*

16. ___G___    Ineffective coping related to anticipated recurrent lesions, embarrassment about appearance of mouth *(1139)*

17. ___L___    Risk for injury related to inadequate circulation to grafted tissue, pressure created by edema or implants, nerve damage *(1153)*

## MULTIPLE-CHOICE QUESTIONS

**R.** Choose the most appropriate answer.

1. Epidermal cells produce a dark pigment that helps determine the color of the skin called: *(1122)*
   1. sebum.
   2. cerumen.
   3. keratin.
   4. melanin.

2. Scalp hair thins in older men and women, but there may be an increase in: *(1124)*
   1. elastic tissue.
   2. facial hair.
   3. subcutaneous tissue.
   4. capillaries.

3. Nevi (moles) are carefully inspected for pigmentation, ulcerations, changes in surrounding skin, and: *(1125)*
   1. vascular irregularities.
   2. amount of edema.
   3. amount of pus.
   4. irregularities in shape.

4. When assessing capillary refill, after applying pressure to cause blanching and then releasing the pressure, the nurse should observe that the color returns to normal within: *(1126)*
   1. 1–2 minutes.
   2. 3–5 seconds.
   3. 30–40 seconds.
   4. 50–60 seconds.

5. The potassium hydroxide (KOH) examination is used in combination with a culture to diagnose infections of the skin, hair, or nails that are: *(1129)*
   1. viral.
   2. bacterial.
   3. caused by parasites.
   4. fungal.

6. When a skin biopsy is scheduled, the physician may advise the patient to avoid which drug before the procedure to reduce bleeding? *(1129)*
   1. Diphenhydramine
   2. Tetracycline
   3. Aminophylline
   4. Aspirin

7. Two assessments of the fingernails and toenails include noting the color of the nail bed and assessing: *(1126)*
   1. capillary refill.
   2. edema.
   3. hemorrhage.
   4. mobility.

8. The most common nursing diagnosis for patients with pruritus is Risk for: *(1132)*
   1. poisoning.
   2. impaired skin integrity.
   3. injury.
   4. infection.

9. Nursing diagnoses for the patient with atopic dermatitis may include impaired skin integrity related to: *(1133)*
   1. decreased resistance to infection.
   2. self-care practices.
   3. hypertension.
   4. excessive dryness.

10. Patients with any break in the skin are at risk for infection because the break in the skin presents a portal for: *(1133)*
    1. pathogens.
    2. blood.
    3. pus.
    4. sweat.

11. The assessment of patients with seborrheic dermatitis includes inspecting affected areas for: *(1133-1134)*
    1. bleeding and exudate.
    2. edema and redness.
    3. scales and crusts.
    4. yellow skin and ascites.

12. An important risk factor for developing candidiasis is: *(1137)*
    1. hypertension.
    2. antibiotic therapy.
    3. emotional stress.
    4. tachycardia.

13. A primary nursing diagnosis for patients with candidiasis is: *(1137)*
    1. Activity intolerance.
    2. Altered oral mucous membrane.
    3. Decreased cardiac output.
    4. Self-care deficit.

14. Acne is caused by: *(1138)*
    1. eating too much chocolate.
    2. fatty foods.
    3. poor hygiene.
    4. blocked hair follicles.

15. The nurse advises the patient with shingles that the condition is communicable to people who have never been exposed to: *(1141)*
    1. measles.
    2. pertussis.
    3. chickenpox.
    4. polio.

16. The most serious form of skin cancer is: *(1143)*
    1. basal cell carcinoma.
    2. melanoma.
    3. squamous cell carcinoma.
    4. cutaneous T-cell lymphoma.

17. Following a burn injury, plasma leaks into the tissue due to increased capillary: *(1146)*
    1. constriction.
    2. dilation.
    3. production.
    4. permeability.

18. After a burn injury, shifts in fluids and electrolytes cause local edema and a decrease in: *(1146)*
    1. respiratory rate.
    2. CNS stimulation.
    3. cardiac output.
    4. red blood cell production.

19. The shift of plasma proteins from the capillaries may result in: *(1146)*
    1. hypoproteinemia.
    2. increased blood volume.
    3. dehydration.
    4. increased urine output.

20. A complication of untreated fluid shifts in burn patients is: *(1146)*
    1. hypovolemic shock.
    2. kidney failure.
    3. pneumonia.
    4. convulsions.

21. A type of therapy used in the treatment of psoriasis, vitiligo, and chronic eczema is: *(1128)*
    1. phototherapy.
    2. soaks.
    3. wet wraps.
    4. débridement.

22. Vitamin A is essential for: *(1127)*
    1. blood clotting.
    2. bone formation.
    3. wound healing.
    4. healthy skin.

23. Food allergies can cause: *(1132)*
    1. scabies.
    2. basal cell carcinoma.
    3. psoriasis.
    4. atopic dermatitis.

24. Which is a topical herbal preparation used as an emollient? *(1129)*
    1. Aloe
    2. Angelica
    3. Balm of Gilead
    4. Ginseng

25. When a patient has an allergic dermatitis, the nurse should be sure to assess for the topical use of: *(1133)*
    1. corticosteroids.
    2. aloe.
    3. antihistamines.
    4. emollients.

26. Acne lesions develop when there is: *(1138)*
    1. increased fatty food intake.
    2. increased sebum production.
    3. increased chocolate intake.
    4. poor hygiene.

27. Which drug, used to remove heavy scales in patients with psoriasis, can stain normal skin and hair? *(1134)*
    1. Tazarotene (Tazorac)
    2. Glucocorticoids
    3. Methotrexate sodium
    4. Anthralin (Anthra-Derm)

28. Cornstarch should not be used in patients with intertrigo because it supports the growth of: *(1135)*
    1. S. aureus.
    2. C. albicans.
    3. E. coli.
    4. streptococci.

29. Which skin disorder, characterized by irritation and redness in body folds, is fairly common among patients in long-term care facilities? *(1135)*
    1. Intertrigo
    2. Impetigo
    3. Candidiasis
    4. Pemphigus

30. Who is at greatest risk for skin cancer? *(1142)*
    1. Caucasians
    2. African-Americans
    3. Native Americans
    4. Hispanics

31. A prominent symptom of psoriasis, dermatitis, eczema, and insect bites is: *(1131)*
    1. fever.
    2. pain.
    3. pruritus.
    4. edema.

32. If one arm and one leg are burned, what is the estimated burn size, according to the rule of nines? *(1145)*
    1. 18%
    2. 27%
    3. 36%
    4. 54%

33. The burn patient is at great risk for: *(1146)*
    1. hyperthermia.
    2. paralysis.
    3. edema.
    4. infection.

**S.  Nursing Care Plan.** Refer to the Nursing Care Plan, The Patient with Psoriasis, p. 1136 in the textbook.

1.  What is the priority nursing diagnosis? *(1136)*

2.  What are data collected in the health history and physical examination that are indicative of a patient with psoriasis? *(1136)*

# CHAPTER 51

# Eye and Vision Disorders

---

## OBJECTIVES

1. Identify the data to be collected in the nursing assessment of the eye and vision.

2. Identify the nursing responsibilities for patients having diagnostic tests or procedures to diagnose eye disorders.

3. List measures to reduce the risk of eye injuries.

4. Describe the nursing care of patients who require common therapeutic measures for eye disorders: irrigation, application of ophthalmic drugs, and surgery.

5. Describe the pathophysiology, signs and symptoms, diagnosis, and treatment of selected eye conditions.

6. Assist in developing a nursing care plan for the patient with an eye disorder.

---

## LEARNING ACTIVITIES

**A. Eye Disorders.** Match the definition in the numbered column with the most appropriate term in the lettered column. Some terms may be used more than once, and some terms may not be used.

1. _____ Measurement of pressure, such as intraocular pressure *(1162)*

2. _____ Agent that causes the pupil to constrict *(1165)*

3. _____ Error of refraction caused by uneven curvature of the cornea or lens; causes visual distortion *(1175)*

4. _____ Inflammation of the cornea *(1172)*

5. _____ Inflammation of the membrane lining the eyelids and the eyeball *(1172)*

6. _____ Clouding or opacity of the normally transparent lens within the eye; causes blurred vision and objects to take on a yellowish hue *(1176)*

7. _____ Agent that paralyzes the ciliary muscle so that the eye does not accommodate *(1165)*

8. _____ Bending of light rays *(1162)*

9. _____ Farsightedness *(1160)*

10. _____ Agent that causes the pupil to dilate *(1165)*

11. _____ Visual impairment associated with older age *(1160)*

12. _____ Nearsightedness *(1174)*

A. Keratitis
B. Myopia
C. Tonometry
D. Cycloplegic
E. Conjunctivitis
F. Refraction
G. Presbyopia
H. Miotic
I. Mydriatic
J. Cataract
K. Astigmatism
L. Hyperopia

B. **Glaucoma.** Complete the statement in the numbered column with the most appropriate term in the lettered column. Some terms may be used more than once, and some terms may not be used.

1. Timolol maleate (Timoptic), used in glaucoma to lower intraocular pressure, is classified as a _____. *(1179)*

2. A condition in which intraocular pressure is increased above normal is _____. *(1179)*

3. Excess pressure impairs blood flow to the optic nerve, resulting in _____. *(1179)*

4. Type of vision that is lost first in glaucoma is _____. *(1179)*

5. Patients with glaucoma have fields of vision that gradually narrow until the patient has _____. *(1179)*

6. A type of acute glaucoma that is considered a medical emergency is _____. *(1180)*

7. Acetazolamide (Diamox), used to reduce intraocular pressure by decreasing the production of aqueous humor, is classified as a _____. *(1179)*

8. A surgical procedure for glaucoma is _____. *(1179)*

9. Chronic glaucoma is also called _____. *(1179)*

10. A person who can only see a small circle, as if looking through a tube, has _____. *(1179)*

11. A surgical procedure in which a window is cut to permit aqueous humor to flow through the pupil normally in patients with angle-closure glaucoma is _____. *(1181)*

12. Open-angle glaucoma is usually treated first with drug therapy, which includes _____. *(1179)*

13. Decreasing the formation of aqueous humor and increasing its outflow, the action of adrenergics is to decrease _____. *(1179)*

A. Open-angle glaucoma
B. Iridotomy
C. Intraocular pressure
D. Miotic(s)
E. Carbonic anhydrase inhibitor(s)
F. Peripheral
G. Phacoemulsification
H. Glaucoma
I. Angle-closure glaucoma
J. Tunnel vision
K. Trabeculoplasty
L. Vision impairment
M. Beta blocker(s)

**C. Cataracts.** Complete the statement in the numbered column with the most appropriate term in the lettered column. Some terms may be used more than once, and some terms may not be used.

1. Cataracts may be congenital, degenerative, or _____. *(1176)*
2. Located behind the iris and changes shape to focus on images of various sizes _____. *(1176)*
3. When the lens becomes opaque so that it is no longer transparent, it is called a _____. *(1176)*
4. Once the lens is removed, the eye is said to be _____. *(1177)*
5. Type of cataracts that are more common with aging but may occur earlier in patients with diabetes or Down syndrome _____. *(1176)*
6. Signs and symptoms of cataracts include cloudy vision, seeing spots, and _____. *(1176)*
7. The only treatment for cataracts is removal of the _____. *(1176)*
8. The surgical treatment for cataracts that involves the use of sound waves to break up the lens is _____. *(1177)*

A.  Floaters
B.  Cataract
C.  Degenerative
D.  Phacoemulsification
E.  Traumatic
F.  Lithotripsy
G.  Aphakic
H.  Lens
I.  Cornea

**D. Drug Therapy.** Match the actions and uses in the numbered column with the most appropriate drug classification in the lettered column.

1. _____   Used to treat or prevent eye infections *(1167)*
2. _____   Used to treat herpes simplex keratitis *(1167)*
3. _____   Dilate pupil; used in open-angle glaucoma; decrease corneal congestion; controls hemorrhage *(1166)*
4. _____   Prevent redness and swelling caused by inflammation due to causes other than bacterial infection *(1167)*
5. _____   Used primarily to treat glaucoma *(1166)*
6. _____   Block sensation in external eye for tonometry; used in removal of sutures or foreign bodies and in some surgical procedures *(1166)*
7. _____   Are effective against some fungal infections of eye *(1167)*
8. _____   Dilate pupil; used before eye exams and for uveitis; decrease lacrimal gland secretion *(1166)*

A.  Antibacterials
B.  Anti-inflammatory agents
C.  Miotics
D.  Antifungals
E.  Topical anesthetics
F.  Anticholinergics
G.  Antivirals
H.  Adrenergics

E. **Eye Surgery.** Match the most appropriate nursing diagnosis for patients following eye surgery in the numbered column with the "related to" statement in the lettered column. *(1167)*

1. _____ Acute pain
2. _____ Anxiety
3. _____ Risk for injury
4. _____ Disturbed sensory perception (visual)

A. Tissue trauma
B. Temporary vision impairment
C. Disease process, trauma to the eye, patching
D. Pressure or trauma

F. **Nursing Interventions.** Which are interventions that relate to lighting for patients who are partially sighted? Select all that apply. *(1170)*

1. _____ Reduce glare because it interferes with vision.
2. _____ Make sure the furniture is a different color from the floors and walls.
3. _____ Use dishes and cups with a solid, single color to facilitate self-feeding and reduce spills.

G. **Drug Therapy for Glaucoma.**

1. Which medications are used in the treatment of glaucoma? Select all that apply. *(1180)*
   1. _____ Anticholinergics
   2. _____ Beta-adrenergic blockers
   3. _____ Adrenergics
   4. _____ Cholinergics
   5. _____ Carbonic anhydrase inhibitors
   6. _____ Antihistamines
   7. _____ Hyperosmotic agents

2. Match the actions and uses in the numbered column with the classification of drugs used to treat glaucoma in the lettered column. Some classifications may be used more than once, and some classifications may not be used.

   1. _____ Treatment of acute glaucoma *(1181)*
   2. _____ Initial treatment of acute and chronic glaucoma *(1179)*
   3. _____ Preoperative preparation for glaucoma surgery *(1181)*
   4. _____ Treatment of chronic glaucoma *(1180)*
   5. _____ Action of these topical drugs is to lower intraocular pressure by decreasing the production of aqueous humor *(1180)*
   6. _____ Action of drugs is to constrict the pupil, facilitating the outflow of aqueous humor *(1179)*
   7. _____ Action of drugs is to decrease intraocular pressure by decreasing the formation of aqueous humor and increasing its outflow *(1180)*

   A. Cholinergic miotics
   B. Osmotic diuretics
   C. Beta-adrenergic blockers
   D. Adrenergics

**H.   Diseases of the Eye.** Match the disease in the numbered column with the effect on the eyes in the lettered
column. *(1160)*

1. _____   Elevated blood glucose in
patients with diabetes

2. _____   Changes in retina due to
diabetes

3. _____   Vision problem in neurologic disorders (brain
tumors, head injuries, and
strokes)

4. _____   Problem with movement
of the eyes in neurologic
disorders (brain tumors,
head injuries, and strokes)

5. _____   Hyperthyroidism

6. _____   Changes in blood vessels
of the eye in patients with
hypertension

A.   May cause bulging eyes (exophthalmos)

B.   Causes temporary blurring of vision

C.   May cause blindness

D.   Inability to move eyes

E.   May be impaired, blurred, diplopia, and loss
of part of visual fields

F.   May lead to vision loss

**I.   Eye Structures.** Using Figure 51-2 (p. 1158) below, label the internal structures of the eye (A–O) by using
the terms (1–15) below. *(1158)*

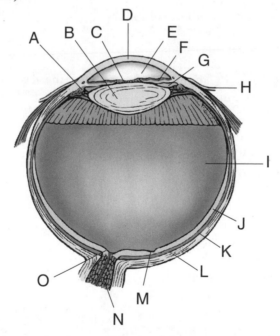

1. _____   Anterior chamber

2. _____   Choroid

3. _____   Ciliary muscle

4. _____   Conjunctiva

5. _____   Cornea

6. _____   Fovea

7. _____   Iris

8. _____   Lens

9. _____   Optic disk

10. _____   Vitreous body

11. _____   Optic nerve

12. _____   Posterior chamber

13. _____   Pupil

14. _____   Retina

15. _____   Sclera

**J. Diagnostic Tests and Procedures.** Refer to Table 51-1 in the textbook. Match the description of diagnostic procedures in the numbered column with the diagnostic test or procedure in the lettered column. Answers may be used more than once and some may not be used. *(1163)*

1. _____ A contact lens electrode is placed, the eye is exposed to flashes of light, and the retinal response is recorded.

2. _____ Identifies refractive errors and corrective lens needed.

3. _____ Pictures of blood vessels in the eye are taken after a dye is injected into a vein in the hand or arm, showing abnormalities in the retina.

4. _____ Examines the inner eye through the pupil to diagnose abnormalities of the retina, optic disk, and blood vessels.

5. _____ Identifies the area a person can see while looking straight ahead.

6. _____ Use of an instrument to measure intraocular pressure.

A. Ophthalmologic exam
B. Refractometry
C. Tonometry
D. Fluorescein angiography
E. Visual fields
F. Electroretinography

**K. Nursing Diagnoses for Eye Disorders.** Match the nursing diagnosis in the numbered column with the eye disorder in the lettered column. Answers may be used more than once.

1. _____ Disturbed sensory perception relate to vision changes caused by disease process, trauma to the eye, patching *(1167)*

2. _____ Ineffective coping related to decreased independence, threat to body image, denial *(1169)*

3. _____ Disturbed sensory perception related to inflammation, rejection of transplanted tissue *(1174)*

4. _____ Anxiety related to temporary vision impairment *(1167)*

5. _____ Disturbed sensory perception related to altered reception, transmission, interpretation of visual stimuli *(1169)*

6. _____ Fear related to actual or potential loss of vision *(1182)*

7. _____ Disturbed sensory perception related to surgical trauma, lens removal, patching *(1177)*

8. _____ Anxiety related to uncertain outcome, lack of knowledge about surgery and surgical routines *(1166)*

9. _____ Acute pain related to acute increase in intraocular pressure, inflammation caused by corrective procedures *(1182)*

10. _____ Self-care deficit (feeding, hygiene, grooming) related to visual impairment *(1169)*

A. Impaired vision
B. Glaucoma
C. Cataract surgery
D. Keratoplasty, postoperative
E. Eye surgery, preoperative
F. Eye surgery, postoperative

## MULTIPLE-CHOICE QUESTIONS

**L.** Choose the most appropriate answer.

1. As light enters the eye, it passes through the transparent cornea, aqueous humor, lens, and: *(1159)*
   1. conjunctiva.
   2. sclera.
   3. vitreous humor.
   4. lacrimal glands.

2. Dark spots that are actually bits of debris in the vitreous are called: *(1160)*
   1. flashes.
   2. floaters.
   3. blind spots.
   4. cataracts.

3. Sensitivity to light is called: *(1160)*
   1. photophobia.
   2. presbyopia.
   3. myopia.
   4. hyperopia.

4. When the nurse is performing a physical assessment of the eyes, the lids should cover the eyeball completely when closed; when the eyes are open, the lower lid should be at the level of the: *(1160)*
   1. conjunctiva.
   2. retina.
   3. iris.
   4. lacrimal gland.

5. The eyeball is inspected for color and moisture; the sclera should be clear: *(1160)*
   1. yellow.
   2. white.
   3. gray.
   4. black.

6. Excessive redness of the sclera may be an indication of: *(1160)*
   1. hypertension.
   2. exophthalmos.
   3. liver dysfunction.
   4. irritation.

7. The pupils are assessed for size, equality, and reaction to light; pupils that are unequal, dilated, or do not respond to light suggest: *(1161)*
   1. diabetes.
   2. liver dysfunction.
   3. inflammation.
   4. neurologic problems.

8. When the nurse asks the patient to focus on the nurse's finger as it is moved slowly toward the patient's nose, the nurse is assessing: *(1161)*
   1. presbyopia.
   2. astigmatism.
   3. accommodation.
   4. refraction.

9. Visual acuity is commonly tested using: *(1161)*
   1. the Snellen chart.
   2. the accommodation test.
   3. tonometry.
   4. fluorescein angiography.

10. If more than one eye medication is being given, the nurse must wait how long between each medication? *(1165)*
    1. 60 seconds
    2. 5 minutes
    3. 30 minutes
    4. 60 minutes

11. Eye surgery may involve surgical incisions, the application of cold probes (cryotherapy), or the use of: *(1165)*
    1. tonometry.
    2. lasers.
    3. fluorescein angiography.
    4. topical dyes.

12. Following eye surgery, the patient is usually positioned: *(1167)*
    1. flat in bed.
    2. prone.
    3. side-lying on affected side.
    4. with the head of bed elevated.

13. An important aspect of the care of postoperative eye patients is to prevent increased: *(1168)*
    1. blood pressure.
    2. cardiac output.
    3. intraocular pressure.
    4. ocular movement.

14. Nurses can teach people how to care for their eyes in order to protect their vision; it is important to tell people that: *(1168)*
    1. burning sensations in the eyes should be reported to the physician.
    2. watching too much television or sitting too close to the television injures the eyes.
    3. eating foods with high vitamin A content will improve vision.
    4. eyes need to be rinsed regularly to protect vision.

15. The most frequently performed eye operation in the United States is: *(1176)*
    1. enucleation.
    2. cryotherapy.
    3. cataract extraction.
    4. vitrectomy.

16. Medications prescribed after cataract surgery usually include antibiotics and: *(1178)*
    1. miotics.
    2. antihistamines.
    3. anticholinergics.
    4. corticosteroids.

17. One of the leading causes of blindness in the United States is: *(1179)*
    1. conjunctivitis.
    2. retinal detachment.
    3. glaucoma.
    4. cataracts.

18. Which drug has a side effect of vision disturbances? *(1160)*
    1. Digitalis
    2. Lasix
    3. Aspirin
    4. Synthroid

19. A vision of 20/30 on the Snellen chart means that the person can: *(1161)*
    1. read at 20 feet from the left eye and 30 feet from the right eye what a normal person reads at these distances.
    2. read at 20 feet what a normal person reads at 50 feet.
    3. read at 30 feet what a person with normal vision reads at 20 feet.
    4. read at 20 feet what a person with normal vision reads at 30 feet.

20. The measurement of pressure in the anterior chamber of the eye is: *(1162)*
    1. refraction.
    2. electroretinopathy.
    3. tonometry.
    4. angiography.

21. The nurse should treat nausea promptly in the postoperative eye surgery patient in order to prevent: *(1168)*
    1. infection.
    2. hemorrhage.
    3. pain.
    4. increased intraocular drainage.

22. Which is correct patient teaching regarding protection of health of the eyes? *(1169)*
    1. Watching too much TV or sitting too close to the TV can injure your eyes.
    2. Gently cleanse your eyelids each time you wash your face.
    3. Eating foods that contain large amounts of vitamin A improves vision.
    4. Eyes need to be rinsed on a daily basis.

23. A primary consideration of the patient with visual impairment is: *(1171)*
    1. safety.
    2. infection.
    3. hemorrhage.
    4. nutrition.

24. Which is an inflammation of hair follicles along the eyelid? *(1171)*
    1. Hordeolum (stye)
    2. Conjunctivitis
    3. Blepharitis
    4. Keratitis

25. Corticosteroids are contraindicated in patients with conjunctivitis caused by: *(1172)*
    1. herpes.
    2. bacteria.
    3. fungi.
    4. chlamydia.

26. Which drug is ordered before surgery for a patient with cataracts? *(1177)*
    1. An analgesic
    2. A mydriatic
    3. A miotic
    4. An anticholinergic

27. Following cataract surgery, the nurse should: *(1178)*
    1. advise the patient to sleep on the affected side.
    2. have the patient cough and deep-breathe.
    3. administer mydriatic agents.
    4. keep the bed low.

28. In which eye condition is peripheral vision lost first? *(1179)*
    1. Cataracts
    2. Macular degeneration
    3. Conjunctivitis
    4. Glaucoma

29. Which drugs are used to treat glaucoma? *(1180)*
    1. Anticholinergics (Atropine)
    2. Carbonic anhydrase inhibitors (Diamox)
    3. Anticonvulsants (Dilantin)
    4. Antihistamines (Benadryl)

30. Which herb should not be taken by patients with glaucoma because it increases intraocular pressure? *(1182)*
    1. Kava kava
    2. Garlic
    3. Ginkgo
    4. Ephedra

31. A patient sees floaters and states: "It is like a curtain has come down across my vision." This is a symptom of: *(1183)*
    1. cataracts.
    2. macular degeneration.
    3. retinal detachment.
    4. glaucoma.

32. Which antioxidant is believed to slow the progression of age-related macular degeneration? *(1184)*
    1. Vitamin A
    2. Vitamin B
    3. Vitamin E
    4. Vitamin K

M. **Nursing Care Plan.** Refer to Nursing Care Plan, The Patient Having Cataract Surgery, on p. 1178 in the textbook.

1. What is the priority nursing diagnosis? *(1178)*

2. Which nursing interventions for the patient are planned to prevent increased intraocular pressure? Select all that apply. *(1178)*
   1. Keep the bed in low position.
   2. Keep head of bed elevated.
   3. Instruct the patient not to rub the operative eye, strain, or lean forward.
   4. Instruct the patient to lie on the affected side.
   5. Administer antiemetics immediately as ordered for nausea and vomiting.
   6. Encourage patient to take stool softeners as ordered to prevent constipation.
   7. Acknowledge fear of vision loss common with eye surgery.

# 52 Ear and Hearing Disorders

---

## OBJECTIVES

1. Identify the data to be collected when assessing a patient with a disorder affecting the ear, hearing, or balance.

2. Describe the tests and procedures used to diagnose disorders of the ear, hearing, or balance.

3. Explain the nursing considerations for each of the tests and procedures.

4. Explain the nursing involvement for patients receiving common therapeutic measures for disorders of the ear, hearing, or balance.

5. For selected disorders, describe the pathophysiology, signs and symptoms, complications, and medical or surgical treatment.

6. Assist in the development of a nursing care plan for a patient with a disorder of the ear, hearing, or balance.

7. Identify measures the nurse can take to reduce the risk of hearing impairment and to detect problems early.

---

## LEARNING ACTIVITIES

A.  **Key Terms.** Match the definition in the numbered column with the most appropriate term in the lettered column.

1. _____ Eardrum; the structure that separates the external and middle portions of the ear *(1187)*

2. _____ Waxy secretion in the external auditory canal; earwax *(1187)*

3. _____ Ringing, buzzing, or roaring noise in the ears *(1189)*

4. _____ State of balance needed for walking, standing, and sitting *(1187)*

5. _____ Feeling of unsteadiness *(1196)*

6. _____ Sensation that one's body or one's surroundings are rotating *(1196)*

7. _____ Capable of injuring the eighth cranial nerve (acoustic) of hearing and balance structures in the ear *(1190)*

8. _____ Pain in the ear *(1189)*

9. _____ Hearing loss associated with age *(1188)*

A.  Tinnitus
B.  Cerumen
C.  Tympanic membrane
D.  Otalgia
E.  Equilibrium
F.  Vertigo
G.  Dizziness
H.  Ototoxic
I.  Presbycusis

**B. Hearing Loss.** Complete the statement in the numbered column with the most appropriate term in the lettered column. Some terms may be used more than once, and some terms may not be used.

1. Patients who hear better in noisy settings than in quiet settings have _____. *(1197)*

2. Congenital problems, noise trauma, aging, Meniere's syndrome, ototoxicity, diabetes, and syphilis may all be causes of _____. *(1197)*

3. A condition in which the stapes in the middle ear does not vibrate is _____. *(1197)*

4. A hearing loss that results from interference with the transmission of sound waves from the external or middle ear to the inner ear is _____. *(1197)*

5. A disturbance of the neural structures in the inner ear or the nerve pathways to the brain results in _____. *(1197)*

6. Patients who either cannot perceive or cannot interpret sounds that are heard may have _____. *(1197)*

7. Otosclerosis can be treated surgically with a procedure called _____. *(1201)*

8. A combination of conductive and sensorineural losses results in _____. *(1197)*

9. People with conductive hearing losses are usually helped to hear by _____. *(1197)*

10. Otosclerosis or obstruction of the external canal or eustachian tube may cause _____. *(1197)*

11. Sensorineural hearing loss is sometimes called _____. *(1197)*

12. Problems in the central nervous system may result in _____. *(1197)*

13. Patients who can hear sounds but have difficulty understanding speech have _____. *(1197)*

A. Mixed hearing loss
B. Otosclerosis
C. Cochlear implants
D. Nerve deafness
E. Central hearing loss
F. Otitis media
G. Cholesteatoma
H. Sensorineural hearing loss
I. Hearing aids
J. Labyrinthitis
K. Conductive hearing loss
L. Bone conduction
M. Stapedectomy

C. **Ear Infections.** Complete the statement in the numbered column with the most appropriate term in the lettered column. Some terms may be use more than once, and some terms may not be used.

1. A type of ear infection that usually develops with colds is _____. *(1200)*

2. The treatment for cholesteatoma is _____. *(1201)*

3. Soreness, headache, malaise, and an elevated white blood cell count are symptoms of _____. *(1200)*

4. If fluid remains in the middle ear following serous otitis media, _____ may develop. *(1200)*

5. A very serious infection that can lead to a brain abscess, meningitis, or paralysis of the facial muscles is _____. *(1201)*

6. The usual treatment for acute otitis media is _____. *(1200)*

7. An infection of the middle ear is called _____. *(1200)*

8. A condition that produces disturbances in both hearing and balance is _____. *(1202)*

9. An ear infection characterized by hearing loss and continuous or intermittent drainage is _____. *(1200)*

10. Sterile fluid accumulates behind the tympanic membrane in _____. *(1200)*

11. _____ is the creation of a small opening in the tympanic membrane to reduce pressure and allow fluid to drain. *(1200)*

12. _____ is characterized by thickening and scarring in the middle ear structures. *(1200)*

13. An ear infection that is usually not painful but in which the eardrum is usually perforated is _____. *(1200)*

14. Edema in acute otitis media leads to blockage of the _____. *(1200)*

15. Inflammation of the labyrinth is _____. *(1202)*

16. A growth in the middle ear is called a _____. *(1201)*

A. Meningitis
B. Mastoiditis
C. Serous otitis media
D. Labyrinthitis
E. Anti-inflammatories
F. Chronic otitis media
G. Eustachian tube
H. Acute otitis media
I. Electronystagmography
J. Antibiotics
K. Adhesive otitis media
L. Cholesteatoma
M. Chemotherapy
N. Surgical removal
O. Myringotomy
P. Otitis media

D. **External Ear Infections.** Complete the statement in the numbered column with the most appropriate term in the lettered column. Some terms may be used more than once, and some terms may not be used. *(1199-1200)*

1. "Swimmer's ear" is also called _____.
2. An inflamed area in the external auditory canal caused by infection of a hair follicle is a _____.
3. Treatment of otitis externa includes topical corticosteroids and _____.
4. Infection or inflammation of the lining of the external ear canal is called _____.
5. Swimming can lead to otitis by washing out protective _____.
6. Drainage in otitis externa may be blood-tinged or _____.
7. _____ may be caused by scratching or cleaning the ear with sharp objects.
8. When infection is present in otitis externa, it is frequently caused by streptococci or _____.
9. The most characteristic symptom of otitis externa is _____.

A. Cerumen
B. Pain
C. Furuncle
D. Otitis media
E. Purulent
F. Antibiotics
G. Redness
H. Staphylococci
I. Otitis externa

E. **Nursing Interventions.** Match the nursing intervention in the numbered column with the nursing diagnoses in the lettered column for patients who have had ear surgery. Answers may be used more than once. *(1205)*

1. _____ Encourage patient to avoid crowds and people with colds for several weeks.
2. _____ Position patient and offer massage to promote relaxation.
3. _____ Instruct patient not to shampoo for 2 weeks.
4. _____ Advise patient to avoid straining; give stool softeners as ordered.
5. _____ Have patient keep ear canal dry for 2–4 weeks.
6. _____ Advise patient to avoid nose blowing, coughing, and sneezing.
7. _____ Raise side rails and leave bed in low position.
8. _____ Encourage balanced diet with adequate protein and vitamin C.
9. _____ Assist with ambulation as long as dizziness occurs.

A. Risk for infection
B. Disturbed sensory perception
C. Pain
D. Risk for injury

F. **Ototoxic Drugs.** Match the ototoxic drugs in the numbered column with their most appropriate classification in the lettered column. Some classifications may be used more than once, and some classifications may not be used. *(1206)*

| | | | |
|---|---|---|---|
| 1. _____ | Aspirin | A. | Antiarrhythmics |
| 2. _____ | Erythromycin estolate | B. | Antibiotics |
| | (Ilosone) | C. | Antineoplastics |
| 3. _____ | Furosemide (Lasix) | D. | Antihistamines |
| 4. _____ | Cisplatin (Platinol-AQ) | E. | Anti-inflammatories/analgesics |
| 5. _____ | Indomethacin (Indocin) | F. | Diuretics |
| 6. _____ | Streptomycin sulfate | | |
| 7. _____ | Ethacrynic acid (Edecrin) | | |
| 8. _____ | Quinidine | | |
| 9. _____ | Tetracycline | | |
| 10. _____ | Bleomycin (Blenoxane) | | |

G. **Meniere's Disease.** Which are potential complications of surgery for Meniere's disease? Select all that apply. *(1204)*

1. _____    Tinnitus

2. _____    Infection

3. _____    Hearing loss

4. _____    Ataxia

5. _____    Loss of cerebral spinal fluid

6. _____    Damage to cranial nerve VII (facial nerve)

H. **Ototoxicity.** Which are signs and symptoms of ototoxicity? Select all that apply. *(1206)*

1. _____    Hearing loss

2. _____    Ataxia

3. _____    Infection

4. _____    Tinnitus

5. _____    Dizziness

6. _____    Drainage

**I.** **Ear.** Using Figure 52-1 (p. 1188) below, label all parts of the ear (A–L) from the terms (1–12) below. *(1188)*

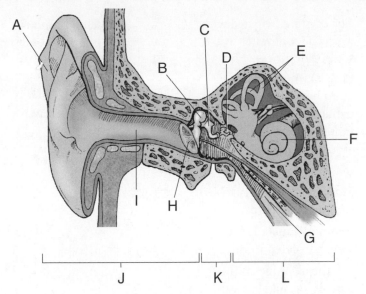

1. _____ Auricle
2. _____ External ear
3. _____ Stapes
4. _____ Malleus
5. _____ Inner ear
6. _____ Semicircular canals

7. _____ Eustachian tube
8. _____ Incus
9. _____ Middle ear
10. _____ Tympanic membrane
11. _____ Cochlea
12. _____ Ear canal

**J.** **Hearing.** Trace the sound waves from the external ear to the brain in Figure 52-3 (p. 1189) below. Label each step (A–F) from the terms (1–6) below. *(1189)*

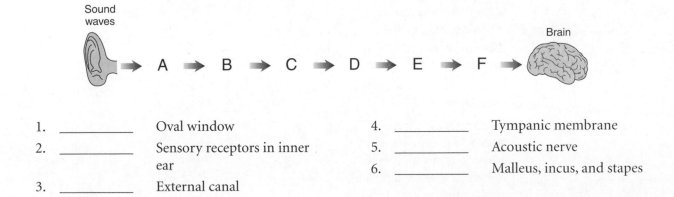

1. _____ Oval window
2. _____ Sensory receptors in inner ear
3. _____ External canal

4. _____ Tympanic membrane
5. _____ Acoustic nerve
6. _____ Malleus, incus, and stapes

**K. Diagnostic Procedures.** Match the description in the numbered column with diagnostic test in lettered column. Answers may be used more than once. *(1191-1192)*

1. _____ The ears are irrigated with warm or cool water to assess for dizziness.

2. _____ Detects hearing impairment by assessing the patient's ability to hear a range of sounds.

3. _____ Used to detect lesions in the vestibule.

4. _____ Measures the ability to hear spoken words.

5. _____ Test is conducted in a sound-isolated room.

6. _____ Tell the examiner if the patient has had central nervous system depressants, alcohol, or barbiturates because they alter test response.

7. _____ Patient listens to simple words through earphones and repeats them.

8. _____ Nothing by mouth for 3 hours before the test. No alcohol or caffeine for 24–48 hours before the test.

9. _____ Test is conducted in a sound-isolated room. A tuning fork is used to measure when vibrating sounds are heard.

10. _____ Examples are the Rinne's test and the Weber's test.

11. _____ Electrodes are placed around the eyes, patient asked to focus on specific targets as ears are irrigated, air is blown in ears, head position is changed.

A. Speech audiometry
B. Pure tone audiometry test
C. Caloric test
D. Electronystagmography
E. Tuning fork tests

L. **Drug Therapy.** Match the description in the numbered column with the drug classification in the lettered column. Answers may be used more than once. *(1194)*

1. _____ Decrease risk of infection by drying the external canal after swimming or bathing.

2. _____ Broad-spectrum antibiotic used to treat infections of the lining of the external auditory canal.

3. _____ Prevent or treat nausea, vomiting, motion sickness.

4. _____ Treat inflammation, pruritus, and allergic response.

5. _____ Soften earwax.

6. _____ Side effects include sedation, drowsiness, dry mouth.

7. _____ Side effects include hypersensitivity: redness, rash, burning.

8. _____ Contraindicated with ear surgery, perforated tympanic membrane, ear drainage, redness, pain.

9. _____ Boric acid is an example.

10. _____ Otocort, neomycin and colistin (Coly-Mycin S Otic), and polymyxin B are examples.

A. Antibiotics
B. Topical corticosteroids
C. Antibacterial and softening agents
D. Drying agents
E. Antiemetics

M. **Nursing Diagnoses.** Match the nursing diagnosis in the numbered column with the ear disorder in the lettered column. Answers may be used more than once.

1. _____ Disturbed sensory perception related to packing and edema in affected ear *(1195)*

2. _____ Impaired verbal communication related to inability to hear *(1198)*

3. _____ Risk for injury related to vertigo *(1203, 1204)*

4. _____ Risk for deficient fluid volume related to vomiting *(1203, 1204)*

5. _____ Social isolation related to inability to communicate verbally *(1198)*

6. _____ Risk for injury related to dizziness or vertigo, fluid accumulation, pressure in ear *(1195)*

A. Hearing impairments
B. Labyrinthitis
C. Meniere's disease
D. Ear surgery, postoperative

## MULTIPLE-CHOICE QUESTIONS

**N.** Choose the most appropriate answer.

1. Age-related changes in the inner ear affect sensitivity to sound, understanding of speech, and: *(1188)*
   1. balance.
   2. infection.
   3. cerumen production.
   4. blood pressure.

2. The type of hearing loss usually associated with aging is: *(1205)*
   1. otitis media.
   2. cholesteatoma.
   3. otosclerosis.
   4. presbycusis.

3. Pain in the ear is called: *(1189)*
   1. otosclerosis.
   2. otitis.
   3. ototoxicity.
   4. otalgia.

4. Ototoxicity means that a drug can damage the eighth cranial nerve or the organs of: *(1206)*
   1. hearing and balance.
   2. vision and sight.
   3. smell and taste.
   4. movement and coordination.

5. Examples of drugs that can have ototoxic effects are: *(1206)*
   1. aspirin and antibiotics.
   2. anticoagulants and corticosteroids.
   3. central nervous system stimulants and adrenergics.
   4. diuretics and antihypertensives.

6. When assessing the position of the auricles, the nurse should observe that the top of the auricle normally will be at about the level of the: *(1190)*
   1. nostrils.
   2. forehead.
   3. eye.
   4. mouth.

7. The external auditory canal is inspected for obvious obstructions or: *(1190)*
   1. edema.
   2. cyanosis.
   3. drainage.
   4. jaundice.

8. The only normal secretion in the external auditory canal is: *(1187)*
   1. sebum.
   2. purulent drainage.
   3. cerumen.
   4. mucus.

9. Otic drops, or ear drops, are intended to be placed directly into the: *(1193)*
   1. middle ear canal.
   2. inner ear canal.
   3. tympanic membrane.
   4. external ear canal.

10. The use of a solution to cleanse the external ear canal or to remove something from the canal is called: *(1193)*
    1. audiometry.
    2. irrigation.
    3. débridement.
    4. electronystagmography.

11. A common indication for irrigation is: *(1193)*
    1. clot formation.
    2. impacted cerumen.
    3. purulent drainage.
    4. bleeding.

12. A device that amplifies sound is: *(1193)*
    1. an audiometer.
    2. a tuning fork.
    3. a hearing aid.
    4. an otoscope.

13. People who benefit the most from hearing aids are those with: *(1193)*
    1. sensorineural loss.
    2. mixed hearing loss.
    3. conductive hearing loss.
    4. hearing loss due to Meniere's disease.

14. Postoperative dizziness or vertigo following ear surgery may put the patient at risk for: *(1196)*
    1. injury.
    2. impaired skin integrity.
    3. infection.
    4. pain.

15. Patients who have had ear surgery may have altered auditory sensory perception as a result of: *(1197)*
    1. dizziness or vertigo.
    2. knowledge deficit.
    3. self-care deficit.
    4. packing and edema in affected ear.

16. Following ear surgery, patients often complain of the sensation that the room is spinning or that their bodies are spinning. This is charted as: *(1196)*
    1. dizziness.
    2. otalgia.
    3. edema.
    4. vertigo.

17. After ear surgery, patients are advised to move slowly and carefully, and to avoid sudden movement, which may cause: *(1196)*
    1. hemorrhage.
    2. vertigo.
    3. infection.
    4. edema.

18. Of all patients with sensory disorders, people who probably suffer the most severe social isolation are those with: *(1197)*
    1. hearing impairment.
    2. sight impairment.
    3. smell impairment.
    4. taste impairment.

19. To prevent one form of congenital hearing impairment, all women of childbearing age should be immunized for: *(1199)*
    1. pertussis.
    2. influenza.
    3. rubella.
    4. hepatitis B.

20. One of the most common causes of obstruction of the external ear canal is: *(1199)*
    1. hemorrhage.
    2. infection.
    3. impacted cerumen.
    4. blood clots.

21. Patients with impacted cerumen may complain of hearing loss or: *(1199)*
    1. sharp pain.
    2. tinnitus.
    3. bloody discharge.
    4. headache.

22. A very common problem after mastoidectomy or middle ear surgery is: *(1201)*
    1. nausea.
    2. constipation.
    3. oliguria.
    4. seizures.

23. Because the fixed stapes cannot vibrate in patients with otosclerosis, sound waves cannot be transmitted to the: *(1201)*
    1. middle ear.
    2. tympanic membrane.
    3. inner ear.
    4. external auditory canal.

24. Slow progressive hearing loss in the absence of infection is the primary symptom of: *(1201)*
    1. acute otitis media.
    2. labyrinthitis.
    3. perforated eardrum.
    4. otosclerosis.

25. The most common treatment for otosclerosis is a surgical procedure called: *(1201)*
    1. myringotomy.
    2. stapedectomy.
    3. mastoidectomy.
    4. incision and drainage.

26. A hereditary condition in which an abnormal growth causes the footplate of the stapes to become fixed is: *(1201)*
    1. cholesteatoma.
    2. otosclerosis.
    3. labyrinthitis.
    4. conductive hearing loss.

27. An inner ear infection that usually follows an upper respiratory infection and that may lead to Meniere's disease is: *(1202)*
    1. otitis media.
    2. otosclerosis.
    3. mastoiditis.
    4. labyrinthitis.

28. The treatment for labyrinthitis is: *(1202)*
    1. antiemetics.
    2. analgesics.
    3. corticosteroids.
    4. beta blockers.

29. A major concern for a patient with vertigo is: *(1202)*
    1. infection.
    2. safety.
    3. nutrition.
    4. edema.

30. The primary symptom of ototoxicity with salicylates is: *(1206)*
    1. vertigo.
    2. tinnitus.
    3. dizziness.
    4. anorexia.

31. A low buzzing sound that sometimes becomes a roar and that is a symptom of Meniere's disease is documented as: *(1203)*
    1. vertigo.
    2. tinnitus.
    3. dizziness.
    4. otitis.

32. When the caloric test or electronystagmography is done in patients with Meniere's disease, they will experience severe: *(1203)*
    1. vertigo.
    2. seizures.
    3. headache.
    4. flushing.

33. Following surgery for Meniere's disease, the nurse needs to assess the patient for: *(1204)*
    1. facial nerve damage.
    2. fluid volume excess.
    3. decreased cardiac output.
    4. urinary retention.

34. Presbycusis is the result of changes in one or more parts of the: *(1205)*
    1. middle ear.
    2. external auditory canal.
    3. eustachian tube.
    4. cochlea.

35. A labyrinth disorder in which there is an accumulation of fluid in the inner ear is: *(1203)*
    1. otosclerosis.
    2. otitis media.
    3. Meniere's disease.
    4. presbycusis.

36. Drugs that can cause permanent hearing loss are: *(1206)*
    1. antihypertensives.
    2. aminoglycosides (antibiotics).
    3. anticholinergics.
    4. diuretics.

37. Patients who are at special risk of developing ototoxicity because their bodies excrete drugs more slowly are those with: *(1206)*
    1. renal failure.
    2. pneumonia.
    3. myocardial infarction.
    4. liver disease.

38. Rinne's and Weber's tests use a tuning fork to assess the: *(1192-1193)*
    1. ability to hear whispers.
    2. presence of lesions in the vestibule.
    3. conduction of sound by air and bone.
    4. function of the eighth cranial nerve.

39. The correct postoperative intervention for a patient who has had ear surgery is as follows: *(1197)*
    1. Position yourself on the unaffected side to promote drainage.
    2. Keep your mouth closed, if you need to cough or sneeze.
    3. Increase vitamin K and protein intake in your diet.
    4. Avoid shampooing for 2 weeks.

40. A nursing intervention related to patients with impaired verbal communication is: *(1198)*
    1. provide adequate lighting away from the patient's face.
    2. raise the tone your voice.
    3. if the patient has a good ear, speak to that side.
    4. explain the use of the call button and bedside intercom.

41. Which problem for patients with inner ear disorders may be worsened by taking certain herbal products? *(1202)*
    1. Sedation
    2. Dry mouth
    3. Confusion
    4. Constipation

42. Which diet may be recommended for patients with Meniere's disease? *(1203)*
    1. Increased calcium
    2. Increased vitamin K
    3. Increased potassium
    4. Low sodium

O. **Nursing Care Plan.** Refer to Nursing Care Plan, The Patient with Meniere's Disease, on p. 1205 in the textbook.

1. What is the priority nursing diagnosis? *(1205)*

2. What data were collected during the health history and physical examination that indicate the presence of Meniere's disease? *(1205)*
   1.

   2.

   3.

   4.

   5.

3. Which tasks may be assigned to unlicensed assistive personnel? *(1205)*
   1.

   2.

   3.

   4.

   5.

   6.

---

## OBJECTIVES

1. Describe the nursing assessment of the nose, sinuses, and throat.

2. Identify nursing responsibilities for patients undergoing tests or procedures to diagnose disorders of the nose, sinuses, or throat.

3. Describe the nurse's role when the following common therapeutic measures are instituted: administration of topical medications, irrigations, humidification, suctioning, tracheostomy care, and surgery.

4. Explain the pathophysiology, signs and symptoms, complications, and medical or surgical treatment of selected disorders of the nose, sinuses, and throat.

5. Assist in developing nursing care plans for patients with disorders of the nose, sinuses, or throat.

---

## LEARNING ACTIVITIES

**A. Key Terms.** Complete the statement in the numbered column with the most appropriate term in the lettered column. Some terms may be used more than once, and some terms may not be used.

1. The terms *maxillary, frontal, ethmoid,* and *sphenoid* refer to _____. *(1209)*

2. Projections that increase the surface area where inspired air moves are called _____. *(1209)*

3. The procedure by which the nurse shines a special light into the patient's mouth to see whether the sinus cavities are filled with air is called _____. *(1210)*

4. Mucus protects the nasal airway because it is _____. *(1209)*

5. Spaces in the bones of the skull are called _____. *(1209)*

6. The sinuses are lined with _____. *(1209)*

7. Particles that are trapped in the mucus are swept toward the throat by _____. *(1209)*

8. Type of cells that line the roof of the nasal cavity are _____. *(1209)*

9. Specialized sensory cells detect odors and relay information about odors to the brain by way of the _____. *(1209)*

10. A layer of mucus covers the membrane inside the nose; this layer traps particles and _____ dry air. *(1209)*

11. The sinuses produce mucus that drains into the _____. *(1209)*

12. Air spaces that act as sound chambers for the voice and reduce the weight of the skull are called _____. *(1209)*

A. Acidic
B. Optic nerve
C. Cilia
D. Nasal cavity
E. Olfactory nerve
F. Turbinates
G. Nares
H. Mucous membrane
I. Moisturizes
J. Sinuses
K. Alkaline
L. Tonsils
M. Transillumination
N. Olfactory

**B. Sinus Disorders.** Complete the statement in the numbered column with the most appropriate term in the lettered column. Some terms may be used more than once, and some terms may not be used.

1. Pain or a feeling of heaviness over the frontal or maxillary area is a common symptom of _____. *(1217)*

2. Sinus infection usually spreads into the sinuses from the _____. *(1217)*

3. Type of sinusitis that follows obstruction of the flow of secretions from the sinus is known as _____. *(1217)*

4. Two findings related to assessment of the sinuses, which may be observed during palpation of the frontal and maxillary sinuses, include _____. *(1217)*

5. Toothache-like pain is a common symptom of sinusitis that involves the _____. *(1217)*

6. Potential complications of sinusitis include brain abscess, osteomyelitis, orbital cellulitis, and _____. *(1218)*

7. Repeated infections often result in _____. *(1218)*

8. Inflammation of the sinuses, usually the maxillary and frontal sinuses, is called _____. *(1217)*

9. The most common causative organisms of sinusitis are staphylococci and _____. *(1217)*

10. Type of sinusitis that is a permanent thickening of the mucous membranes in the sinuses is known as _____. *(1217)*

11. The possibility of brain infection exists in patients with sinusitis because the sinuses are located in the _____. *(1217)*

12. Allergic rhinitis, deviated septum, nasal polyps, tumors, airborne pollution, and inhaled drugs such as cocaine are causes of _____. *(1217)*

A. Pain and tenderness
B. Chronic
C. Meningitis
D. Pharynx
E. Nasal passages
F. Chronic sinusitis
G. Redness and fever
H. Acute
I. Skull
J. Acute sinusitis
K. Sinusitis
L. Streptococci
M. Maxillary sinuses

**C. Nose Disorders.** Complete the statement in the numbered column with the most appropriate term in the lettered column. Some terms may be used more than once, and some terms may not be used.

1. To decrease the patient's reaction to offending allergens, the allergist may recommend injections for _____. *(1219)*

2. Nasal polyps tend to grow, and they eventually obstruct the _____. *(1218)*

3. Medical treatment for epistaxis includes the use of silver nitrate or _____. *(1221)*

4. The priority assessment when a patient has severe epistaxis is for evidence of excessive _____. *(1221)*

5. A common respiratory condition, which is classified as acute (seasonal) or chronic (perennial), is _____. *(1219)*

6. The drugs used to treat allergic rhinitis are primarily decongestants and _____. *(1219)*

7. Two methods used to apply pressure in patients with epistaxis include placement of a nasal balloon catheter and _____. *(1221)*

8. Three symptoms that are normal following the Caldwell-Luc operation are swelling, bruising, and _____. *(1218)*

9. Following nasal polyp surgery, the patient is advised not to take _____. *(1218)*

10. Complications related to posterior packing include infection, blockage of the eustachian tube, and _____. *(1221)*

11. Chronic allergic rhinitis is often due to exposure to allergens in the environment such as _____. *(1219)*

12. Nursing care of patients with epistaxis includes monitoring vital signs to detect signs of _____. *(1221)*

A. Numbness
B. Allergic rhinitis
C. Hypovolemia
D. Nasal airways
E. Antihistamines
F. Airway obstruction
G. Nasal packing
H. Electric cautery
I. Desensitization
J. Coryza
K. Aspirin
L. House dust
M. Blood loss

**D. Nose Disorders.** Complete the statement in the numbered column with the most appropriate term in the lettered column. Some terms may be used more than once, and some terms may not be used.

1. Complications of the common cold include sinusitis and _____. *(1219)*

2. The release of chemicals, including histamine, following exposure to an allergen causes increased capillary permeability and _____. *(1219)*

3. Structures that resemble white grapes in size and shape are _____. *(1218)*

4. Acute allergic rhinitis is most often due to exposure to _____. *(1219)*

5. Patients with triad disease have asthma, aspirin allergy, and _____. *(1218)*

6. Removing allergens or treating the allergic responses may reduce the size of _____. *(1218)*

7. The overuse of decongestant nose drops or sprays may result in _____. *(1219)*

8. A condition that follows exposure to an allergen is _____. *(1219)*

9. Swelling of the nasal mucosa occurs as a result of fluid leaks from the _____. *(1219)*

10. The cause of nasal polyps is unknown, but patients often have a history of infections or _____. *(1218)*

A. Allergic rhinitis
B. Vasodilation
C. Vasoconstriction
D. Capillaries
E. Pollens
F. Rhinitis
G. Coryza
H. Nasal polyps
I. Otitis media

**E. Nose Disorders.** Complete the statement in the numbered column with the most appropriate term in the lettered column.

1. Growths that may develop in the nasal passages and sinuses and that may be benign or malignant are called _____. *(1220)*

2. The primary symptom of nasal tumors is _____. *(1220)*

3. Carcinomas that are external nasal tumors are usually either basal cell or _____. *(1220)*

4. The common cold is known as _____. *(1219)*

5. Acute viral coryza is contagious and spread by _____. *(1219)*

6. Signs and symptoms of the common cold include fever, fatigue, sore throat, and _____. *(1219)*

7. Complications of acute viral coryza include otitis media, sinusitis, bronchitis, and _____. *(1219)*

8. Septal deviations are corrected by a surgical procedure called a submucosal resection or nasal _____. *(1220)*

9. The two major complications of submucosal resection are tears of the septum and _____. *(1220)*

10. A diagnosis of cancer of the nose is made by taking a _____. *(1220)*

11. The nose is divided into two passages by a cartilaginous wall called the _____. *(1220)*

12. Complications of acute viral coryza are more common in people with lowered _____. *(1219)*

13. Drug therapy for acute common coryza includes antipyretics, antihistamines, and _____. *(1219)*

14. Antibiotics are not effective against infections caused by _____. *(1219)*

15. Inappropriate use of antibiotics promotes the development of resistant strains of _____. *(1219)*

A. Nasal discharge
B. Resistance
C. Septoplasty
D. Biopsy
E. Squamous cell
F. Viruses
G. Droplet infection
H. Acute viral coryza
I. Septum
J. Nasal obstruction
K. Bacteria
L. Pneumonia
M. Decongestants
N. Tumors
O. Saddle deformity

**F.  Pharyngitis.** Complete the statement in the numbered column with the most appropriate term in the lettered column. *(1222-1223)*

1.  Pharyngitis is treated with rest, fluids, analgesics, and _____.

2.  As long as the patient has a fever, the level of activity that is often recommended is _____.

3.  A soft or liquid diet may be ordered because of _____.

4.  A treatment that may be ordered to increase moisture in the room air is _____.

5.  The recommended daily fluid intake for patients with pharyngitis is _____.

6.  Fluids must be increased slowly in older adults because they do not adjust well to sudden changes in _____.

7.  Inflammation of the mucous membranes of the throat is called _____.

8.  _____ is a complication of bacterial pharyngitis that occurs 7–10 days after the throat infection.

9.  A usual course of antibiotic therapy is _____.

10. If bacterial infection is confirmed, the antibiotic is usually continued for _____ after all signs and symptoms disappear.

11. The physician often orders antibiotics for pharyngitis, usually erythromycin or _____.

12. Before an antibiotic is ordered, a _____ should be taken.

13. _____ is a complication of bacterial pharyngitis that occurs 3–5 weeks after the initial throat infection.

A.  48 hours
B.  Humidification
C.  Acute glomerulonephritis
D.  Dysphagia
E.  Blood volume
F.  Culture specimen
G.  Rheumatic fever
H.  Bed rest
I.  10 days
J.  Pharyngitis
K.  Throat gargles (irrigations)
L.  Penicillin
M.  2000–3000 mL

G. **Tonsillitis.** Complete the statement in the numbered column with the most appropriate term in the lettered column. *(1223)*

1. Common causative organisms of tonsillitis include streptococcus, staphylococcus, *Haemophilus influenzae*, and _____ .

2. Tonsillitis is a contagious infection spread by food or _____.

3. A patient with tonsillitis usually reports a sore throat, difficulty swallowing, fever, chills, muscle aches, and _____.

4. If swollen tissue blocks the eustachian tubes in patients with tonsillitis, there may also be pain in the _____.

5. An elevated white blood cell count in patients with tonsillitis suggests a _____.

6. The medical treatment of tonsillitis usually includes the use of _____.

7. A serious complication of tonsillitis caused by streptococcus is _____.

A. Headache
B. Peritonsillar abscess
C. Airborne routes
D. Bacterial infection
E. Ears
F. Antibiotics
G. Pneumococcus

H. **Obstructive Sleep Apnea (OSA).** Refer to Figure 53-6 (p. 1226) below. *(1226)*

1. _____  Which figure shows the nasal CPAP in place?

2. _____  Which figure shows a patient predisposed to obstructive sleep apnea (OSA) with a small pharyngeal airway?

3. _____  Which figure shows the relaxation of the pharyngeal muscles, allowing the airway to close, resulting in repeated apneic episodes?

4. Which of the following are symptoms of OSA? Select all that apply. *(1225-1226)*

   1. _____  Sore throat
   2. _____  Epistaxis
   3. _____  Irritable and sleepy during the day
   4. _____  Impaired concentration and memory
   5. _____  Muscle aches
   6. _____  Loud snoring
   7. _____  Hypotension
   8. _____  Cardiac dysrhythmias

A

B

C

5.  Which diagnostic test is done to confirm obstructive sleep apnea? *(1226)*
    1.  Laryngoscopy
    2.  Bronchoscopy
    3.  Polysomnography
    4.  Blood gases

**I.   Laryngectomy.** Complete the statement in the numbered column with the most appropriate term in the lettered column.

1.  Following laryngectomy, many patients are able to learn to control and use air to produce sounds, which is called _____. *(1231)*
2.  Following laryngectomy, some patients use an electronic device to produce sound, which is called a(n) _____. *(1231)*
3.  A procedure used for small tumors of the larynx is _____. *(1229)*
4.  Surgery in which the voice is preserved is _____. *(1229)*

A.  Laser surgery
B.  Artificial larynx
C.  Esophageal speech
D.  Hemilaryngectomy

**J.   Drug Therapy.** Match the actions and uses of the drugs in the numbered column with the classification of drugs in the lettered column.

1.  _____   Anesthetic effect on skin and mucous membranes *(1215)*
2.  _____   Reduce body temperature, treat fever *(1214)*
3.  _____   Decongestion, vasoconstriction *(1215)*
4.  _____   Treat allergic reactions, prevent motion sickness *(1215)*
5.  _____   Reduce pain *(1214)*
6.  _____   Kill or suppress growth of microorganisms *(1214)*
7.  _____   Decrease salivary and respiratory secretions *(1215)*

A.  Sympathomimetics
B.  Anticholinergics
C.  Antihistamines
D.  Antipyretics
E.  Analgesics
F.  Topical anesthetics
G.  Anti-infectives

**K.   Bacterial Pharyngitis.** Indicate for each characteristic below whether it refers to (A) viral or (B) bacterial pharyngitis. *(1222)*

1.  _____   Positive culture
2.  _____   Dysphagia
3.  _____   Normal CBC
4.  _____   Rhinorrhea
5.  _____   Abrupt onset of symptoms
6.  _____   Malaise
7.  _____   Mild elevation of temperature
8.  _____   Gradual onset of symptoms
9.  _____   Joint and muscle pain
10. _____   Rare complications

**L.  Age-Related Changes.**  Which are age-related changes of the nose, throat, and sinuses? Select all that apply. *(1210-1212)*

1. _____    Decreased nasal obstruction
2. _____    Cartilage of the external nose hardens
3. _____    Increased, more serious side effects of nasal decongestants
4. _____    Production of mucus increases
5. _____    Mucous membrane becomes thinner
6. _____    Sense of smell declines
7. _____    Occurrence of epistaxis (nosebleed) increases
8. _____    Esophageal sphincter may weaken, causing gastric content to flow back into the throat when patients lie down
9. _____    Tissues of the larynx becomes drier and less elastic

**M.  Nose and Throat.**  Using Figure 53-2 (p. 1211) below, label the structures of the nose and throat (A–J) by using the terms (1–10) below. *(1211)*

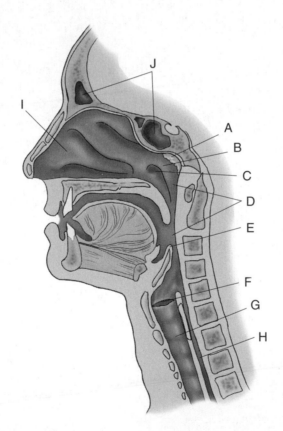

1. _____    Nasal cavity
2. _____    Sinuses
3. _____    Area of pharynx
4. _____    Auditory tube orifice
5. _____    Vocal cord
6. _____    Esophagus
7. _____    Pharyngeal tonsils (adenoids)
8. _____    Epiglottis
9. _____    Nasopharynx
10. _____    Larynx

**N.  Nursing Diagnoses.**  Match the nursing diagnosis in the numbered column with the disorder in the lettered column. Answers may be used more than once.

1. _____  Ineffective airway clearance related to increased pulmonary secretions or weak cough *(1230)*

2. _____  Decreased cardiac output related to hypovolemia secondary to hemorrhage *(1221)*

3. _____  Risk for injury related to excision of muscles in the neck or altered upper airway *(1230)*

4. _____  Impaired verbal communication related to aphonia or prescribed voice rest *(1227)*

5. _____  Risk for injury related to pressure (of packing, balloon) and possible airway obstruction *(1221)*

6. _____  Impaired verbal communication related to surgical excision of larynx *(1230)*

7. _____  Risk for infection related to presence of nasal packing *(1221)*

8. _____  Decreased cardiac output related to blood loss from vascular nasal passageways *(1216)*

9. _____  Disturbed body image related to facial bruising *(1216)*

A.  Epistaxis
B.  Laryngitis
C.  Nasal surgery, postoperative
D.  Tonsillectomy
E.  Total laryngectomy, postoperative

## MULTIPLE-CHOICE QUESTIONS

**O.**  Choose the most appropriate answer.

1.  The mucous membranes and tonsils of the throat are inspected for redness, drainage, swelling, or: *(1210)*
    1.  cyanosis.
    2.  lesions.
    3.  pallor.
    4.  coolness.

2.  Inspection and palpation of the neck may reveal enlarged: *(1210)*
    1.  lymph nodes.
    2.  tonsils.
    3.  adenoids.
    4.  vocal cords.

3.  Epistaxis (nosebleed) is more common in older people, especially in those taking: *(1212)*
    1.  antibiotics.
    2.  analgesics.
    3.  anticoagulants.
    4.  diuretics.

4.  A weakened esophageal sphincter allows gastric contents to flow back into the throat when the patient lies down. The patient experiences a burning sensation in the: *(1212)*
    1.  larynx.
    2.  nares.
    3.  trachea.
    4.  stomach.

5.  Following laryngoscopy, the patient takes nothing by mouth until: *(1212)*
    1.  respirations are normal.
    2.  vomiting has stopped.
    3.  the gag reflex returns.
    4.  24 hours after surgery.

6.  Before suctioning a patient, it is important to: *(1215)*
    1.  administer antiemetics as ordered.
    2.  ambulate the patient.
    3.  oxygenate the patient.
    4.  administer antibiotics as ordered.

7.  A key point to remember when suctioning a patient is to: *(1214)*
    1.  keep the vent closed when inserting the catheter.
    2.  apply suction continuously as the catheter is withdrawn.
    3.  suction for no longer than 30 seconds.
    4.  use sterile procedure.

8.  A key point to remember when providing tracheostomy care is to: *(1216)*
    1.  use standard precautions.
    2.  suction the tracheostomy after removing the old dressings.
    3.  use a sterile solution of iodine to clean the inner cannula.
    4.  cut a new pad to fit around the tracheostomy site.

9.  After nasal surgery, the nurse assesses for pain, pressure, anxiety, and: *(1216)*
    1.  tachycardia.
    2.  dyspnea.
    3.  hypotension.
    4.  pallor.

10. After nasal surgery, the patient's vital signs are monitored to detect signs of: *(1216)*
    1.  hypokalemia.
    2.  hypernatremia.
    3.  hypovolemia.
    4.  inadequate circulation.

11. The patient who has had nasal surgery may be at risk for decreased cardiac output because of: *(1216)*
    1.  blood loss from nasal passageways.
    2.  nasal packing.
    3.  airway obstruction.
    4.  facial bruising.

12. Because the nasal cavity has an extensive blood supply, following nasal surgery there is a risk of: *(1216)*
    1.  hemorrhage.
    2.  infection.
    3.  hypertension.
    4.  confusion.

13. Laxatives or stool softeners may be ordered for patients after nasal surgery in order to prevent: *(1216)*
    1.  diarrhea.
    2.  vomiting.
    3.  hypertension.
    4.  straining.

14. The best position for patients after nasal surgery to help control swelling is: *(1216)*
    1.  lying flat in bed.
    2.  lying with the head of bed elevated.
    3.  side-lying.
    4.  supine.

15. When the nasal cavity is packed following surgery, the patient breathes through the mouth; a measure that helps decrease dryness of the mucous membranes is use of: *(1216)*
    1.  frequent oral hygiene.
    2.  humidifiers.
    3.  oral fluids high in vitamin C.
    4.  ice packs.

16. Patients may experience disturbed body image following nasal surgery due to: *(1216)*
    1.  airway obstruction.
    2.  blood loss.
    3.  hypovolemia.
    4.  facial bruises.

17. Serious neurologic complications should be suspected in patients with sinusitis if the patient develops: *(1218)*
    1. tachycardia and restlessness.
    2. high fever and seizures.
    3. confusion and cyanosis.
    4. dyspnea and anxiety.

18. The type of surgery performed for chronic maxillary sinusitis is: *(1218)*
    1. laryngoscopy.
    2. tonsillectomy and adenoidectomy.
    3. the Caldwell-Luc operation.
    4. nasal septoplasty.

19. Desensitizing injections, or "allergy shots," are composed of dilute solutions of: *(1219)*
    1. allergens.
    2. histamines.
    3. antihistamines.
    4. plasma.

20. A deviated septum may obstruct the nasal passage and block: *(1220)*
    1. sinus drainage.
    2. eustachian tube drainage.
    3. pharyngeal drainage.
    4. jugular vein drainage.

21. Patients with a deviated septum may complain of epistaxis, sinusitis, and: *(1220)*
    1. palpitations.
    2. headaches.
    3. insomnia.
    4. sweating.

22. When epistaxis occurs, the patient should sit down and lean forward and direct pressure should be applied for: *(1220)*
    1. 1–2 minutes.
    2. 3–5 minutes.
    3. 7–10 minutes.
    4. 15–20 minutes.

23. With facial trauma or nasal fracture, the recommended treatment initially is application of: *(1220)*
    1. an ice pack.
    2. a warm compress.
    3. direct pressure.
    4. heat.

24. Patients with severe epistaxis may be at high risk for infection due to: *(1221)*
    1. possible airway obstruction.
    2. nasal packing.
    3. hypotension.
    4. hypovolemia.

25. The two major problems that may develop in the postoperative phase of tonsillectomy are respiratory distress and: *(1224)*
    1. infection.
    2. hemorrhage.
    3. hypersensitivity reaction.
    4. cardiac dysrhythmia.

26. Early signs of inadequate oxygenation in the postoperative tonsillectomy patient include restlessness, increased pulse rate, and: *(1224)*
    1. cyanosis.
    2. pallor.
    3. numbness.
    4. confusion.

27. Following a tonsillectomy, a treatment that may be applied to the neck to decrease swelling and pain is: *(1224)*
    1. a heating pad.
    2. a TENS unit.
    3. antibiotic ointment.
    4. an ice collar.

28. Which foods should be avoided in patients after a tonsillectomy? *(1224)*
    1. Frozen liquids
    2. Ice cream
    3. Applesauce
    4. Citrus juices

29. Which symptoms should be reported to the physician if the nurse observes them in the postoperative tonsillectomy patient who is ready to be discharged? *(1225)*
    1. Bleeding
    2. Earache
    3. White patches in the throat (surgical site)
    4. Sore throat

30. In order to reduce irritation of the larynx in patients with laryngitis, a treatment usually prescribed is: *(1227)*
    1. surgery.
    2. voice rest.
    3. intravenous fluids.
    4. application of heat.

31. A primary nursing diagnosis for patients with laryngitis due to aphonia is: *(1227)*
    1. Risk for infection.
    2. Risk for injury.
    3. Impaired verbal communication.
    4. Altered tissue perfusion.

32. Benign masses of fibrous tissue that result primarily from overuse of the voice but that can also follow infections are called: *(1227)*
    1. nodules.
    2. myomas.
    3. fibromas.
    4. tumors.

33. The only symptom of laryngeal nodules is: *(1227)*
    1. pain.
    2. fever.
    3. dysphagia.
    4. hoarseness.

34. A swollen mass of mucous membrane attached to the vocal cord is called a: *(1227)*
    1. nodule.
    2. tumor.
    3. cancer.
    4. polyp.

35. Individuals who both smoke and use alcohol are at particularly high risk for: *(1228)*
    1. tonsillitis.
    2. pneumonia.
    3. cancer of the larynx.
    4. nasal polyps.

36. Malignancies in the larynx tend to spread fairly early; the most common site of metastasis is the: *(1228)*
    1. liver.
    2. colon.
    3. lung.
    4. brain.

37. Total laryngectomy causes permanent loss of: *(1229)*
    1. the voice.
    2. cough.
    3. the sternocleidomastoid muscle.
    4. the swallow reflex.

38. A total laryngectomy involves removal of the entire larynx, vocal cords, and: *(1229)*
    1. pharynx.
    2. epiglottis.
    3. tonsils.
    4. esophagus.

39. Gently closing one naris at a time and instructing the patient to breathe through the other naris is a way to assess: *(1210)*
    1. lung sounds.
    2. aphonia.
    3. sense of smell.
    4. patency of the nostrils.

40. Normally, the frontal and maxillary sinuses are filled with: *(1209)*
    1. fluid.
    2. air.
    3. polyps.
    4. cysts.

41. In the immediate postoperative period after total laryngectomy, the nurse's assessment focuses on comfort, circulation, and: *(1230)*
    1. fluid balance.
    2. oxygenation.
    3. infection.
    4. hypovolemia.

42. In the patient with a laryngectomy, the nurse assesses the need for suctioning by observing audible or visible mucus, increased pulse, and: *(1230)*
    1. pallor.
    2. swelling.
    3. pain.
    4. restlessness.

43. Factors that affect the respiratory status of patients with laryngectomies include positioning, fluids, and: *(1230)*
    1. nutrition.
    2. verbal communication.
    3. humidification.
    4. personal hygiene.

44. A position that promotes maximal lung expansion in the patient with a laryngectomy is: *(1230)*
    1. semi-prone.
    2. flat.
    3. semi-Fowler's.
    4. side-lying.

45. To prevent pooling of secretions in the lungs of patients with laryngectomies, the nurse should encourage: *(1230)*
    1. coughing and deep breathing.
    2. increased fluid intake.
    3. early ambulation.
    4. avoidance of dusty places.

46. Which herb is used to boost the immune system and is taken by some to decrease the severity of a cold? *(1220)*
    1. Ginseng
    2. Ephedra
    3. Echinacea
    4. St. John's wort

47. Suctioning is limited to 10 seconds because prolonged suctioning may lead to: *(1214-1215)*
    1. hypoxia.
    2. hypertension.
    3. increased intracranial pressure.
    4. bradycardia.

P. **Nursing Care Plan.** Refer to Nursing Care Plan, The Patient Having Tonsillectomy, on p. 1225 in the textbook.

1. What is the priority nursing diagnosis? *(1225)*

2. What were this patient's signs and symptoms listed in the health history that indicate a need for a tonsillectomy? *(1225)*
   1.

   2.

   3.

   4.

   5.

3. Which nursing intervention will you perform first? *(1225)*

4. Which data in the physical examination indicate the need to watch for excessive bleeding in this patient? *(1225)*
   1.

   2.

5. In what position should this patient be placed? *(1225)*

6. Which of the following should be included in this patient's discharge teaching? Select all that apply. *(1225)*
   1. Consume soft, high-calorie, high-protein diet for 10 days.
   2. Drink 6–8 8-ounce glasses of fluids daily.
   3. Avoid strenuous activity or straining for 2 weeks.
   4. Do not take aspirin.
   5. Headaches are common following surgery.

## OBJECTIVES

1. Define mental health.

2. Discuss the concepts of stress, anxiety, adaptation, and homeostasis.

3. Discuss how age and cultural and spiritual beliefs affect an individual's ability to cope with illness.

4. Identify some basic coping strategies (defense mechanisms).

5. Discuss the concepts of anxiety, fear, stress, loss, grief, hopelessness, and powerlessness in relation to illness.

6. Describe several factors that may precipitate adaptive or maladaptive coping behaviors in response to illness.

7. Discuss implementation of the nursing process to enhance a patient's mental health as the patient deals with the stresses of illness.

## LEARNING ACTIVITIES

A. **Defense Mechanisms.** Complete the statement in the numbered column with the most appropriate term in the lettered column. Some terms may be used more than once. *(1240)*

1. When a woman finds a suspicious lump in her breast and does not keep appointments for a breast biopsy, this action could be called _____.

2. When anxiety intensifies to an excessive level, perception of reality becomes solely focused on the _____.

3. When a student fails to complete an assignment correctly and complains about the objectives for the assignment, this action is _____.

4. Transferring feelings associated with one person or event to another that is considered less threatening is _____.

5. An attempt to make up for real or imagined weakness is _____.

6. The use of logic, reasoning, and analysis to avoid unacceptable feelings is _____.

7. A painful emotion that results from one's perception of danger is _____.

8. Internalizing or taking on the values and beliefs of another person is _____.

9. A boy who is angry with a teacher comes home and yells at his dog; this is an example of _____.

10. When a man appears apathetic as he discusses a firefight in which he participated in Vietnam, it is an example of _____.

11. When a child dresses and uses mannerisms similar to those of a movie star, this action is called _____.

12. Refusal to acknowledge a real situation is _____.

13. When an adolescent perceived as unattractive becomes an outstanding athlete, this action could be called _____.

14. When a child takes on the values and beliefs of a parent, it is called _____.

15. Emulation of admirable qualities in another to enhance one's self-esteem is _____.

16. The separation of emotion from an associated thought or memory is _____.

A. Introjection
B. Rationalization or intellectualization
C. Compensation
D. Denial
E. Identification
F. Isolation
G. Displacement
H. Crisis
I. Anxiety

**B. Defense Mechanisms.** Complete the statement in the numbered column with the most appropriate term in the lettered column. Some terms may be used more than once.

1. The transformation of unacceptable impulses or drives into constructive or more acceptable behavior is _____. *(1241)*
2. Actually or symbolically attempting to cancel out an action that was unacceptable is _____. *(1241)*
3. When the individual who witnesses a murder then experiences sudden blindness without an organic cause, it is called _____. *(1240)*
4. When a patient who unconsciously hates his father continuously tells the nurses how great his father is, it is an example of _____. *(1240)*
5. Unacceptable feelings or impulses are transferred to another in _____. *(1240)*
6. _____ is a conscious or voluntary inhibition of unacceptable ideas, impulses, and memories. *(1241)*
7. Sprinkling salt over one's left shoulder to prevent bad luck after spilling salt on the table is an example of _____. *(1241)*
8. When the person who has a strong unconscious sexual attraction to a parent marries someone who resembles that parent, it is called _____. *(1241)*
9. When a child starts sucking her thumb when her new baby brother comes home from the hospital, it is an example of _____. *(1240)*
10. When a child who fails an algebra class forgets to show his report card to his parents, this action is called _____. *(1241)*
11. An emotional conflict is turned into a physical symptom, which provides the individual with some sort of benefit (secondary gain), is _____. *(1241)*
12. Avoidance of unacceptable thoughts and behaviors by expressing opposing thoughts or behaviors is _____. *(1240)*
13. When a wife who is jealous of her husband accuses him of jealousy, this is called _____. *(1240)*
14. An unconscious defense mechanism in which unacceptable ideas, impulses, and memories are kept out of consciousness is _____. *(1240)*
15. In _____, an individual replaces a highly valued, unattainable object with a less valued, attainable object. *(1241)*
16. _____ is withdrawing to an earlier level of development to benefit from the associated comfort levels. *(1240)*
17. When a person cannot remember a sexual assault, it is an example of _____. *(1240)*
18. When a person who has aggressive tendencies becomes a football star, it is an example of _____. *(1241)*

A. Substitution
B. Projection
C. Sublimation
D. Repression
E. Regression
F. Reaction formation
G. Undoing
H. Suppression
I. Isolation
J. Conversion

C. **Coping Strategies.** Match the descriptions in the numbered column with the coping strategy in the lettered column. Some strategies may be used more than once, and some strategies may not be used. *(1241)*

1. _____ Imagery, therapeutic touch, and music therapy

2. _____ The use of imagination to develop sensory pictures that focus away from the stressful experience and emphasize other sensory experiences and pleasant memories

3. _____ Use of earphones with audiocassettes

4. _____ Discussion with clients about a higher power or their beliefs

5. _____ Biofeedback, meditation, yoga, and Zen practices

6. _____ A process by which the therapist acts as a channel for environmental and universal energy through the therapist's mental concentration

A. Therapeutic touch
B. Relaxation techniques
C. Spiritual dimension
D. Music therapy
E. Art therapy
F. Role-playing
G. Imagery

D. **Mental Health Definition.** Which are characteristics of healthy individuals, according to Maslow? Select all that apply. *(1235-1236)*

1. _____ Positive self-esteem
2. _____ Accurate perception of reality
3. _____ Sense of spirituality
4. _____ Ability to accept oneself and others
5. _____ Ability to be spontaneous
6. _____ Need for privacy
7. _____ Need for isolation
8. _____ Independence or autonomy
9. _____ Frequent "peak experiences"
10. _____ Sense of ethics
11. _____ Sense of conformity
12. _____ Identification with humankind

E. **Powerlessness.** Which of the following are characteristics of powerlessness? Select all that apply. *(1242)*

1. _____ Loss of motivation
2. _____ Passivity
3. _____ Nonparticipation in care and decision-making
4. _____ Dependence on others, which may lead to anger, resentment, or guilt

F. **Nursing Diagnoses.** Which of the following are nursing diagnoses often identified in a person with inadequate coping? Select all that apply. *(1242)*

1. _____ Activity intolerance
2. _____ Interrupted family process
3. _____ Ineffective role performance
4. _____ Acute confusion
5. _____ Disturbed body image
6. _____ Fear
7. _____ Low self-esteem
8. _____ Deficient fluid volume
9. _____ Disturbed sleep pattern
10. _____ Sedentary lifestyle

## MULTIPLE-CHOICE QUESTIONS

G. Choose the most appropriate answer.

1. Defense mechanisms are adopted by the individual as protective measures to allow the ego relief from: *(1239)*
   1. rationalization.
   2. denial.
   3. anxiety.
   4. repression.

2. A factor that is basic to helping the patient cope with illness is the nurse's: *(1237)*
   1. caring attitude.
   2. educational background.
   3. professionalism.
   4. organization.

3. Effective nursing interventions can be made only after patients have been assessed as: *(1238)*
   1. members of a particular culture.
   2. members of a particular sex.
   3. members of a certain race.
   4. unique individuals.

4. A group's affiliation because of a shared language, race, and values is: *(1237)*
   1. culture.
   2. behavior.
   3. morality.
   4. ethnicity.

5. People subjected to prolonged stressors eventually become: *(1239)*
   1. defensive.
   2. exhausted.
   3. cognitive.
   4. emotional.

6. An early response to illness is often: *(1239)*
   1. grief.
   2. depression.
   3. anxiety.
   4. loss.

7. When a person with a severe illness is forced to relinquish original hopes, this process is called: *(1240)*
   1. mourning.
   2. grief.
   3. anxiety.
   4. fear.

8. The experience of loss is related to the individual's: *(1240)*
   1. self-concept.
   2. sense of belonging.
   3. anxiety.
   4. depression.

9. Any changes in a person's life create: *(1236)*
   1. fear.
   2. anxiety.
   3. stress.
   4. mourning.

10. Unconscious coping mechanisms are referred to as: *(1240)*
    1. stressors.
    2. defense mechanisms.
    3. self-concepts.
    4. illusions.

11. Passivity and verbal expression of loss of control over situations are characteristics of: *(1242)*
    1. gratification.
    2. denial.
    3. intellectualization.
    4. powerlessness.

12. Denial of obvious problems and weaknesses is related to the nursing diagnosis of: *(1242)*
    1. Ineffective individual coping.
    2. Activity intolerance.
    3. Altered growth and development.
    4. Ineffective management of therapeutic regimen: individual.

13. Passivity and dependence on others are characteristics of: *(1242)*
    1. helplessness.
    2. powerlessness.
    3. denial.
    4. displacement.

14. Minimizing the severity of an illness by a patient is an example of: *(1242)*
    1. denial.
    2. repression.
    3. compensation.
    4. regression.

15. Ineffective coping mechanisms may evolve from a sense of: *(1242)*
    1. isolation.
    2. projection.
    3. powerlessness.
    4. reaction formation.

H. **Nursing Care Plan.** Refer to Sample Nursing Care Plan for a Patient Ineffectively Coping with Illness (Box 54-1, p. 1243 in the textbook). Which are nursing interventions for this patient? Select all that apply. *(1243)*
    1. Use confrontational techniques to help the patient accept the problem of coping.
    2. Give the patient an opportunity to verbalize feelings of powerlessness by approaching patient care in an unhurried manner.
    3. Establish a no-harm contract with the patient.
    4. Collect data about the patient's and family's current coping strategies and behaviors.
    5. Involve dietitian in planning adequate diet.
    6. Implement stress-reduction strategies, such as music therapy, to help patient deal with stressful moments.

# Psychiatric Disorders

---

## OBJECTIVES

1. Describe the differences between social relationships and therapeutic relationships.

2. Describe key strategies in communicating therapeutically.

3. Describe the components of the mental status examination.

4. Identify target symptoms, behaviors, and potential side effects for the following types of medications: antianxiety (anxiolytic), antipsychotic, and antidepressant drugs.

5. Summarize current thinking about the etiology of schizophrenia and the mood disorders.

6. Identify key features of the mental status examination and their relevance in: anxiety disorders, schizophrenia, mood disorders, cognitive disorders, and personality disorders.

7. Identify common nursing diagnoses, goals, and interventions for people with: anxiety disorders, schizophrenia, mood disorders, cognitive disorders, and personality disorders.

---

## LEARNING ACTIVITIES

**A.  Key Terms.** Match the definition or description in the numbered column with the most appropriate term in the lettered column.

1. _____ Frequently irreversible side effect of antipsychotic medication that develops after years of use; symptoms include involuntary movements of face, jaw, and tongue, leading to grimacing; jerky movements of upper extremities; and tonic contractions of neck and back *(1253)*

2. _____ A state in which a person's perception of reality is impaired, thereby interfering with the capacity to function and to relate to others *(1252)*

3. _____ Assumes that mental disorders are related to physiologic changes within the central nervous system *(1245)*

4. _____ Level of consciousness and orientation to time, place, person, and self *(1249)*

5. _____ Based on the theory that people function at different levels of awareness (conscious to unconscious) and that ego defense mechanisms, such as denial and repression, are used to prevent anxiety *(1245)*

6. _____ A defense mechanism in which particular feelings or specific aspects of reality are excluded from awareness *(1245)*

7. _____ A defense mechanism in which one sees others as a source of one's own unacceptable thoughts, feelings, or impulses *(1245)*

8. _____ Side effects of antipsychotic drugs on the portion of the central nervous system controlling involuntary movements *(1253)*

9. _____ Refers to behaviors and symptoms of masklike face, rigid posture, shuffling gait, and resting tremors *(1253)*

10. _____ A state of feeling outside of oneself; that is, watching what is happening as if it were happening to someone else *(1251)*

11. _____ The patient learns new ways to behave in a therapeutic relationship built on trust *(1246)*

12. _____ A term used when a definite organic cause, such as delirium or dementia, is established for behaviors and symptoms *(1261)*

A.  Sensorium
B.  Depersonalization
C.  Projection
D.  Psychosis
E.  Parkinsonian yndrome
F.  Psychoanalytic approach
G.  Disorder
H.  Tardive dyskinesia
I.  Extrapyramidal effects
J.  Interpersonal approach
K.  Biologic approach
L.  Denial

B. **Mental Health Disorders.** Match the definition or description in the numbered column with the most appropriate term in the lettered column.

1. _____ Uses behavior modification (positive and negative reinforcement) and recognizes that particular thoughts influence emotional states *(1246)*

2. _____ Observations and descriptions regarding appearance, mood and effect, speech and language, thought content, perceptual disturbances, insight and judgment, sensorium, and memory and attention *(1247-1248)*

3. _____ Involves deficits in orientation, memory, language comprehension, and judgment *(1261)*

4. _____ Class of antidepressant drugs; patients taking these drugs must be carefully monitored to avoid life-threatening food and drug interactions *(1257)*

5. _____ Briefly occurring feelings such as happiness, sadness, or worry; when inappropriate, there is incongruence between the feeling appropriate to the situation and the way the feeling is expressed *(1248)*

6. _____ A very serious group of usually chronic thought disorders in which patients' ability to interpret the world around them is severely impaired *(1252)*

7. _____ A mental disorder that involves a change in identity, memory, or consciousness that enables patients to remove themselves from anxiety-provoking situations *(1251)*

8. _____ Periods of elevated mood (manic episodes) and depression *(1255-1256)*

9. _____ Fear of situations outside the home *(1249)*

10. _____ Possible side effect after years of antipsychotic drug therapy; patient exhibits mask-like face, shuffling gait, resting tremor, and rigid posture *(1254)*

11. _____ A mental state that is characterized by cognitive and intellectual deficits severe enough to impair social or occupational functioning (memory, abstract thinking, and judgment) *(1261)*

12. _____ Patient experiences intense episodes of apprehension to the point of terror *(1249)*

13. _____ Patient exhibits unstable relationships, unstable self-image, and unstable mood *(1261-1262)*

14. _____ Feeling state experienced by the patient over a period of time *(1248)*

15. _____ Controversial therapy that uses electric current to the brain to evoke a grand mal seizure *(1256)*

A. Dissociative disorder
B. Dementia
C. Organic mental disorder
D. Borderline personality disorder
E. Parkinsonian syndrome
F. Monoamine oxidase inhibitor
G. Electroconvulsive therapy
H. Bipolar disorder
I. Mood
J. Mental status examination
K. Panic disorder
L. Affect
M. Cognitive behavioral approach
N. Agoraphobia
O. Schizophrenia

C. **Mental Health Disorders.** Match the definition or description in the numbered column with the most appropriate term in the lettered column.

1. _____ Person exhibits two or more distinct personalities *(1251)*

2. _____ Effect of medication that can develop after one dose or after years of drug therapy; the first symptom usually is muscular rigidity accompanied by akinesia and respiratory distress; the cardinal sign is hyperthermia (body temperature 101–103° F or higher) *(1253)*

3. _____ Incessant behaviors, such as handwashing, that interfere with normal functioning *(1249)*

4. _____ Loss of body function (e.g., paralysis) without physiologic cause *(1250)*

5. _____ A disorder that is characterized by vague, multiple, recurring physical complaints that are not caused by real physical illness *(1250)*

6. _____ Pervasive, chronic, and maladaptive personality characteristics that interfere with normal functioning *(1261)*

7. _____ A psychological disorder experienced following a traumatic event that is characterized by flashbacks, detachment, and sleeping and eating difficulties *(1250)*

8. _____ A reversible condition of restlessness manifested as an urge to pace *(1253)*

9. _____ Emotional responsiveness and feeling state *(1248)*

10. _____ Recurrent intrusive thoughts that interfere with normal functioning *(1249)*

11. _____ Recurrent obsessions or compulsions, or both, that produce distress and interfere with daily functioning *(1249)*

12. _____ Belief that a serious medical condition exists when medical findings are absent *(1250)*

13. _____ Persistent depressed mood *(1256)*

14. _____ Disorder that occurs after exposure to a recent distressing event that is characterized by detachment, derealization, depersonalization, and dissociative amnesia *(1250)*

15. _____ State of being uneasy, apprehensive, or nervous in response to a vague, nonspecific threat *(1249)*

A. Post-traumatic stress disorder
B. Major depression
C. Dissociative identity disorder
D. Hypochondriasis
E. Obsessions
F. Anxiety
G. Affect
H. Neuroleptic malignant syndrome
I. Somatoform disorder
J. Personality disorder
K. Compulsions
L. Akathisia
M. Obsessive-compulsive disorder
N. Conversion disorder
O. Acute stress disorder

**D. Mental Status Examination.** Complete the statement in the numbered column with the most appropriate term in the lettered column. Some terms may be used more than once, and some terms may not be used.

1. A mechanism frequently utilized by patients with borderline personality disorder that is caused by problems with separation-individuation is called _____. *(1262)*

2. Asking the patient to interpret proverbs, such as asking "What does 'a rolling stone gathers no moss' mean?" is a way to assess _____. *(1249)*

3. The four levels of consciousness are alert, drowsy, stuporous, and _____. *(1249)*

4. When a spot on the wall is perceived as a bug, this is called _____. *(1248)*

5. Asking a patient to spell the word *world* backwards is a way to measure _____. *(1249)*

6. Paranoid, schizoid, antisocial, borderline, avoidant, obsessive-compulsive, and passive-aggressive are examples of _____. *(1261)*

7. Important factors in relation to suicide potential are insight and _____. *(1248)*

8. Asking the patient "What day is today?" is a way to assess _____. *(1249)*

9. The person with borderline personality disorder has patterns involving unstable relationships, unstable self-image, and marked _____. *(1261)*

10. Asking a patient what was eaten at the previous meal is one way to measure _____. *(1249)*

11. The ability to assess a situation accurately and determine the appropriate course of action is _____. *(1248)*

12. When a person sees nonexistent bugs crawling on the floor or feels nonexistent bugs crawling on the skin, this is called _____. *(1248)*

13. A clear understanding of the correct cause or meaning of a situation is _____. *(1248)*

A. Illusion
B. Multiple personality disorder(s)
C. Sensorium
D. Comatose
E. Recent memory
F. Personality disorder(s)
G. Insight
H. Hallucination
I. Splitting
J. Impulsivity
K. Attention
L. Remote memory
M. Judgment
N. Abstract thinking
O. Phobia(s)

**E.  Therapeutic Relationship.** Match the description in the numbered column with (A) therapeutic or (B) social relationship. *(1246)*

1. _____     May or may not have clear boundaries and a clear ending

2. _____     Focus is on personal and emotional needs of patient

3. _____     Purpose is to benefit both participants in the relationship

4. _____     Participants are not formally responsible for evaluating their interaction

5. _____     Helper has responsibility for evaluating the interaction and the changing behavior

6. _____     Relationship has some boundaries (purpose, place, time) and clear ending

7. _____     Relationship develops spontaneously

**F.  Therapeutic Relationship.** Match the description in the numbered column with the appropriate interpersonal strategy in the lettered column. Some strategies may be used more than once, and some strategies may not be used.

1. _____     "Experiencing" the patient and refraining from thinking of responses to the patient when the patient is speaking *(1246)*

2. _____     When with the patient, the nurse's attention should be directed completely toward him or her *(1246)*

3. _____     The nurse asks the patient, "What do you mean when you say, 'The world is falling apart'?" *(1246)*

4. _____     This approach allows patients time to consider their own thoughts as well as the communication of the nurse *(1247)*

5. _____     Patients benefit from knowing what nurses see and hear while listening *(1246)*

6. _____     If nurses are aware of their own feelings, they will be able to control their own responses *(1246)*

7. _____     The nurse makes a statement that lets the patient know that verbal and nonverbal behaviors are not congruent *(1247)*

8. _____     The nurse says, "You are saying that your life is falling apart, and you are also smiling." *(1247)*

9. _____     Asking questions of the patient *(1246)*

A.  Sharing observations
B.  Accepting silence
C.  Listening
D.  Clarifying
E.  Being available

**G. Communication Terms.** Match the description in the numbered column with the most appropriate term in the lettered column. *(1248)*

1. _____ A continual shifting from topic to unrelated topic

2. _____ Minimal or very little speech

3. _____ A patient starts out toward a particular point but veers away and never reaches the point

4. _____ Stopping speaking before reaching the point

5. _____ Loud and insistent speech

6. _____ Shifting topics to the point of incoherence

7. _____ Not speaking

A. Tangential
B. Word salad
C. Pressured speech
D. Paucity
E. Loose associations
F. Mutism
G. Thought blocking

**H. Schizophrenia.** Match the nursing intervention in the numbered column with the appropriate nursing diagnosis for the patient with schizophrenia in the lettered column. Some diagnoses may be used more than once, and some diagnoses may not be used. *(1255)*

1. _____ Encourage involvement in activities

2. _____ Focus on reality

3. _____ Make brief, frequent contacts with the patient to interrupt hallucinatory experiences

4. _____ Let the patient know that the nurse does not share the delusion

5. _____ Connect delusions with anxiety-provoking situations

6. _____ Encourage the patient to pay attention to what is occurring in the environment (instead of internal stimuli)

7. _____ Inform the patient that hallucinations are part of the disease process

8. _____ Encourage the patient to express feelings and anxiety

A. Disturbed thought processes
B. Self-care deficit
C. Disturbed senory perception
D. Impaired verbal communication

**I.  Mental Status Examination.** Which features are assessed during the mental status examination? Select all that apply. *(1247)*

1. _____     Heart rate
2. _____     Blood pressure
3. _____     Appearance
4. _____     Mood and affect
5. _____     Speech and language
6. _____     Thought content

7. _____     Respirations
8. _____     Perceptual disturbances
9. _____     Insight and judgment
10. _____    Sensorium
11. _____    Emotional responses
12. _____    Memory and attention

**J.  Anxiety.** Which of the following are common physical signs and symptoms of anxiety? Select all that apply. *(1249)*

1. _____     Decreased heart rate
2. _____     Elevated blood pressure
3. _____     Sweaty palms
4. _____     Drowsiness
5. _____     Urinary frequency
6. _____     Diarrhea

7. _____     Ataxia
8. _____     A tight sensation in the chest
9. _____     Difficulty breathing
10. _____    Confusion

**K.  Drug Therapy.** What are side effects of antianxiety medications that are associated with sedation? Select all that apply. *(1251)*

1. _____     Nausea
2. _____     Drowsiness
3. _____     Fatigue

4. _____     Dizziness
5. _____     Confusion
6. _____     Fever

**L.  Anxiety Management.** In addition to counseling the patient, what are ways to prevent and manage increasing anxiety in patients? Select all that apply. *(1252)*

1. _____     Rise slowly from sitting position
2. _____     Relaxation techniques
3. _____     Warm baths
4. _____     Positive self-talk
5. _____     Physical exercise

**M.  Schizophrenia.** Which of the following are typical symptoms of schizophrenia? Select all that apply. *(1252)*

1. _____     Feelings of panic
2. _____     Disturbed thought processes
3. _____     Delusions

4. _____     Hallucinations
5. _____     Bizarre behavior
6. _____     Disturbed emotional responses

**N.  Drug Therapy.** Which of the following are side effects of drug therapy (antipsychotic and antiparkinsonian medications) used for patients with schizophrenia? Select all that apply. *(1254)*

1. _____     Agitation
2. _____     Akathisia (restlessness and inability to sit still)
3. _____     Orthostatic hypotension
4. _____     Extrapyramidal effects

5. _____     Neuroleptic syndrome
6. _____     Hypertensive crisis
7. _____     Agranulocytosis

**O. Mood Disorders.** Which are probable etiologic factors of mood disorders? Select all that apply. *(1256)*

1. _____ Childhood trauma
2. _____ Neuroendocrine dysfunction
3. _____ Genetic factors
4. _____ Learned helplessness
5. _____ Loss of significant others

**P. Drug Therapy.** Which are types of antidepressant medications used for mood disorders? Select all that apply. *(1256)*

1. _____ Benzodiazepines
2. _____ Tricyclic antidepressants
3. _____ Second-generation antidepressants
4. _____ Monoamine oxidase (MAO) inhibitors

**Q. Drug Therapy.** Refer to Table 55-2 in the textbook. Match the descriptions in the numbered column with the drug classification in the lettered column. Answers may be used more than once.

1. _____ Antidepressant drug that affects serotonin and epinephrine/norepinephrine; may cause cardiac complications *(1257)*

2. _____ Used in the treatment of bipolar disorders with narrow therapeutic range; may cause toxicity signs, including tremors *(1258)*

3. _____ Antipsychotic agent that is helpful in the treatment of schizophrenia; may cause drowsiness, hypotension, dry mouth, EPS (extrapyramidal symptoms), and tardive dyskinesia *(1254)*

4. _____ Antidepressants that can be taken once a day without being cardiotoxic; useful in treatment of panic disorder and obsessive-compulsive disorder *(1257)*

5. _____ Antipsychotic agents that treat both positive and negative symptoms of schizophrenia; examples are Clozaril, Zyprexa, and Seroquel *(1254)*

6. _____ Important to maintain hydration, and monitor renal function and serum blood levels of drug *(1258)*

7. _____ Antidepressant drugs that require strict diet restriction to avoid hypertensive crisis *(1257)*

8. _____ Mood-stabilizer used in the treatment of bipolar disorders *(1258)*

A. Typical neuroleptics
B. Atypical neuroleptics
C. SSRIs
D. Tricyclics
E. MAOIs
F. Lithium
G. Valproic acid (Depakote)

**R.  Nursing Diagnoses.** Match the nursing diagnosis in the numbered column with the disorder in the lettered column. Answers may be used more than once.

1. _____    Altered thought processes related to delusions, loose associations, concrete thinking *(1255)*

2. _____    Altered nutrition: less than body requirements related to hyperactivity *(1259)*

3. _____    Risk for self-directed violence related to episodes of anger and impaired judgment *(1262)*

4. _____    Risk for self-directed violence related to hopelessness, increased energy level associated with treatment *(1258)*

5. _____    Disturbed personal identity related to splitting *(1262)*

6. _____    Chronic or situational low self-esteem related to negative feelings about self *(1258)*

7. _____    Anxiety related to severe stress *(1252)*

8. _____    Sensory perception alteration related to hallucinations, illusions *(1255)*

9. _____    Risk for violence directed at others related to impaired judgment, low frustration tolerance, and emotional lability *(1259)*

10. _____    Ineffective coping related to dissociation, amnesia in stressful situations *(1252)*

A.  Borderline personality disorder
B.  Manic episodes
C.  Depression
D.  Schizophrenia
E.  Anxiety, somatoform, and dissociative disorders

## MULTIPLE-CHOICE QUESTIONS

**S.**  Choose the most appropriate answer.

1.  Intense episodes of apprehension, at times to the point of terror, that are often accompanied by the feeling of impending doom are characteristic of: *(1249)*
    1.  panic disorder.
    2.  obsessive-compulsive disorder.
    3.  somatoform disorder.
    4.  personality disorder.

2.  A type of anxiety disorder in which the individual is extremely fearful of situations outside the home from which escape may be difficult is: *(1249)*
    1.  somatoform disorder.
    2.  borderline personality disorder.
    3.  agoraphobia.
    4.  hypochondriasis.

3.  Repeated checking to see whether the door is locked is an example of: *(1249)*
    1.  obsessions.
    2.  hallucinations.
    3.  delusions.
    4.  compulsions.

4.  Many people with obsessive-compulsive disorders have become symptom-free once therapeutic levels of which drug have been reached? *(1249)*
    1.  Analgesics
    2.  Antihistamines
    3.  Antidepressants
    4.  Anticonvulsants

5. Conversion disorders and hypochondriasis are examples of: *(1249)*
   1. mood disorders.
   2. somatoform disorders.
   3. panic disorders.
   4. obsessive-compulsive disorders.

6. Amnesia and multiple personality disorder are examples of: *(1251)*
   1. somatoform disorders.
   2. dissociative disorders.
   3. panic disorders.
   4. post-traumatic stress disorders.

7. A symptom of dissociative disorders is: *(1251)*
   1. depersonalization.
   2. hypochondriasis.
   3. agitation.
   4. hallucinations.

8. Most patients with multiple personality disorder report severe: *(1251)*
   1. agoraphobia.
   2. hallucinations.
   3. delusions.
   4. childhood abuse.

9. The primary antianxiety medications are the: *(1251)*
   1. benzodiazepines.
   2. antihistamines.
   3. thiazides.
   4. salicylates.

10. Withdrawal from antianxiety medications should be medically supervised because of the effect(s) of: *(1251)*
    1. amnesia and confusion.
    2. negative feedback.
    3. hormones and histamines.
    4. physical and psychological dependence.

11. The two key nursing diagnoses for patients with anxiety disorders are Anxiety and: *(1249)*
    1. Disturbed body image.
    2. Powerlessness.
    3. Spiritual distress.
    4. Ineffective coping.

12. One of the most common psychiatric disorders is: *(1256)*
    1. bipolar disorder.
    2. major depression.
    3. post-traumatic stress disorder.
    4. conversion disorder.

13. As patients respond to antidepressant medications and their energy level increases, what risk may increase? *(1257)*
    1. Mutism
    2. Panic
    3. Suicide
    4. Hypertension

14. A type of therapy that may be used for patients with severe depression when other forms of therapy have failed is: *(1256)*
    1. antidepressants.
    2. electroconvulsive therapy.
    3. psychotherapy.
    4. isolation therapy.

15. Possible side effects of electroconvulsive therapy are temporary memory loss and: *(1256)*
    1. orthostatic hypotension.
    2. confusion.
    3. tardive dyskinesia.
    4. parkinsonian syndrome.

16. A patient who exhibits psychomotor retardation, no spontaneous movements, a downcast gaze, and occasional agitated movements of hand wringing is exhibiting signs of: *(1002)*
    1. major depression.
    2. agoraphobia.
    3. schizophrenia.
    4. post-traumatic stress syndrome.

17. Frequently assessing a patient's suicidal potential and maintaining continuous one-to-one contact, if indicated, are interventions for depressed patients who are at risk for: *(1257)*
    1. sleep pattern disturbance.
    2. anxiety.
    3. self-directed violence.
    4. self-esteem disturbance.

18. Learning to limit self-criticism and to give and receive compliments are interventions for the nursing diagnosis of: *(1258)*
    1. Risk for self-directed violence.
    2. Chronic low self-esteem.
    3. Anxiety.
    4. Dysfunctional grieving.

19. Offering small snacks and warm baths and teaching relaxation exercises to be used before retiring for the evening are interventions for patients with: *(1259)*
    1. Chronic low self-esteem.
    2. Risk for self-directed violence.
    3. Hopelessness.
    4. Disturbed sleep pattern.

20. The key medication for patients with manic episodes is: *(1256)*
    1. alprazolam (Xanax).
    2. fluoxetine hydrochloride (Prozac).
    3. lithium.
    4. benztropine mesylate (Cogentin).

21. The key problems for people with organic mental disorders stem from: *(1261)*
    1. speech and language impairments.
    2. anxiety disorders.
    3. conversion disorders.
    4. cognitive impairments.

22. Which herbal preparation is used by many people to relieve depression? *(1256)*
    1. Ephedra
    2. Ginkgo
    3. Ginseng
    4. St. John's wort

T. **Nursing Care Plan.** Refer to Nursing Care Plan, The Patient with Major Depression, p. 1260 in the textbook.

1. What is the priority nursing diagnosis? *(1260)*

2. Which data were collected in the health history and physical examination that indicate the presence of major depression? *(1260)*
   1.

   2.

   3.

   4.

   5.

3. Which are nursing interventions related to the nursing diagnosis: Risk for self-violence related to suicidal feelings? Select all that apply. *(1260)*
   1. Encourage patient to improve hygiene.
   2. Provide sleep-producing measures such as small snacks, warm baths, and relaxation exercises before going to bed.
   3. Establish a no-harm contract.
   4. Take necessary suicide precautions.
   5. Remove dangerous objects from the environment
   6. Maintain continuous one-to-one contact.
   7. Assist in identifying symbols of hope in this patient's life.
   8. Involve dietitian in planning adequate diet.

# 56 Substance-Related Disorders

## OBJECTIVES

1.  Discuss the biologic, sociocultural, behavioral, and interpersonal theories of the etiology of substance abuse or dependence.

2.  Describe the components of the nursing assessment of a patient with substance abuse or dependence.

3.  Describe alcohol dependence, alcohol withdrawal syndrome, medical complications of alcohol dependence, and treatment of alcohol abuse and dependence.

4.  Discuss the pathophysiologic effects of frequently abused drugs.

5.  Describe disorders associated with substance abuse and dependence.

6.  Differentiate between drug abuse treatment and alcohol abuse treatment.

7.  Describe the nursing diagnoses and interventions associated with substance abuse and dependence.

8.  Discuss populations who present special problems in relation to drug abuse and dependency.

## LEARNING ACTIVITIES

**A. Key Terms.** Match the definition in the numbered column with the most appropriate term in the lettered column.

1. _____ Maladaptive pattern of substance use that differs from generally accepted cultural norms; sometimes referred to as *chemical abuse* or *drug abuse* (**1265**)

2. _____ Self-help support process outlining 12 steps to overcoming a physical or psychological dependence on something outside oneself that has a destructive impact on one's life (**1270-1271**)

3. _____ Intense cravings for the substance on which one is dependent without physical withdrawal symptoms (**1274**)

4. _____ Effect of habitual ingestion of a substance to the point of physical dependence; used interchangeably with the term *dependence* (**1269**)

5. _____ Occurs when body cells are dependent on alcohol to carry out metabolic processes (**1269**)

6. _____ Ingestion of substances in gradually increasing amounts due to a physical need; used interchangeably with the terms *chemical dependence* and *drug dependence* (**1265**)

7. _____ Unpleasant and sometimes life-threatening physical substance-specific syndrome occurring after stopping or reducing the habitual dose or frequency of an abused drug (**1269**)

8. _____ Simultaneous existence of a major psychiatric condition and a medical condition (**1283**)

9. _____ Lifelong process of maintaining abstinence from the substance to which one is addicted; a return to moderate substance use is never the end result (**1272**)

10. _____ Exaggerated dependent pattern of self-defeating behaviors, beliefs, and feelings learned as a result of pathologic relationship to a chemically dependent, or otherwise dysfunctional, person (**1270**)

11. _____ Need for increasing amounts of a substance to achieve the same effect brought about by the original amount (**1265**)

A. Substance dependence
B. Substance abuse
C. Tolerance
D. Physical addiction
E. Dual diagnosis
F. Codependence
G. Psychological dependence
H. Withdrawal
I. Twelve-step program
J. Recovery
K. Addiction

B. **Complications.** Complete the statement in the numbered column with the most appropriate term in the lettered column. Some terms may be used more than once, and some terms may not be used.

1.  A recent addition to the methods for the detection of abused substances is _____. *(1268)*

2.  A complication of chronic alcoholism that is due to thiamine and niacin deficiencies, which contribute to the degeneration of the cerebrum and the peripheral nervous system, is _____. *(1269)*

3.  The preferred way of screening for the recent use of an unknown drug is _____. *(1268)*

4.  Occurs when alcohol becomes integrated into physiologic processes at the cellular level _____. *(1269)*

5.  Legal intoxication in most states occurs when a person's blood alcohol level is _____. *(1268)*

6.  Requires sensitive technology and can detect drugs for up to 1 year after use _____. *(1268)*

7.  Bugs, snakes, and rats are commonly described by patients with _____. *(1269)*

8.  A critical sign of withdrawal in substance abusers is _____. *(1269)*

9.  A medical complication that may cause low birth weight and heart defects in newborn babies _____. *(1269)*

10. The detection of amphetamines, barbiturates, marijuana, narcotics, and benzodiazepines can be identified with _____. *(1268)*

11. The most accurate type of test available to measure the degree of intoxication on initiation of treatment for alcohol abuse is _____. *(1268)*

A.  Urine drug screening
B.  Hypertension
C.  0.1%
D.  Withdrawal
E.  Hair analysis
F.  Fetal alcohol syndrome
G.  Hallucinations
H.  Physical addiction
I.  0.05%
J.  Korsakoff's psychosis
K.  Blood alcohol
L.  1.0%

C. **Psychoactive Substances.** Complete the statement in the numbered column with the most appropriate term in the lettered column. Some terms may be used more than once, and some terms may not be used. *(1274-1278)*

1. Oversedation, respiratory depression, impaired coordination, and brain damage are symptoms of overdose of _____.

2. Amphetamines and cocaine are _____.

3. Once a person is dependent on depressants, such as barbiturates, abruptly stopping any of these drugs may trigger _____.

4. Runny nose, sniffles, weight loss, and hyperactivity are symptoms of chronic inhalation of _____.

5. A substance of which an overdose is life-threatening because no drug is available to counteract the overstimulation, resulting in respiratory failure is _____.

6. Regular use of depressants results in _____.

7. A drug that may cause strokes, seizures, and heart attacks, even in first-time users, is _____.

8. There are no physical withdrawal symptoms following amphetamine use, but the user typically experiences a profound depression and sense of exhaustion commonly called _____.

9. Hyperactivity, irritability, combativeness, and paranoia are symptoms of use of _____.

10. Depressants that are misused include the sedatives, hypnotics, and _____.

11. A stimulant that is commonly misused among middle- to upper-socioeconomic classes owing to its status and expense and is typically inhaled nasally or mixed with other drugs is _____.

12. LSD, PCP, MDMA, and marijuana are examples of _____.

13. A form of methamphetamine ingested by smoking with effects that last as long as 14 hours is _____.

14. A smokable form of cocaine is called _____.

A. Psychosis
B. "Ice"
C. Crack
D. Amphetamines
E. "Bad trip"
F. Stimulants
G. "Snow"
H. Physical dependence
I. Narcotics
J. Depressants
K. Anxiolytics
L. Cocaine
M. Hallucinogens
N. "Crashing"

**D. Defense Mechanisms.** Match the description in the numbered column with the appropriate defense mechanism in the lettered column. Some mechanisms may be used more than once, and some mechanisms may not be used. *(1267)*

1. _____ Drug abusers insist that they became addicted to alcohol as a result of pressure to drink socially with colleagues so that colleagues would not think they were prudes

2. _____ Abusers attempt to justify the reasons for their abuse of substances, making an excuse for their addiction

3. _____ Abusers focus only on objective facts as a way of avoiding dealing with unconscious conflicts and the emotions they evoke

4. _____ Patients state that they do not have a problem with drug abuse despite evidence to the contrary

5. _____ Patients state that they must use heroin because the drugs their doctor gave them for their back injuries were not working

6. _____ People shift blame for their behavior on someone else

7. _____ Individuals may minimize their substance abuse problems by maintaining that they can stay sober by themselves

A. Intellectualization
B. Rationalization
C. Denial
D. Regression
E. Projection

**E.**   **Substance Abuse.** Match the description in the numbered column with the most appropriate drug in the lettered column. Some drugs may be used more than once, and some drugs may not be used. *(1275)*

1. _____    Abusers may possess enormous strength and may feel no pain

2. _____    When this drug is smoked, the inner experience of patients is altered so that individuals have a sense of heightened awareness, distortion of space and time, heightened sensitivity to sound, and depersonalization

3. _____    Individuals taking this drug often experience depersonalization

4. _____    Very high temperature, hypertensive crisis, and renal failure, in addition to the risk of injuring oneself or others, are symptoms of its use

5. _____    Chronic smoking of this drug irritates the lungs and may lead to lung cancer

6. _____    This drug produces physical symptoms of altered perceptions that are dream-like

7. _____    Abusers experience a psychotic state similar to that observed in schizophrenics

8. _____    Psychosis, depression, and flashbacks are chronic long-term effects

9. _____    Acute adverse reactions are most often described as a "bad trip"

10. _____    This drug is likely to have a sedative rather than stimulant effect and is unlikely to produce true hallucinations

11. _____    Paranoia, depression, frightening hallucinations, and confusion may be acute adverse reactions

12. _____    Users' emotions are intensified and labile

A.   LSD
B.   Amphetamines
C.   PCP
D.   Heroin
E.   Marijuana

F.    **Common Mood-altering Chemicals.**

1.    Refer to Table 56-1, p. 1277 in the textbook. Match the classification of common mood-altering chemicals in the numbered column with the most appropriate effects in the lettered column. Some effects may be used more than once, and some classifications may have more than one effect.

| | | | |
|---|---|---|---|
| 1. _____ | Hallucinogens *(1276)* | A. | Stimulation |
| 2. _____ | Cannabinoids *(1276)* | B. | Emotional swings/lability |
| 3. _____ | Opioids *(1276)* | C. | Dilated pupils |
| 4. _____ | Sedative-hypnotics and anxiolytics *(1276)* | D. | Increased blood pressure |
| | | E. | Analgesia |
| 5. _____ | Stimulants *(1276)* | F. | Restlessness |
| 6. _____ | Phencyclidines *(1277)* | G. | Illusions of superhuman strength |
| 7. _____ | Inhalants *(1277)* | H. | Paranoia |
| 8. _____ | Alcohol *(1277)* | I. | Euphoria |
| 9. _____ | Xanthines *(1277)* | J. | Pupillary constriction |
| 10. _____ | Nicotine *(1277)* | K. | Sexual arousal |
| | | L. | Sedation |

2.    Refer to Table 56-1 in the textbook. Which is a common effect of xanthines (caffeine) and nicotine? *(1277)*
1.    Euphoria
2.    Poor judgment
3.    Stimulation
4.    Relaxation

3.    Which substance produces euphoria? *(1276)*
1.    Alcohol
2.    Caffeine
3.    Nicotine
4.    Amphetamine

4.    Refer to Table 56-1 in the textbook. Match the objective signs that are effects in the numbered column with the drug classification in the lettered column. Answers may be used more than once. *(1276-1277)*

| | | | | |
|---|---|---|---|---|
| 1. _____ | Dilated pupils | 12. _____ | Dysrhythmias and damage to kidneys | |
| 2. _____ | Constricted pupils | | | |
| 3. _____ | Liver abnormalities | 13. _____ | Confusion, hallucinations, and violence | |
| 4. _____ | Flushing | | | |
| 5. _____ | Tremors | | | |
| 6. _____ | Diarrhea and gastric disorders | A. | Hallucinogens | |
| 7. _____ | Constipation | B. | Cannabinoids | |
| 8. _____ | Increased blood pressure | C. | Opioids | |
| | | D. | Sedative-hypnotics and anxiolytics | |
| 9. _____ | Increased heart rate | E. | Stimulants | |
| 10. _____ | Insomnia | F. | Phencyclidines | |
| 11. _____ | Incoordination, slurred speech, nausea and vomiting | G. | Inhalants | |
| | | H. | Alcohol | |
| | | I. | Xanthines | |
| | | J. | Nicotine | |

G. **Withdrawal.** A few patients may not experience any physical withdrawal symptoms despite a history of prolonged, frequent, and heavy substance abuse. Which factors may affect the incidence of withdrawal effects? Select all that apply. *(1279)*

1. _____ Weight of the patient

2. _____ Stage of addiction

3. _____ Baseline physical status of the patient

4. _____ Type of drugs being misused

5. _____ Defense mechanisms used

H. **Signs Of Abuse.** Which of the following are physical characteristics of the appearance of the average substance abuser? Select all that apply. *(1267)*

1. _____ Obese

2. _____ Malnourished

3. _____ Poorly cared for

4. _____ Evidence of physical trauma

5. _____ Peripheral neuropathy

I. **Neurologic Signs of Abuse.** Which are significant neurologic signs that may be associated with nutritional deficits in the substance abuser? Select all that apply. *(1268)*

1. _____ Paranoia

2. _____ Euphoria

3. _____ Confusion

4. _____ Memory loss

5. _____ Tremors

6. _____ Lack of coordination

J. **Older Adults.** Which of the following are typical stressors of aging that may cause older adults to use or abuse alcohol for the first time? Select all that apply. *(1282)*

1. _____ Cognitive decline

2. _____ Retirement

3. _____ Losses of significant others

4. _____ Confusion

5. _____ Family conflict

6. _____ Health problems

7. _____ Social isolation

8. _____ Loss of self-worth

K. **Impaired Nurse.** Which are goals of an intervention for an impaired nurse? Select all that apply. *(1283)*

1. _____ Assist the impaired nurse to receive treatment

2. _____ Protect the public from an untreated nurse

3. _____ Terminate employment of the impaired nurse

4. _____ Help the recovering nurse reenter nursing in a planned, safe way

5. _____ Assist in monitoring the continued recovery of the nurse for a period of time

**L. Impaired Nurse.** Usually there is a 2-year time period after intervention for an impaired nurse to comply with the peer assistance process. Which are steps to be accomplished by the impaired nurse in this 2-year period? Select all that apply. *(1283)*

1. _____ The nurse is required to attend AA or NA groups regularly.

2. _____ The nurse participates in peer support groups.

3. _____ The nurse meets routinely with an identified support person representing the peer assistance program.

4. _____ The nurse must report how substance abuse impaired his/her practice to the state board of nursing.

5. _____ The nurse submits random urine drug screens to ensure that no relapse has occurred.

**M. Drug Therapy.** Match the description in the numbered column with the drug in the lettered column. Answers may be used more than once. *(1279)*

1. _____ Synthetic opioid analgesic that is sometimes prescribed for chronic severe pain

2. _____ Used for opioid detoxification

3. _____ Opioid antagonist

4. _____ Non-opiate antihypertensive drug

5. _____ Partially blocks withdrawal symptoms of heroin use

6. _____ Counteracts respiratory depressant effects of heroin and other opioid overdose

7. _____ Controversial substance as it constitutes substituting another addictive drug for the one misused by the patient

8. _____ Side effects include constipation and sweating

A. Methadone
B. Naloxone (Narcan)
C. Clonidine hydrochloride (Catapres)

**N.  Nursing Diagnoses.** Match the description in the numbered column with the nursing diagnosis in the lettered column. Answers may be used more than once. *(1281)*

1. _____ Related to ineffective problem-solving and series of self-perpetuating crises

2. _____ Related to refusal to acknowledge actual consequences of substance abuse

3. _____ Related to excessive use of the drug and risk for relapse

4. _____ Related to driving while under the influence

5. _____ Related to returning to places where one used drugs

6. _____ Related to using substances to deal with anxiety, emotional discomfort, and stress

A.  Ineffective coping
B.  Ineffective denial
C.  Risk for injury
D.  Family processes, altered: alcoholism

## MULTIPLE-CHOICE QUESTIONS

**O.**  Choose the most appropriate answer.

1. The least likely way to alienate an already defensive patient is to use a manner that is matter-of-fact and: *(1267)*
   1. nonjudgmental.
   2. assertive.
   3. reassuring.
   4. positive.

2. It is believed that the cause of hangover symptoms is related to the buildup of acetaldehyde and lactic acid in the blood and to: *(1269)*
   1. hyperkalemia.
   2. hyponatremia.
   3. hypoglycemia.
   4. hyperthyroidism.

3. When patients abusing alcohol state that they can quit easily and that they do not have a problem, they may be experiencing: *(1267)*
   1. Chronic low self-esteem.
   2. Ineffective denial.
   3. Risk for injury.
   4. Impaired verbal communication.

4. Substance abusers who are overly sensitive and use critical self-talk may be experiencing: *(1281)*
   1. Ineffective coping.
   2. Risk for injury.
   3. Knowledge deficit.
   4. Chronic low self-esteem.

5. Substance abusers who have driven under the influence of drugs and who engage in excessive drug use are at risk for: *(1281)*
   1. infection.
   2. injury.
   3. aspiration.
   4. activity intolerance.

6. The biggest issue to be addressed at first during rehabilitation is: *(1267)*
   1. rationalization.
   2. sublimation.
   3. denial.
   4. compensation.

7. Overtiredness, argumentativeness, depression, self-pity, and decreased participation in AA or NA meetings are symptoms that often lead to: *(1281)*
   1. relapse.
   2. detoxification.
   3. withdrawal.
   4. rehabilitation.

8. Older individuals who abuse substances over an extended period of time may experience significant medical problems as a result of decreased ability to: *(1282)*
   1. circulate and absorb drugs.
   2. utilize and react to drugs.
   3. metabolize and excrete drugs.
   4. transport and detoxify drugs.

9. Intravenous drug use and the likelihood of sexual activity without precautions in the adolescent age group have led to an increased risk of: *(1282)*
   1. injuries and falls.
   2. IIIV infection.
   3. altered self-esteem.
   4. ineffective individual coping.

10. Dually diagnosed patients usually have psychiatric illnesses of schizophrenia, bipolar illness, or: *(1283)*
    1. depression.
    2. panic.
    3. conversion disorder.
    4. somatoform disorder.

11. Patients taking antianxiety or antidepressant agents with alcohol may risk accidental overdose due to: *(1283)*
    1. antagonist effects.
    2. idiosyncratic effects.
    3. stimulant effects.
    4. additive effects.

12. Programs designed to offer a supportive alternative to health professionals addicted to a substance so that they do not have to have their licenses revoked are called: *(1283)*
    1. Alcoholics Anonymous.
    2. peer assistance programs.
    3. Codependents Anonymous.
    4. Al-Anon.

13. Substance abusers frequently have erratic and unprovoked mood swings, blackouts, significant work problems, and damaged: *(1267)*
    1. relationships.
    2. circulation.
    3. grieving.
    4. activity levels.

14. Individuals with chronic alcoholism may require supplements of: *(1268)*
    1. vitamin C.
    2. vitamin K.
    3. vitamin $B_6$.
    4. vitamin E.

15. Which findings should be reported to the physician because they may indicate physical withdrawal from alcohol abuse? *(1269)*
    1. Mental status changes
    2. High blood pressure
    3. Tachycardia
    4. Nausea and vomiting

16. A patient who has abused alcohol or a benzodiazepine must be monitored for signs of physical withdrawal, since the patient may be at risk for: *(1269)*
    1. paranoia.
    2. seizures.
    3. violence.
    4. euphoria.

17. Which drug is not identified in urine drug screening? *(1268)*
    1. Methadone
    2. Amphetamines
    3. Benzodiazepines
    4. Cocaine

18. Which supplements may be given to individuals with chronic alcoholism? *(1268)*
    1. Beta carotene and vitamin E
    2. Iron and vitamin C
    3. Folate and vitamin $B_6$
    4. Calcium and vitamin D

P. **Nursing Care Plan.** Refer to Nursing Care Plan, the Patient Abusing Alcohol, on p. 1273 in the textbook.

1. What is the priority nursing diagnosis for this patient? *(1273)*

2. Which data were collected in the health history and the physical examination that indicate a problem of alcohol abuse? Select all that apply. *(1273)*
   1. Blood pressure 128/72
   2. Found lying on the floor at home, passed out
   3. Long history of alcohol abuse, but claims he does not have a problem, since he only drinks beer
   4. Lost his job due to tardiness at work
   5. Children are afraid of him when he drinks
   6. Pulse 80
   7. Respirations 20
   8. Yellowish tinge to eyes and skin
   9. Appears thin and wasted
   10. Age 37 years old

3. Which physical characteristics of this patient show evidence of substance abuse? Select all that apply. *(1273)*
   1. Malnourished
   2. Poorly cared for
   3. Evidence of physical trauma
   4. Jaundice

4. Which of the following is evidence of ineffective denial in this patient? *(1273)*
   1. Found lying on the floor at home
   2. Long history of alcohol abuse
   3. States he does not have problem with alcohol since he drinks beer
   4. Recently lost his job for not reporting to work on time